Adverse Drug Reactions

Edited by

Anne Lee

MPhil, MRPharmS

Principal Pharmacist
Area Medicines Information Centre
Glasgow Royal Infirmary
Glasgow, UK

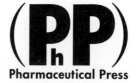

Pharmaceutical Press

Published by the Pharmaceutical Press
1 Lambeth High Street, London SE1 7JN, UK

First published 2001

© Pharmaceutical Press 2001

Text design by Barker/Hilsdon, Lyme Regis, Dorset
Typeset by Mackreth Media Services, Hemel Hempstead
Printed in Great Britain by TJ International, Padstow, Cornwall

ISBN 0 85369 460 5

A catalogue record for this book is available from the British Library

This book is for Patrick and Philip, for all the evenings and weekends when I wasn't around to do all those 'mummy' things because I was in my office bashing away at the computer keyboard. And for Michael, too, for making sure he was there to do the needful!

Contents

Preface

Adverse drug reactions are a massive problem. All over the world, they lead to illness and death and are a burden on limited healthcare resources. There is a huge amount of published literature on adverse reactions and this book does not attempt to summarise it. Instead, it is intended as a resource for students and healthcare professionals who want to know more about the subject. There is a brief introduction to the problem of adverse reactions followed by twelve chapters on reactions affecting particular organ systems. We have concentrated on the most common types of reaction, how to recognise them, and on the drugs implicated most often. Where possible, we have tried to give practical guidance on the most appropriate management of suspected adverse reactions. We hope the book will be helpful to pharmacists, doctors and nurses who are striving to ensure that medicines are used safely.

Acknowledgements

I want to thank lots of people for making this book happen, especially all the authors who worked extremely hard to contribute chapters in time to meet deadlines – Professor Sir Michael Rawlins and Dr Jim Smith for inspiring my interest in adverse reactions, Jo Lumb for her patience and encouragement with the series of articles in the *Pharmaceutical Journal,* and Paul Weller, Linda Horrell and colleagues at the Pharmaceutical Press. Special thanks also to my mum and dad for all those years of support and guidance and keeping me (more or less) on the straight and narrow as a student.

Anne Lee
January 2001

About the editor

Anne Lee graduated in 1984 with a BSc in pharmacy from Heriot Watt University in Edinburgh and went on to do her preregistration year at Edinburgh Royal Infirmary. In 1986 she took up a post at the Regional Drug Information Centre in the Wolfson Unit at the University of Newcastle upon Tyne, which is also a regional monitoring centre for the Committee on Safety of Medicines. At that time, working together with Professor Sir Michael Rawlins, Dr Jim Smith, Dr Robin Ferner and others with a long-standing interest in the problem of adverse drug reactions, she began an MPhil on causality assessment of adverse reactions, which was completed in 1991. She was later involved in the Northern Region's successful pilot study of hospital pharmacist reporting of adverse reactions to the Committee on Safety of Medicines. Since 1996 Anne has been principal pharmacist in the Area Medicines Information Centre at Glasgow Royal Infirmary. She has continued to develop her interest in drug safety issues and has also edited a textbook on *Therapeutics in Pregnancy and Lactation*, published in 2000. She is currently an honorary lecturer at both Strathclyde University and Caledonian University in Glasgow.

Contributors

Keith Beard BSc, FRCP
Consultant Physician
Victoria Infirmary
South Glasgow University Hospitals NHS Trust
Glasgow

Karen Belton BPharm, DipClinPharm, MRPharmS
Senior Pharmacist, Pharmacovigilance Research
Wolfson Unit of Clinical Pharmacology
University of Newcastle
Newcastle upon Tyne

Susan Bishop BSc, DipClinPharm, MRPharmS
Chief Pharmacist
Forth Valley Primary Care NHS Trust
Old Denny Road
Larbert

Mike Daly BSc, PhD, MRPharmS
Chief Pharmacist
Royal Wolverhampton NHS Trust Hospitals
Wolverhampton

Sharon Hems BSc, DipClinPharm, MRPharmS
Formulary Pharmacist
Pharmacy Department
St John's Hospital at Howden
Livingston, West Lothian

Fiona MacLean BSc, MSc, MRPharmS
Senior Clinical Pharmacist, Oncology
Pharmacy Department
Western General Hospital
Lothian University Hospitals NHS Trust
Edinburgh

Moira McMurray BSc, MSc, Cert Health Economics, MRPharmS
Formulary Pharmacist
Area Medicines Information Centre
Glasgow Royal Infirmary
North Glasgow University Hospitals NHS Trust
Glasgow

John Morris MB, ChB, FRCP
Consultant Gastroenterologist
Glasgow Royal Infirmary
North Glasgow University Hospitals NHS Trust
Glasgow

Fiona Thomson BPharm, MSc, MRPharmS
Senior Pharmacist
(Medicines Information and Neurology)
Pharmacy Department
Southern General Hospital
South Glasgow University Hospitals NHS Trust
Glasgow

John Thomson MD, FRCP (Glas & Edin), FChS, DObst, RCOG
Consultant Dermatologist
Glasgow Royal Infirmary
North Glasgow University Hospitals NHS Trust
Glasgow

Fiona Ward BSc, DipClinPharm, MRPharmS
Senior Pharmacist
Hepatology and Clinical Teaching
Pharmacy Department
St James's Hospital
Leeds Teaching Hospitals Trust
Leeds

Janice Watt BSc, MSc, MRPharmS
Senior Clinical Pharmacist
Pharmacy Department
Inverclyde Royal Hospital
Greenock

Philip Young BSc, MSc, MRPharmS
Consultant Pharmacist
GMCPC Ltd
William Brown Centre
Peterlee
County Durham

1

Introduction

Keith Beard

Adverse drug reactions (ADRs) are unwanted or unintended effects of medicines which occur during proper use. The safe use of medicines is an important issue for prescribers, pharmacists, nurses, regulatory authorities, the pharmaceutical industry and the public. Although prescribers aim to use medicines that help patients and do no harm, no drug is administered without risk. Healthcare professionals have a responsibility to their patients, who themselves are increasingly aware of problems associated with drug therapy. It is increasingly important that healthcare professionals have knowledge of the adverse effects of medicines. Minimising the occurrence of ADRs is the main challenge; to do this effectively requires an understanding of their frequency, severity, predictability and reversibility. It is also helpful to have an appreciation of the patient groups that are predisposed to drug toxicity (Lee and Rawlins, 1999).

ADRs have been known to cause significant morbidity and mortality for centuries (D'Arcy, 1986; Davies, 1999). In 400 BC, Hippocrates recommended that drugs should never be prescribed unless the patient had been thoroughly examined. In 1785, when William Withering described the benefits of digitalis, he also identified almost all its adverse effects and demonstrated how its toxicity could be minimised by careful dose titration (Rawlins, 1995). With the development of new synthetic drugs in the early 20th century, governments became involved in some aspects of medicines control. In 1922, the Medical Research Council carried out a formal inquiry into jaundice following the use of arsenic to treat syphilis. In the US, the Food, Drug and Insecticide Administration (later the Food and Drug Administration) was established in 1927. It was the thalidomide disaster in the early 1960s, with the discovery of a large number of cases of phocomelia (a major congenital limb defect) in infants exposed *in utero*, that provided the catalyst for the development of drug safety legislation worldwide. In 1963, the UK Committee on Safety of Drugs was formed and the following year it established the world's first ADR reporting system. In 1971 it became the Committee on Safety of Medicines.

Epidemiology

Many authors have studied the incidence of ADRs in a variety of settings. The estimates of incidence of ADRs in these studies vary widely and this reflects differences in the methods used to detect suspected reactions and differences in the definition of an ADR. Nevertheless, several important studies in the 1960s helped establish the epidemiological basis of drug-induced disease (Seidl et al., 1966a, b; Smith et al., 1966; Ogilvie and Reudy, 1967; Hurwitz, 1969a, b) . The Boston Collaborative Drug Surveillance Program (BCDSP) made great impact in this field (Borda et al., 1968); those investigators collected data on consecutive patients admitted to medical wards over a 10-year period. During that time, information was collected on over 50 000 patients, allowing much original research on the association between short-term drug exposures and acute ADRs to be carried out. In an interim analysis of 19 000 patients monitored, there were approximately 171 000 drug exposures and an adverse reaction rate of 30% (Jick, 1974). Many ADRs were, however, minor and the author concluded that drugs were 'remarkably non-toxic'. Detailed analysis of the data provided much information on patient characteristics predisposing to ADRs and allowed some established adverse effects of drugs, such as excessive drowsiness or 'hangover' with flurazepam, to be quantified (Greenblatt et al., 1977; Jick, 1977).

The Harvard Medical Practice study showed that 3.7% of 30 195 patients admitted to acute non-psychiatric hospitals in 1984 experienced adverse reactions during their stay (Brennan et al., 1991). Further data from this group suggested a 6% incidence of adverse drug events and 5% incidence of potential adverse drug events among 4031 medical and surgical admissions over a six-month period (Bates et al., 1995). Of all events observed, 1% were fatal, 12% life-threatening, 30% serious and 57% significant. A total of 28% of observed adverse drug events were considered preventable, with a greater proportion of the life-threatening and serious reactions in that category. The drug classes most frequently implicated in those reactions were analgesics, antibiotics, sedatives, cytotoxics, cardiovascular drugs, anticoagulants, antipsychotics, antidiabetics and electrolytes.

A recently published study of adverse events in hospital inpatients in Colorado and Utah in 1992 found a similar frequency and type of adverse events to those observed in the Harvard study (Thomas *et al.*, 2000). A review of data on nearly 15 000 patients discharged from 28 hospitals in the two states identified adverse events (not necessarily drug-related) associated with 2.9% of hospitalisations in each state. ADRs were the second most common type of adverse event, accounting for 19.3% of those identified. A quarter (24.9%) of the ADRs were associated with antibiotics, 17.4% with cardiovascular agents, 8.9% with analgesics and 8.6% with anticoagulants. More than a third of the ADRs were considered avoidable and nearly one in ten caused irreversible harm. UK data from a study carried out in Oxford suggested that 7% of over 20 000 medical inpatients experienced an ADR during their stay in hospital (Smith *et al.*, 1996).

Adverse reactions to drugs are responsible for a significant number of hospital admissions, with reported rates ranging from 0.3% to as high as 11% (Beard, 1992; Lazarou *et al.*, 1998). Overall, the incidence of ADR-induced admissions, as estimated from large early studies, is of the order of 3% of medical admissions. For ADRs occurring in the community, the reported incidence ranges from 2.6% to 41% of patients, but this is a much more difficult area to study and there are fewer well-designed studies (Mulroy, 1973; Jick, 1974; Martys, 1979). Despite the problems with definition and incidence studies, ADRs undoubtedly increase hospital admission rates, increase morbidity and mortality and have a significant impact on healthcare costs. Two recent case-control studies carried out in the USA have shown that the length of hospital stay was significantly greater in patients who experienced an ADR while in hospital (Bates *et al.*, 1997; Classen *et al.*, 1997). Both studies estimated direct costs associated with ADRs and, not surprisingly, concluded that such costs may be substantial. Classen *et al.* estimated that the occurrence of an ADR increased the cost of patient care by US$2262 per patient. Bates *et al.* estimated the cost of preventable ADRs in a 700-bed hospital to be US$2.8 million per annum.

Classification

An ADR has been defined by the World Health Organization as 'any response to a drug which is noxious, unintended and occurs at doses used for prophylaxis, diagnosis, or therapy' (WHO, 1970). The simplest classification is into types A and B (Rawlins and Thompson, 1991).

Type A reactions

Type A reactions include normal and augmented, but undesirable, responses to the drugs in question. Examples include hypoglycaemia with a sulphonylurea and orthostatic hypotension with an antihypertensive drug. Many type A reactions arise from secondary pharmacological effects of a drug, such as anticholinergic effects with antihistamines and tricyclic antidepressants. Type A reactions are usually dose-dependent and predictable and are often recognised before a drug is marketed. Type A reactions may occur after a long latency, such as carcinogenesis or effects on reproduction. An example is vaginal adenocarcinoma in the daughters of women exposed to diethylstilbestrol during pregnancy.

Type B reactions

Type B reactions are unrelated to the known pharmacological action of the drugs in question. These reactions are often caused by immunological and pharmacogenetic mechanisms. Type B reactions are generally unrelated to dosage and, although comparatively rare, they are more likely to cause serious illness or death. Immunological reactions such as anaphylaxis with penicillins fall into this category. Other examples include aplastic anaemia with chloramphenicol and malignant hyperthermia with anaesthetic agents. Because of their nature, type B reactions are more likely to result in withdrawal of marketing authorisation.

The main differences between type A and B reactions are shown in Table 1.1.

Table 1.1 Comparison between type A (augmented response) and type B (bizarre response) adverse drug reactions

	Type A reaction	*Type B reaction*
Pharmacologically predictable	Yes	No
Dose-dependent	Yes	No
Incidence	High	Low
Morbidity	High	Low
Mortality	Low	High
Management	Dose adjustment may be sufficient	Stop drug

Predisposing factors

Factors predisposing to ADRs may relate to the properties of the drug or the characteristics of the patient.

Multiple drug therapy

The incidence of ADRs and interactions has been shown to increase sharply with the number of drugs taken (Smith *et al.*, 1966; Cadieux, 1989). This suggests that the effects of multiple drug use are not simply additive. There is likely to be a synergistic effect, but the concept of confounding by multiple disease states must be borne in mind.

Age

The very old and the very young are more susceptible to ADRs. The elderly often have multiple and chronic diseases and are major consumers of medicines. They are particularly vulnerable to the adverse effects of drugs because of the physiological changes that accompany ageing. Most studies have shown a positive correlation between age and the number of ADRs, but this is a complex issue (Hurwitz and Wade, 1969; Greenblatt *et al.*, 1977; Castleden and Pickles, 1988; Gurwitz and Avorn, 1991; Thomas and Brennan, 2000). It is difficult to determine whether age alone renders these patients more susceptible to ADRs or whether this simply reflects increased drug exposure, multiple disease states and age-related pharmacokinetic changes. There is, however, evidence that age-related pharmacodynamic changes make the elderly more sensitive to the effects of some drugs (Jacobs *et al.*, 1995). Adverse reactions in elderly patients often present in a vague, non-specific fashion. Mental confusion, constipation, hypotension and falls may be the presenting features of illness but may also suggest ADRs. Drugs which commonly cause problems in elderly patients include hypnotics, diuretics, non-steroidal anti-inflammatory drugs, antihypertensives, psychotropics and digoxin (Lindley *et al.*, 1992; Cumming and Kineberg, 1993; Willcox *et al.*, 1994).

All children, and particularly neonates, differ from adults in the way they handle and respond to drugs. Some drugs are particularly likely to cause problems in neonates but are generally well tolerated in older children, e.g. morphine. Other drugs are associated with an increased risk of problems in children of any age, e.g. sodium valproate. Hazardous drugs for neonates include chloramphenicol, morphine and antiarrhythmics (Knight, 1994). Specific examples of concern in children are Reye's syndrome with aspirin and hepatotoxicity with sodium valproate (Choonara *et al.*, 1996).

Gender

In general, women appear to be at greater risk of ADRs than men. Increased drug exposure does not completely account for the difference. Women are reputed to be more susceptible to blood dyscrasias with phenylbutazone and chloramphenicol, to histaminoid reactions to neuromuscular blocking drugs, and to reactions involving the gastrointestinal tract (Lawson, 1991; Kando *et al.*, 1995; McKinnon and Wildsmith, 1995).

Intercurrent disease

Drug handling may be altered in patients with renal, hepatic and cardiac disease and this has implications for practical therapeutics. When faced with a possible ADR, one may have difficulty in attributing causality in view of other diseases and alternative explanations for the observed event. There are, however, specific disease states which may predispose to ADRs, such as human immunodeficiency virus (HIV)-positive patients who suffer an increased incidence of the adverse effects of co-trimoxazole (van der Ven *et al.*, 1995; Ellis and Leung, 1996). Immune deficiency is a complex clinical area with multiple drug exposures, multiple illness events and consequent difficulty in interpreting drug toxicity data.

Pharmacokinetic variables

There is great variation in how the body handles and metabolises drugs. The dose required to produce a given pharmacological effect varies between individuals, as does the response to a defined dose. Patients with decreased hepatic or renal function may show considerable changes in drug disposition, leading to ADRs unless dose adjustments are made. Even in a normal population, there may be great variation in drug metabolism because of genetic and environmental influences. Such variability may lead to subtherapeutic response or drug toxicity. Sound knowledge of a given drug's pharmacokinetics and the patient's individual characteristics may help prevent such ADRs.

Race

Ethnic differences may affect drug handling and render some individuals more at risk of ADRs. Genetic factors are often responsible. For example, glucose-6-phosphate dehydrogenase (G6PD) deficiency is more prevalent in African, Middle Eastern and South East Asian populations. The acute porphyrias, attacks of which can be precipitated by certain drugs, are more prevalent in South African than UK populations.

Pharmacogenetics

Heredity and genetic heterogeneity have a direct effect on pharmacokinetics and pharmacodynamics. Genetic polymorphisms altering drug metabolism and disposition are important causes of type A reactions. This genetically determined variability in drug response defines the research area known as pharmacogenetics (Roland Wolf *et al.*, 2000). The most important pathways of drug metabolism subject to genetic variability are acetylation and oxidation (Lennard, 1993). The most common of these are shown in Table 1.2. Qualitative differences in response to drugs usually have a genetic or immunological basis. A well-known example is G6PD deficiency, which affects about 100 million people worldwide. Erythrocytes deficient in this enzyme have weakened cell membranes which predisposes to haemolysis by certain oxidant drugs. The number of medicines proven to cause problems in G6PD deficiency is small, but those most likely include methylthioninium chloride (methylene blue), nalidixic acid, nitrofurantoin, quinolones, primaquine and sulfamethoxazole (Beutler, 1994).

Pharmacogenetics research has identified polymorphisms in more than 20 human drug-metabolising enzymes, several with substantial ethnic differences in their frequencies (Roland Wolf *et al.*, 2000). Polymorphisms in the cytochrome P450 enzymes in the liver can have a profound effect on drug efficacy. In 'poor metabolisers' the genes encoding specific cytochrome P450 enzymes often contain inactivating mutations, which result in a complete lack of active enzyme and a severely compromised ability to metabolise drugs. Thus, mutations in the gene encoding cytochrome P450 CYP2C9, which metabolises warfarin, affects patients' dose requirements.

Interindividual variability in debrisoquine metabolism is well recognised. Poor metabolisers of debrisoquine tend to have reduced first-pass metabolism, increased plasma levels and exaggerated pharmacological

Table 1.2 Genetic polymorphisms influencing drug metabolism

Pathway	Marker drug	Incidence of defect in UK population (%)	Examples of drugs involved	Potential adverse effects
Acetylation	Isoniazid	50	Isoniazid	Peripheral neuropathy
			Hydralazine	Lupus-like syndrome
			Sulfasalazine	Haemolysis
Oxidation	Debrisoquine (enzyme CYP2D6)	5–10	Antidepressants, e.g. nortriptyline, clomipramine, paroxetine, venlafaxine	Accumulation of parent compound in poor metabolisers
			Antipsychotics, e.g. clozapine, haloperidol, olanzapine, risperidone, thioridazine, zuclopenthixol	
			Cardiovascular drugs, e.g. amiodarone, flecainide, mexiletine, metoprolol, oxprenolol, propranolol, timolol	
	Mephenytoin (enzyme CYP2C19)	3	Omeprazole	Accumulation of parent compound in poor metabolisers
			Proguanil	

response to this drug, resulting in postural hypotension. By contrast, rapid metabolisers may require considerably higher doses for a standard effect. The antidepressants nortriptyline and desipramine are metabolised by similar mechanisms to those of debrisoquine and as a result the steady-state plasma levels reached with these drugs are dependent on the individual's phenotype. The enzyme showing polymorphism in this situation is debrisoquine hydroxylase or CYP2D6. This enzyme is inactive in about 6% of white people. In the UK several million people are thus at risk of compromised metabolism or ADRs when prescribed drugs that are CYP2D6 substrates. Many such drugs are used in the treatment of psychiatric, neurological and cardiovascular diseases (see Table 1.2). Clinical problems can also arise from the coadministration of drugs that inhibit or compete for CYP2D6. A drug may interact with and inhibit CYP2D6 to the extent that it is no longer functionally active, resulting in a patient responding like a poor metaboliser, even though he or she has an extensive metaboliser genotype. Thus quinidine, a powerful CYP2D6 inhibitor, may exaggerate the effects of other drugs that are prescribed concomitantly or may prevent the metabolic activation of drugs such as codeine by CYP2D6. Genotyping the CYP2D6 enzyme to assist individual dose selection for psychiatric drugs is currently the most widely accepted application of pharmacogenetic testing.

Another clinically important polymorphism occurs in the enzyme thiopurine methyltransferase (TPMT), which is responsible for the metabolism of the antitumour agents mercaptopurine and tioguanine. Genetic polymorphism at this gene locus is associated with difficulty in achieving an effective dose of these drugs in children with leukaemia. Although the TPMT polymorphism is relatively rare, individuals with inherited deficiency of the enzyme exhibit severe haematopoietic toxicity when exposed to drugs such as mercaptopurine. Some specialist centres provide a diagnostic genotyping service for this enzyme.

Other important examples of situations in which genetic polymorphism is the basis of drug toxicity include the hepatic porphyrias, malignant hyperthermia and glucocorticoid glaucoma. It is likely that the genetic basis of pharmacological action, including ADRs, will become increasingly important as the human genome is fully described.

Allergy

True allergic reactions are immunologically mediated effects. The features of these reactions are:

- no relation to the usual pharmacological effects of the drug

- often a delay between the first exposure to the drug and the occurrence of the subsequent adverse reaction
- very small doses of the drug may elicit the reaction once allergy is established
- the reaction disappears on drug withdrawal
- the illness is often recognisable as a form of immunological reaction

Allergic reactions vary from rash, serum sickness and angioedema to life-threatening bronchospasm and hypotension associated with anaphylaxis. Many factors influence the development of allergic reactions. Patients with a history of allergic disorders are at greatest risk. Drug allergy appears to be less common and less severe in infants and the aged.

Pharmaceutical factors

Predictable adverse reactions can occur due to the pharmaceutical characteristics of a formulation, because of alterations either in the quantity of drug present or in its release characteristics. As a result of stringent requirements laid down by regulatory authorities, reactions due to variability in the quantity of drug present are now rare in developed countries. In 1983, a rate-controlled preparation of indometacin (Osmosin) was withdrawn after reports of localised intestinal bleeding and perforation which occurred as a consequence of the delayed-release mechanism. Pharmaceutical factors may also lead to type B reactions. These reactions can arise from the presence of contaminants or degradation products, or because of the excipients used in formulation. The potentially fatal eosinophilia-myalgia syndrome associated with L-tryptophan was probably due to a contaminant (Kilbourne *et al.*, 1996) (see Chapter 8).

Pharmacovigilance

By the time a medicine is granted a product licence, on average only about 1500 patients will have taken it and clinical trials will have detected only the most common adverse effects. Type B reactions, particularly those with an incidence of less than one in 500, are unlikely to have been identified. Exclusion criteria for most trials mean that patients with multiple disease states, children, the elderly and pregnant women are not well studied and the effect of long-term use is often unknown. Post-marketing surveillance or 'pharmacovigilance' is therefore essential for detecting rare reactions.

Published case reports

Case reports have been vital in alerting healthcare professionals to serious ADRs, such as oculomucocutaneous syndrome with practolol (Wright, 1975). This beta-blocker was withdrawn from use with the recognition of a practolol syndrome comprising a psoriasiform rash, dry eyes (due to lacrymal gland fibrosis), fibrinous peritonitis and a lupus-like syndrome. The pathogenesis is unknown and the syndrome appears unique to practolol. Such case reports are valuable in hypothesis generation and are complementary to spontaneous reporting systems and formal epidemiological studies.

Spontaneous reporting schemes

In the UK, a system of spontaneous reporting of suspected adverse reactions to the Committee on Safety of Medicines (the 'yellow card' scheme) has now been operating for more than 30 years. Its purposes are to provide early warnings or signals of possible ADRs and to enable study of factors associated with them. Spontaneous reporting schemes cannot provide estimates of risk because the true number of cases is invariably underestimated and the denominator (i.e. total number of patients exposed) is unknown (Waller, 1992, 1999).

Formal studies

These may be either of cohort or case-control design, and are important epidemiological tools for establishing causation and quantification of the magnitude of any risk. These are often carried out using large multi-purpose databases linking drug exposure and illness events.

The case-control method involves comparing drug exposure among cases of a particular condition which may be drug-induced, with a control group. A significant excess of drug takers in the case group suggests that there may be an association with the drug. This is a useful retrospective method which can provide valuable information on a suspected link between a drug and a disease. However, these studies must be carefully designed to eliminate bias or confounding and should be interpreted with caution.

A cohort study is a longitudinal investigation of a group of patients exposed to a particular product. Comparison of event rates in exposed and non-exposed groups allows estimation of the risk of developing an ADR.

Causality assessment

ADRs often mimic other diseases and may therefore go unrecognised. It is also known that many healthy people who are not taking medicines complain of symptoms typical of minor ADRs (Reidenberg and Lowenthal, 1968). Placebos also cause side-effects. When an adverse reaction is suspected, it may be helpful to try to assess how likely it is that the symptom has occurred because of a drug. Such causality assessment has many limitations. A large number of decision tools have been developed specifically for causality assessment of ADRs but these methods do not give consistent probability estimates of the likelihood that reactions are drug-induced (Lee *et al.*, 1992; Frick *et al.*, 1997).

The patient's role

An increasing proportion of patients and their carers wish to be involved in decisions about medication (Anon, 1995a). In an investigation of the attitudes of patients with ankylosing spondylitis, 47% reported serious ADRs associated with their medication. They regarded insufficient information and inadequate monitoring by the doctor as important causes of ADRs (O'Brien *et al.*, 1990). It seems reasonable to expect that providing education for patients about their drug therapy could assist in preventing or minimising ADRs. Such intervention needs to be carefully constructed and balanced, with risks and benefits being kept in perspective. This type of educational initiative is costly, but it could turn out to be money well spent in the long term by reducing ADRs and associated morbidity (Lazarou *et al.*, 1998).

The prescriber's role

For every medicine a patient takes there is a balance between risk and benefit. Before giving any treatment the prescriber should consider this relationship. Wherever possible, the safest drug among those of similar efficacy should be chosen. The prescriber must explain to the patient the nature, purpose and risks associated with the treatment and ensure that patient consent is based on an adequate understanding of the likely risks and benefits (Anon, 1995b). Risk : benefit information is essential for prescribers, who must constantly make treatment choices. Prescribers must have access to good data and be able to interpret them and relate them to the patient. Some information is provided by textbooks, published literature and electronic databases. In the UK the *British National*

Formulary is a very useful source of information. Medicines Information Centres, usually located in major hospitals, are another useful source of information and advice. All prescribers need to be aware of the importance of ADR reporting to the public health (Pirmohamed *et al.*, 1998). They must be familiar with local or national guidance on which suspected reactions to report and when to do so.

Some ways in which healthcare professionals can contribute to improving drug safety are summarised in Table 1.3.

Table 1.3 Key points for prescribers and pharmacists on the safe use of medicines

- Consider whether drug therapy is really necessary. In all cases, consider the benefit of administering the medicine in relation to the risk involved
- Always consider whether any new symptom(s) the patient is experiencing could indicate an adverse drug reaction (particularly important for rash, constipation, CNS effects)
- Be aware of 'at-risk' patient groups, particularly the elderly, children, patients with renal or liver impairment and women who are pregnant, of child-bearing age or breast-feeding
- Take care with drugs known to produce predictable dose-related adverse effects; avoid their use where an equally effective and safer alternative exists
- When possible use a familiar drug. Consult an appropriate source of information before prescribing any drug with which you are not thoroughly familiar. With a new drug, be particularly alert for ADRs or unexpected events
- Check the patient's history of idiosyncratic reactions or drug allergy. Avoid the use of drugs known to cause problems
- Ask if the patient is taking other medicines, including self-medication with over-the-counter medicines or complementary therapies
- Ensure that patients are not exposed to unnecessary risk through unnecessary drug use, disregard for warnings, special precautions or contraindications, or through drug interactions
- Ensure that patients are informed about the risks : benefits of their medicines. Warn the patient if serious reactions are liable to occur
- Identify patients who may have a compromised ability to take or use medicines. Ensure that the dosage form and treatment regimen are appropriate and that patients are given clear instructions on how to take their medicines
- Try to ensure that there is true concordance between prescriber and patient
- Check whether there are any specific monitoring requirements (e.g. liver function tests, blood counts, therapeutic drug monitoring, etc.) and ensure that they are carried out
- Be vigilant for suspected ADRs and report them to the appropriate regulatory authority

The pharmacist's role

Ensuring that medicines are used safely is fundamental to the pharmacist's role. Pharmacists' involvement in patient care should result in prevention of some and early detection of other ADRs. Recent studies have demonstrated that pharmacist involvement with patients averted a large number of potential adverse reactions (Lesar *et al.*, 1997; Leape *et al.*, 1999). Based on knowledge of relevant patient and medication factors, pharmacists can ensure that prescribing is as safe as reasonably possible. Medication counselling should include alerting the patient to potential adverse effects, although there is a balance between giving important information and causing unnecessary alarm. The pharmacist also has a significant role to play in the education of other healthcare professionals about the prevention, detection and reporting of ADRs.

Regulatory authorities in many countries accept reports of adverse reactions from pharmacists. In the US, pharmacists initiate most reports submitted to the Food and Drug Administration via the Medwatch system (Anon, 1993). Several UK studies have explored the role of pharmacists in ADR monitoring and reporting (Edwards *et al.*, 1989; Winstanley *et al.*, 1989; Whittlesea *et al.*, 1993; Wolfson *et al.*, 1993). The involvement of hospital pharmacists has been shown to increase the number of yellow cards submitted to the Committee on Safety of Medicines. A pilot study, in which pharmacists were able to complete yellow card reports, demonstrated that there was no difference in the quality of reports submitted from hospital doctors and hospital pharmacists (Lee *et al.*, 1997). Similarly, yellow card reports from community pharmacists were shown to be comparable to those received from GPs (Davis and Coulson, 1999). All pharmacists in the UK are now able to contribute to yellow card reporting. Community pharmacists are well placed to assist in monitoring for problems with over-the-counter medicines, complementary therapies and new medicines (indicated with an inverted black triangle symbol in prescribing information).

References

Anon. (1993). Medwatch update: pharmacists submit over half of product problem reports. *Am J Hosp Pharm* 50: 2478.

Anon. (1995a). The NHS: what's the verdict? *Which? Way to Health* June: 80–83.

Anon. (1995b). Risk:benefit analysis of drugs in practice. *Drug Ther Bull* 33: 33–35.

Bates D W, Cullen D J, Laird N *et al.* (1995). Incidence of adverse drug events and potential adverse drug events. Implications for prevention. *JAMA* 274: 29–34.

Bates D W, Spell N, Cullen D J *et al.* (1997). The costs of adverse drug events in hospitalized patients. *JAMA* 277: 307–311.

Beard K (1992). Adverse reactions as a cause of hospital admission in the aged. *Drugs Aging* 2: 356–367.

Beutler E (1994). G6PD deficiency. *Blood* 84: 3613–3636.

Borda I T, Slone D, Jick H (1968). Boston Collaborative Drug Surveillance Program. Assessment of adverse reactions within a drug surveillance program. *JAMA* 205: 645–647.

Brennan T A, Leape L L, Laird N *et al.* (1991). The nature of adverse events in hospitalized patients. The results of the Harvard medical practice study II. *N Engl J Med* 324: 377–384 .

Cadieux R J (1989). Drug interactions in the elderly. *Postgrad Med J* 86: 179–186.

Castleden C M, Pickles H (1988). Suspected adverse drug reactions in elderly patients reported to the Committee on Safety of Medicines. *Br J Clin Pharmacol* 26: 347–353.

Choonara I, Gill A, Nunn A (1996). Drug toxicity and surveillance in children. *Br J Clin Pharmacol* 42: 407–410.

Classen D C, Pestotnik S L, Evans R S *et al.* (1997). Adverse drug events in hospitalized patients: excess length of stay, extra costs, and attributable mortality. *JAMA* 277: 301–306.

Cumming R G, Kineberg R J (1993). Psychotropics, thiazide diuretics and hip fractures. *Med J Aust* 158: 414–417.

D'Arcy P F (1986). Epidemiological aspects of iatrogenic disease. In: D'Arcy P F, Griffin J P, eds. *Iatrogenic Diseases*, 3rd edn. Oxford: Oxford University Press, chapter 4.

Davies D M (1999). 2000 years of adverse drug reactions. *Adverse Drug React Bull* 199: 759–762.

Davis S, Coulson R (1999). Community pharmacist reporting of suspected ADRs: the first year of the yellow card demonstration scheme. *Pharm J* 263: 786–788.

Edwards C, Smith J M, Bateman D N *et al.* (1989). Adverse drug reaction monitoring in hospitals; a study of a pharmacy (green card) monitoring scheme in the Northern region. *Pharm J* 243: R48.

Ellis C J, Leung D (1996). Adverse drug reactions in patients with HIV infection. *Adverse Drug React Bull* 178: 675–678.

Frick P A, Cohen L G, Rovers J P (1997). Algorithms used in adverse drug event reports: a comparative study. *Ann Pharmacother* 31: 164–167.

Greenblatt D J, Allen M D, Shader R I (1977). Toxicity of high-dose flurazepam in the elderly. *Clin Pharmacol Ther* 21: 355.

Gurwitz J H, Avorn J (1991). The ambiguous relation between aging and adverse drug reactions. *Ann Intern Med* 114: 956–966.

Hurwitz N (1969a). Admissions to hospitals due to drugs. *Br Med J* i: 539–540.

Hurwitz N (1969b). Predisposing factors in adverse reactions to drugs. *Br Med J* i: 536–539.

Hurwitz N, Wade O L (1969). Intensive monitoring of adverse reactions to drugs. *Br Med J* i: 531–533.

Jacobs J R, Reves J G, Marty J *et al.* (1995). Aging increases pharmacodynamic sensitivity to the hypnotic effects of midazolam. *Anesth Analg* 80: 143–148.

Jick H (1974). Drugs – remarkably non-toxic. *N Engl J Med* 291: 824.

Jick H (1977). The discovery of drug-induced illness. *N Engl J Med* 296: 481–485.

Kando J C, Yonkers K A, Cole J O (1995). Gender as a risk factor for adverse events to medications. *Drugs* 50: 1–6.

Kilbourne E M, Philen R M, Kamb M L, Falk H (1996). Tryptophan produced by Showa Denko and epidemic eosinophilia–myalgia syndrome. *J Rheumatol* 23 (suppl 46): 81–88.

Knight M (1994). Adverse drug reactions in neonates. *J Clin Pharmacol* 34: 128–135.

Lawson D H (1991). Epidemiology. In: Davies D M, ed. *Textbook of Adverse Drug Reactions*, 4th edn. Oxford: Oxford Medical Publications, chapter 2.

Lazarou J, Pomeranz B H, Corey P N (1998). Incidence of adverse drug reactions in hospitalised patients: a meta-analysis of prospective studies. *JAMA* 279: 1200–1205.

Leape L L, Cullen D J, Clapp M D *et al.* (1999). Pharmacist participation on physician rounds and adverse drug events in the intensive care unit. *JAMA* 282: 267–270.

Lee A, Rawlins M D (1999). Adverse drug reactions. In: Edwards C, Walker R, eds. *Clinical Pharmacy and Therapeutics*, 2nd edn. London: Churchill Livingstone, chapter 3.

Lee A, Rawlins M D, Smith J M (1992). A study of expert judgements on adverse drug reaction reports and comparison with algorithmic methods. *Br J Clin Pharmacol* 34: 157P.

Lee A, Bateman D N, Edwards C *et al.* (1997). Reporting of adverse drug reactions by hospital pharmacists: pilot scheme. *Br Med J* 315: 519.

Lennard M S (1993). Genetically determined adverse drug reactions involving metabolism. *Drug Safety* 9: 60–77.

Lesar T S, Briceland L, Stein D S *et al.* (1997). Factors related to errors in medication prescribing. *JAMA* 277: 312–317.

Lindley C M, Tully M P, Paramsothy V, Tallis R C (1992). Inappropriate medication is a major cause of adverse drug reactions in elderly patients. *Age Aging* 21: 294–300.

Martys C R (1979). Adverse reactions to drugs in general practice. *Br Med J* ii: 1194–1197.

McKinnon R P, Wildsmith J A W (1995). Histaminoid reactions in anaesthesia. *Br J Anaesth* 74: 217–228.

Mulroy R (1973). Iatrogenic disease in general practice: its incidence and effects. *Br Med J* ii: 407–410.

O'Brien B J, Ellswood J, Calin A (1990). Perception of prescription drug risks: a survey of patients with ankylosing spondylitis. *J Rheumatol* 17: 503–507.

Ogilvie R J, Reudy J (1967). Adverse drug reactions during hospitalisation. *Can Med Assoc J* 97: 1450–1455.

Pirmohamed M, Breckenridge A M, Kitteringham N R *et al.* (1998). Adverse drug reactions. *Br Med J* 316: 1295–1298.

Rawlins M D (1995). Pharmacovigilance: paradise lost, regained or postponed? *J R Coll Physicians Lond* 29: 41–49.

Rawlins M D, Thompson J W (1991). Mechanisms of adverse drug reactions. In: Davies D M, ed. *Textbook of Adverse Drug Reactions*, 4th edn. Oxford: Oxford Medical Publications, chapter 3.

Reidenberg M M, Lowenthal D T (1968). Adverse non-drug reactions. *N Engl J Med* 279: 678.

Roland Wolf C, Smith G, Smith R L (2000). Pharmacogenetics. *Br Med J* 320: 987–990.

Seidl L G, Friend D, Sadusk J (1966a). Meeting the problem. Panel discussion of experiences and problems involved in reporting adverse drug reactions. *JAMA* 196: 421–428.

Seidl L G, Thronton G F, Smith J W, Cluff L E (1966b). Studies on the epidemiology of adverse drug reactions, III. Reactions in patients on a general medical service. *Bull Johns Hopkins Med J* 119: 299–315.

Smith J W, Seidl L G, Cluff L E (1966). Studies on the epidemiology of adverse drug reactions. *Ann Intern Med* 65: 629–634.

Smith C C, Bennett P M, Pearce H M *et al.* (1996). Adverse drug reactions in a hospital general medical unit meriting notification to the Committee on Safety of Medicines. *Br J Clin Pharmacol* 42: 423–429.

Thomas E J, Brennan T A (2000). Incidence and types of preventable adverse events in elderly patients: population based review of medical records. *Br Med J* 320: 741–744.

Thomas E J, Studdert D M, Burstin H R *et al.* (2000). Incidence and types of adverse events and negligent care in Utah and Colorado. *Med Care* 38: 261–271.

van der Ven A J, Vree T B, Koopmans P P *et al.* (1995). Adverse reactions to co-trimoxazole in HIV infection: a reappraisal of the glutathione-hydroxylamine hypothesis. *J Antimicrob Chemother* 37 (suppl B): 55 –60.

Waller P C (1992). Measuring the frequency of adverse drug reactions. *Br J Clin Pharmacol* 33: 249–252.

Waller P C (1999). Pharmacovigilance: evaluating and improving the safety of medicines. *Medicine* 27: 26–28.

Whittlesea C, Walker R, Houghton J *et al.* (1993). Development of an adverse drug reaction reporting scheme for community pharmacists. *Pharm J* 251: 21–24.

Willcox S M, Himmelstein D U, Woolhandler S (1994). Inappropriate drug prescribing for the community dwelling elderly. *JAMA* 272: 292–296.

Winstanley P A, Irvin L E, Smith J C *et al.* (1989). Adverse drug reactions: a hospital pharmacy-based reporting scheme. *Br J Clin Pharmacol* 28: 113–116.

Wolfson D J, Booth T G, Roberts P I (1993). The community pharmacist and adverse drug reaction monitoring: (2) an examination of the potential role in the United Kingdom. *Pharm J* 251: 21–24.

World Health Organization (1970). International drug monitoring – the role of the hospital. A WHO report. *Drug Intell Clin Pharm* 4: 101–110.

Wright P (1975). Untoward effects associated with practolol administration: oculomucocutaneous syndrome. *Br Med J* 1: 595–598.

2

Drug-induced skin reactions

Anne Lee and John Thomson

The skin is the organ most frequently affected by adverse reactions to drug therapy so these problems are extremely common. It is difficult to determine their incidence but hospital studies suggest that up to 3% of inpatients will experience some sort of drug-induced cutaneous reaction (Breathnach and Hintner, 1992; Wolkenstein and Revuz, 1995). Almost any drug can induce skin reactions and, although most are not serious, some are severe and potentially life-threatening. Serious reactions include angioedema, erythroderma, the Stevens–Johnson syndrome (SJS) and toxic epidermal necrolysis. Drug eruptions can also occur as part of a spectrum of multiorgan involvement, for example in drug-induced systemic lupus erythematosus (see Chapter 8). For these reasons, healthcare professionals should carefully evaluate all drug-associated rashes. It is important that possible cutaneous reactions to medicines are identified and documented in the patient record so that steps may be taken to prevent their recurrence.

Skin reactions may be due to any drug that the patient is currently taking or has recently been exposed to, including prescribed and over-the-counter medicines, herbal or homoeopathic preparations, vaccines and contrast media. It is important to remember that the non-drug components of a medicine, i.e. the pharmaceutical excipients, may cause hypersensitivity reactions in some patients (Golightly *et al.*, 1988).

Skin reactions

Classification and mechanism

The mechanism of skin reactions is often unknown, although most have an immunological (allergic) or toxic basis. Toxic reactions are dose-dependent and the symptoms usually resolve soon after the causative agent is withdrawn. In contrast, allergic hypersensitivity reactions are usually independent of dose and can persist long after drug withdrawal.

With penicillins, for example, maculopapular rashes, erythema multiforme and urticaria may not appear until a week or more after the course
of treatment has finished (Ryan, 1995). It is especially important that
allergic skin reactions are correctly identified, since subsequent exposure
to the drug may cause a more severe reaction. Patients with a reliable
history of drug allergy should always be carefully monitored when any
new drug is started, but particularly with drugs known to cause skin reactions. The route of administration is a factor in drug allergy; in general,
topical application has the greatest propensity to induce allergy, followed
by parenteral then oral administration (Nowakowski *et al.*, 1997). The
problem of contact dermatitis (which may be due to any external irritant
including drugs and excipients) is not discussed in this chapter.

Several patient groups appear to be predisposed to cutaneous reactions. Systemic lupus erythematosus, Sjögren's syndrome and human
immunodeficiency virus (HIV) infection are disease states associated
with an increased risk. As for adverse reactions in general, conditions
that lead to alterations in drug handling such as hepatic and renal
disease are important. Genetic factors may also have an influence; for
example, acetylator status may predispose to sulphonamide reactions
(Malinverni *et al.*, 1996). The role of atopy in predisposing to drug reactions is controversial. It may be important in reactions to iodinated contrast material but not in reactions to penicillins or reactions during
anaesthesia (Vervloet and Durham, 1998).

Diagnosis

It can be difficult to diagnose a drug eruption with confidence. Most
drugs are associated with a spectrum of skin reactions, and the dictum
'any rash, any drug' has been used. A few drugs seldom cause skin reactions; these include antacids, corticosteroids, digoxin, ferrous sulphate,
paracetamol, potassium chloride, salbutamol and vitamins (Jick and
Derby, 1995; Ryan, 1995). Some types of skin rash are very rarely drug-
induced, for example, eczema. Many drug reactions cannot be distinguished from naturally occurring eruptions so misdiagnosis is common.
For example, there may be uncertainty about whether a morbilliform
rash is due to a viral infection or an antibiotic and this may unnecessarily
limit the future use of a particular medication. Furthermore, patients
may be taking many medicines, making it difficult to establish the one
responsible. Some drugs are more likely to be the cause of a particular
type of eruption than others. For example, if a patient taking both demeclocycline and chlorpromazine develops a photosensitivity reaction, the

chances are that demeclocycline is the cause, although both drugs are capable of producing the reaction. However, if the patient develops skin hyperpigmentation then chlorpromazine is more likely to be implicated.

The timing of skin reactions is often a useful diagnostic tool. In general, the onset occurs within a few weeks of the introduction of the causative drug. If a drug has been taken for many years without a problem then the likelihood of it being responsible is low. When examining a list of drugs taken by a patient with a rash, drugs added within the previous month are the most likely cause. There are some notable exceptions to this rule of thumb. Hypersensitivity reactions to penicillins often occur several weeks after the drug has been discontinued and the typical psoriasiform skin eruption seen with the beta-blocker practolol (withdrawn in the 1970s) generally occurred after many months of treatment.

Drugs suspected of causing skin reactions should usually be withdrawn and not used again in that patient. Symptomatic treatment may be needed. Calamine lotion or systemic antihistamines may relieve pruritus and topical corticosteroids may help inflammation and itch. For more serious reactions, systemic corticosteroids may be indicated. The main clinical features that are suggestive of a more severe reaction include mucous membrane involvement, blisters or skin detachment, high fever, angioedema or tongue swelling, facial oedema, skin necrosis, lymphadenopathy or dyspnoea. In general, drug rashes are reversible, resolving gradually after the causative drug is withdrawn.

Although skin prick or blood tests may be used in the diagnosis of some reactions (e.g. those dependent on immunoglobulin E such as immediate-type reactions to penicillin), they are not usually helpful in skin manifestations of an allergy (DeLeo, 1998). Skin prick tests can be dangerous and should only be carried out close to intensive care facilities. Rechallenge is not normally advised in the diagnosis of skin reactions because of the inherent risks to the patient.

Management points

When a skin rash is potentially drug-induced:

- Take an accurate medication history. Note details of all current and recent medication, including over-the-counter medicines, herbal (e.g. St John's wort, echinacea) and homoeopathic preparations, and injections, including vaccines or contrast media.
- Note the times when each medicine was first taken relative to the onset of the reaction and check whether the patient has taken these medicines previously.

- Some skin reactions, particularly urticaria, may be due to sensitivity to pharmaceutical excipients. If this type of reaction is present, it is worth noting the proprietary (brand) name of medicines taken as well as the generic name.
- Ask the patient if he or she has a previous history of drug sensitivity, contact dermatitis or atopic disease with asthma or eczema.
- Examine the rash to determine what type it is and whether it appears to be a drug eruption.
- Record clearly in the patient's notes any known or suspected adverse drug reaction. Tell the patient or relatives and preferably give a written note. This should help to prevent any medical or medicolegal disasters.
- Take great care in prescribing (see Chapter 1). Check the *British National Formulary* for potential cross-reactions if you are not sure. Clarify that compound preparations do not contain potentially harmful constituents.
- Notify suspected adverse drug reactions to the relevant regulatory authority. This information is essential for identifying new drug safety hazards and enables the study of factors associated with adverse drug reactions.

Exanthematous (erythematous) reactions

The term 'exanthema' is an umbrella term for skin reactions that literally burst forth on the skin. Enanthematous reactions similarly occur on the mucous membranes. Typical characteristics of skin exanthemas include erythema (redness) or morbilliform (resembling measles) or maculopapular lesions (Ryan, 1995). Macules are small, distinct, flat areas and papules are small, raised lesions. This is the most common type of drug-induced cutaneous reaction. The eruption often starts on the trunk; the extremities and intertriginous areas are often involved, but the face may be spared. The rash is usually bright red in colour and the skin may feel hot, burning or itchy.

These reactions can occur with almost any drug at any time up to 2–3 weeks after treatment is started, but they are most common within the first 10 days. If the causative drug is continued, exfoliative dermatitis may develop. These eruptions usually resolve within a few weeks of stopping the causative drug and occasionally while it is still being taken. Penicillins and sulphonamides frequently cause these rashes. With all the penicillins almost every type of exanthematous eruption may occur. A common type for ampicillin and amoxicillin is a generalised morbilliform eruption. Ampicillin almost always causes a severe morbilliform eruption when given to a patient with infectious mononucleosis or lymphatic leukaemia. The exact mechanism involved is unknown. Ampicillin and its derivatives should be avoided in these patients.

Drugs that commonly cause exanthematous reactions are shown in Table 2.1.

Table 2.1 Some drugs that commonly cause exanthematous reactions

Allopurinol	Isoniazid
Antituberculous drugs	Nalidixic acid
Barbiturates	Nitrofurantoin
Carbamazepine	Penicillins
Cephalosporins	Phenothiazines
Chloramphenicol	Phenylbutazone
Erythromycin	Phenytoin
Furosemide (frusemide)	Sulphonamides
Gold salts	Thiazides

Erythroderma and exfoliative dermatitis

A widespread confluent erythematous rash (erythroderma), often associated with desquamation (exfoliative dermatitis), is one of the most severe patterns of cutaneous reaction to drugs. It may follow exanthematous eruptions or may develop as erythema and exudation in the flexures. There may be systemic symptoms such as fever, lymphadenopathy and anorexia. Possible complications include hypothermia, fluid and electrolyte loss and infection. The main drugs implicated are sulphonamides, chloroquine, penicillin, phenytoin and isoniazid. Other drugs recently implicated include teicoplanin and pentostatin (Paul *et al.*, 1992; Ghura *et al.*, 1999).

Fixed drug eruption

A fixed drug eruption is solely caused by drugs or chemicals. It consists of erythematous round or oval lesions of a dusky purple or brown colour, sometimes featuring blisters or vesicles. Initially, one lesion appears, although others may follow. The patient may complain of itching or burning in the affected area but systemic involvement is usually absent. The eruption generally appears within 24 hours of drug ingestion and can occur on any part of the skin or mucous membranes. The hands, feet, tongue, penis or perianal areas are most frequently affected. The site of the eruption is fixed, i.e. whenever the individual takes the causative drug the eruption occurs within 8 hours at exactly the same site. Healing occurs over 7–10 days after the causative drug is stopped, although there may be residual hyperpigmentation (Korkij and Soltani, 1984; Kauppinen and Stubbs, 1985; Mahboob and Haroon, 1998).

The pathogenesis of fixed drug eruption is not well understood. Many agents, including food additives and pharmaceutical excipients, are capable of causing fixed eruptions. Phenolphthalein, sulphonamides, tetracyclines and analgesics are frequently implicated. Where a fixed drug eruption is suspected, oral challenge to confirm the diagnosis is accepted and safe practice. Table 2.2 lists some drugs that may cause fixed drug eruption.

Table 2.2 Some drugs that may cause fixed drug eruption

Barbiturates	Penicillins
Carbamazepine	Phenolphthalein
Chlordiazepoxide	Phenylbutazone
Clindamycin	Quinine
Co-trimoxazole	Salicylates
Metronidazole	Tetracyclines
Non-steroidal anti-inflammatories	Trimethoprim

Urticaria and angioedema

Urticaria and angioedema are both common features of hypersensitivity reactions. Chronic urticaria may have many different causes or may be idiopathic. The mechanisms involved in drug-induced urticaria are believed to include immunological mechanisms, and release of inflammatory mediators such as histamine, bradykinin and leukotrienes. Drugs that release histamine from mast cells include opioids, d-tubocurarine, amphetamines, quinine, vancomycin and contrast media. Pharmaceutical excipients such as benzoates and tartrazine may be implicated in urticaria. Acute urticaria, known as nettle rash or hives, is a common drug reaction, usually occurring within 36 hours of drug exposure. It presents as raised, itchy, red blotches or wheals that are pale in the centre and red around the outside. Individual lesions rarely persist for more than 24 hours. On rechallenge, lesions may develop within minutes. Individual susceptibility to urticaria is variable and a genetic predisposition is well recognised (absence of C1 esterase inhibitor). Management of drug-induced acute urticaria involves stopping the causative agent and treatment with systemic antihistamines (Breathnach and Hintner, 1992).

Angioedema is a vascular reaction resulting in increased perme-ability and fluid leakage, leading to oedema of the deep dermis, subcu-taneous tissue or submucosal areas. It has a lower incidence than urticaria. The tongue, lips, eyelids or genitalia are generally affected and the oedema may be either unilateral or symmetrical. Angioedema of the upper respiratory tract can result in serious acute respiratory distress, airway obstruction and death. The mechanisms responsible are poorly understood. Treatment depends on the severity of the reaction; adrena-line (epinephrine), antihistamines and corticosteroids may be required. Angioedema is a serious reaction that should always be reported to the appropriate regulatory authority if drug therapy is suspected to be the cause.

Angioedema is a recognised problem with all angiotensin-convert-ing enzyme (ACE) inhibitors. The estimated incidence is 0.1–0.5% in Caucasians but may be higher in other racial groups (Gibbs *et al.*, 1999). In most cases, the reaction occurs in the first week of treatment, often within hours of the initial dose. However, in some cases it has developed after prolonged therapy of up to several years (Sabroe and Black, 1997; Vleeming *et al.*, 1998). The mechanism of ACE inhibitor-induced angioedema is thought to involve bradykinin, but angiotensin II receptor antagonists, which do not affect this substance, can also induce angioedema (Pylypchuk, 1998; Cha and Pearson, 1999; Rivera, 1999). ACE inhibitors should be withdrawn immediately in any patient who presents with angioedema. An alternative drug from a different class (not an angiotensin II antagonist) should be substituted. ACE inhibitors are contraindicated in patients with a history of idiopathic angioedema. Table 2.3 lists some drugs which may cause urticaria or angioedema.

Table 2.3 Some drugs that may cause urticaria/angioedema

N-acetylcysteine	Non-steroidal anti-inflammatory
Anaesthetics (local and general)	drugs
Angiotensin-converting enzyme inhibitors	Opioids
Angiotensin II receptor antagonists	Penicillins
Contrast media	Proton pump inhibitors
Dextrans	Radiocontrast media
Enzymes (e.g. streptokinase)	Salicylates
Hydralazine	Sulphonamides
Insulin	Tetracyclines
Muscle relaxants	Vaccines containing egg protein

Acne

Some drugs can cause or exacerbate acne. The term 'acneiform' is applied to drug eruptions that resemble acne vulgaris. The lesions are papulopustular but comedones are usually absent (Chu, 1997). Corticotropin (adrenocorticotrophic hormone or ACTH), corticosteroids, androgens (in females), oral contraceptives, isoniazid and lithium are among the most frequently implicated drugs.

Psoriasis and psoriasiform eruptions

Psoriasiform eruptions typically consist of erythematous plaques surmounted by large dry silvery scales. A number of drugs can induce psoriasis in patients with no previous history or can worsen pre-existing psoriasis, although many reports are anecdotal and causality is unknown. One fairly definite trigger is lithium which can unveil psoriasis in susceptible patients or aggravate existing psoriasis (Tsankov *et al.*, 1998). Several investigators have confirmed that interferon alfa may either induce or worsen psoriasis (Wolfe *et al.*, 1995; Vial and Descotes, 1996). The lesions were shown to improve on withdrawal of interferon and to recur on reintroduction or rechallenge. In patients with pre-existing psoriasis, symptoms usually developed within the first month of treatment but in those with no previous history they developed after at least 2 months' treatment. Other interferons have also been implicated (Kowalzick, 1997; Webster, 1997). There are several recent case reports of the development of psoriasis, or its exacerbation, in patients taking terbinafine (Gupta *et al.*, 1998; Wilson and Evans, 1998; Pauluzzi and Boccucci, 1999). The eruption tended to develop within 2 months of starting treatment and it generally resolved on discontinuation of terbinafine.

The effect of chloroquine and hydroxychloroquine on psoriasis is variable; in some studies, most patients treated noted no change in their condition (Katugampola and Katugampola, 1990) while in others symptoms worsened in a large proportion of patients (Kuflik, 1980). It is clear that psoriasis may worsen in some patients and this may make treatment decisions difficult in some situations. For example, chloroquine may not be an appropriate drug for antimalarial prophylaxis in a patient with psoriasis. However, a decision on whether or not to use chloroquine will need to take into account the relative efficacy of other agents in the area to be visited. Care should be taken with the use of hydroxychloroquine in patients with psoriatic arthropathy.

Over the past 20 years, skin eruptions have been described with numerous beta-blockers. Practolol was withdrawn worldwide following a serious syndrome termed the oculomucocutaneous syndrome, featuring a psoriasiform rash, xerophthalmia due to lacrymal gland fibrosis, otitis media, sclerosing peritonitis and a lupus-like syndrome (Wright, 1975). The pathogenesis of this problem remains unknown, but it appears to have been unique to practolol. Psoriasiform eruptions have since been reported with cardioselective and non-cardioselective beta-blockers (Tsankov *et al.*, 1998). Ophthalmic preparations (e.g. timolol) have also been implicated (Puig *et al.*, 1989). Cross-reactivity has been noted among propranolol, oxprenolol and atenolol.

Beta-blockers may also transform psoriasis into pustular psoriasis or erythrodermatous psoriasis. The time to onset of the reaction can vary between days to up to a year after initiation of therapy. The underlying mechanism is unknown but it is notable that beta-2 receptors are present in the epidermis. Psoriasis induced by beta-blockers is reported to be resistant to antipsoriatic therapy until the beta-blocker has been stopped.

Table 2.4 lists some drugs that may cause psoriasiform eruptions or exacerbate psoriasis.

Table 2.4 Drugs that may cause psoriasiform eruptions or exacerbate psoriasis

Angiotensin-converting enzyme inhibitors	Interferons
Beta-blockers	Lithium
Chloroquine and hydroxychloroquine	Non-steroidal anti-inflammatory
Gold	drugs
Granulocyte colony-stimulating factor	Terbinafine
(GCSF)	Tetracyclines

Purpura

Purpura describes small cutaneous extravasations of blood. It is an occasional feature of drug-induced skin eruptions and in some cases it is the main characteristic. The main causes are thrombocytopenia or platelet dysfunction (drug-induced thrombocytopenia and platelet dysfunction are discussed in Chapter 9). However, a similar picture can be caused by damage to small blood vessels either by immunological mechanisms or changes in vascular permeability. Tests of haemostasis including platelet function are usually within normal limits. Drugs associated with non-thrombocytopenic purpura include aspirin, quinine, sulphonamides, atropine and penicillin.

Henoch–Schönlein purpura is a type of vasculitis which frequently involves the skin, joints, gastrointestinal system, kidneys, heart and central nervous system.

Vasculitis

The term 'vasculitis' refers to inflammation of the blood vessels. The vasculitides comprise a diverse group of conditions which may be manifest mainly as a systemic or cutaneous disorder; both types may be due to drug therapy (Jain, 1993; García-Porrúa *et al.*, 1999). Several drugs can induce both systemic vasculitis with cutaneous manifestations or cutaneous vasculitis without other organ involvement. About 10% of cases of acute cutaneous vasculitis are believed to be drug-induced. Cutaneous vasculitis commonly presents with raised purpuric (purple) lesions on the legs, ranging in size from a pinpoint to several centimetres. Characteristically the margins are irregular or stellate. Other lesions include erythematous macules, haemorrhagic blisters and ulceration. Occasionally the buttocks, upper extremities or even the trunk may be involved. Systemic symptoms, such as malaise, arthralgia and fever, are unusual.

Leukocytoclastic vasculitis is the most common type of cutaneous vasculitis. Skin biopsy is required for accurate diagnosis. The histopathological picture is characterised by necrosis of cutaneous blood vessel walls, polymorphonuclear leukocyte infiltration, endothelial cell swelling and extravasation of red blood cells (Jain, 1993).

Vasculitis typically develops 7–21 days after the initiation of a new drug. The skin lesions may persist for up to 4 weeks or longer and in some cases become yellow-brown upon healing. The mechanism is believed to be immunological. It is often difficult to identify the cause of cutaneous vasculitis; infection and collagen vascular disease need to be excluded. Drug therapy should be stopped at the first suspicion and the condition usually subsides thereafter (Mackel, 1982). Systemic corticosteroids may be of some benefit in severe reactions.

Propylthiouracil is associated with a hypersensitivity syndrome that typically manifests as a vasculitis involving one or more organ systems (Chastain *et al.*, 1999). In some cases the clinical features may be limited almost entirely to the skin, although involvement of the joints has frequently been noted. The time to onset of the reaction has varied between 1 week and several years. Most affected patients recover quickly when the drug is withdrawn but some have required prolonged treatment with high-dose corticosteroids and immunosuppressants.

Other drugs frequently implicated in cutaneous vasculitis are shown in Table 2.5.

Table 2.5 Some drugs that may cause vasculitis

Allopurinol	Methotrexate
Beta-lactam antibiotics	Minocycline
Carbimazole	Non-steroidal anti-inflammatory
Co-trimoxazole	drugs
Furosemide (frusemide)	Penicillamine
Haemopoietic growth factors (granulocyte and granulocyte–macrophage colony-stimulating factors)	Propylthiouracil
	Retinoids
	Thiazides
Hydralazine	Thrombolytic agents
Interferons	

Erythema multiforme

Erythema multiforme is a cutaneous response triggered by various infections and drugs (Table 2.6). As the name implies, it can present in a variety of patterns. The classic pattern affects the hands and feet and limbs more than the trunk. There may be blisters, papular lesions or erythematous areas. A characteristic lesion is one of concentric rings, variously described as target, iris or bullseye shaped. Involvement of the mucosa is common, so the mouth, eyes and genitalia may be affected.

Infections are a more common cause of erythema multiforme than drugs and many cases have been wrongly blamed on drugs. Erythema

Table 2.6 Some drugs that may cause erythema muliforme or Stevens–Johnson syndrome

Barbiturates	Macrolides
Beta-lactam antibiotics	Mefloquine
Carbamazepine	Non-steroidal anti-inflammatory drugs
Co-trimoxazole	Phenothiazines
Chlorpropamide	Phenytoin
Gold	Rifampicin
Histamine H_2-antagonists	Sulphonamides
Lamotrigine	Tetracyclines
Leflunomide	Thiazides

multiforme may be due to vaccination, a variety of topical medications and some environmental substances (e.g. nickel) (Breathnach and Hintner, 1992; Smith, 1994). When the condition is suspected, all drugs, especially those introduced within the past month, should be discontinued since there is a risk of progression to SJS or toxic epidermal necrolysis.

Stevens–Johnson syndrome

SJS comprises fever, malaise, myalgia, arthralgia and extensive erythema multiforme of the trunk and face. It is frequently drug-induced. There may be skin blistering and erosions covering less than 10% of the body's surface area. This syndrome is distinct from toxic epidermal necrolysis (TEN), but there is a degree of overlap as severe forms of SJS can evolve into TEN and several drugs can produce both entities (Roujeau and Stern, 1994; Wolkenstein and Revuz, 1995). The estimated incidence of SJS ranges between 1.2 and 6 per million population per year. In about 50% of cases the cause is not known. The fatality rate is believed to be about 5%.

A large number of drugs have been implicated as a cause of SJS. Penicillins, tetracyclines, sulphonamides and non-steroidal anti-inflammatory drugs (NSAIDs) are among the most common. Patients with HIV infection seem to be at increased risk of developing SJS with co-trimoxazole. Drugs that may be responsible for the reaction should be stopped immediately in all patients. Management involves systemic corticosteroids, fluid replacement and antibiotics, if required. Drug rechallenge is never justified.

Toxic epidermal necrolysis

TEN, or Lyell's syndrome, is a rare variety of erythema with acute epithelial necrosis affecting all areas of the skin. The estimated incidence ranges from 0.4 to 1.2 per million population per year (Wolkenstein et al., 1998). It has a high associated mortality of about 30%. In TEN, sheet-like skin erosion affects more than 10% of the body surface and there is severe involvement of the mucous membranes (oropharynx, eyes and genitalia). The main cause in adults is drugs (Table 2.7). Patients with HIV infection, systemic lupus erythematosus and bone marrow transplant recipients seem to be predisposed to this disorder. Elderly patients and those with extensive TEN have a worse prognosis. Drug-induced TEN is rare in children, in whom the diagno-

Table 2.7 Some drugs that may cause toxic epidermal necrolysis

Allopurinol	Non-steroidal anti-inflammatory drugs
Barbiturates	(especially oxicam derivatives)
Carbamazepine	Penicillins
Gold	Phenytoin
Griseofulvin	Salicylates
Lamotrigine	Sulphonamides
Leflunomide	Tetracyclines
Nitrofurantoin	

sis must be distinguished from staphylococcal 'scalded skin syndrome' (Becker, 1998; Wolkenstein *et al.*, 1998).

TEN presents with a prodromal period of fever, conjunctivitis, pharyngitis, pruritus and, occasionally, difficulty in urination. These symptoms generally last 2–3 days and can resemble an upper respiratory tract infection. The burning or painful skin rash generally begins on the face or upper trunk and is characterised by poorly defined erythematous or dark coloured macules, irregular target-like bullae or diffuse ill-defined erythema. The affected skin may develop flaccid bullae or may detach irregularly, sometimes in large sheets. The lesions generally progress and extend in waves over a 3–4-day period, but can progress rapidly in a few hours, or more slowly. In most cases, mucosal lesions are present, particularly of the buccal mucosa, with the ocular and genital mucosa affected less often. The consequences of such a massive loss of epidermis include dehydration, increased energy expenditure and local or systemic infection such as septicaemia. In severe cases, other organ systems can be involved: hepatocellular damage, pneumonia, nephritis and myocardial damage may occur. Skin sloughing can extend into the oesophagus and bronchial tree.

The mechanisms responsible for TEN are unknown, although a hypersensitivity–immunological basis is suspected. A TEN-like eruption has occurred in patients with a graft-versus-host reaction after bone marrow transplant. Identification of the causative drug is often difficult. In general, most drugs causing TEN have been given in the previous 1–3 weeks. Drugs started less than 7 days or more than 2 months before the onset of the reaction are unlikely to be responsible. Phenytoin-induced TEN can occur at any time between 2 and 8 weeks after initiation of therapy and may progress despite discontinuation of the drug.

There has been debate about where this serious condition should be managed. Most experts now agree that management in a specialist burns unit is preferred. Treatment involves the careful protection of exposed dermis and eroded mucosal surfaces, managing fluid and electrolyte balance, nutritional support and close monitoring for evidence of infection. Antibiotic therapy should be reserved for treatment rather than given prophylactically. The place of systemic corticosteroids in the management of TEN is controversial. It has been suggested that long-term high-dose therapy may be associated with higher rates of morbidity and mortality. The benefits of short-term high doses of steroids prior to skin blistering have not been determined in prospective trials (Smoot, 1999). A recent study described the sucessful use of high-dose intravenous immunoglobulins in ten patients with TEN (Roujeau, 1999). The potential benefits of this treatment require further evaluation.

There is a risk of serious skin reactions with the antiepileptic lamotrigine (Committee on Safety of Medicines, 1997). About 1 in 1000 adults treated develop these reactions, including SJS and TEN. Children are at increased risk; the frequency of these problems may be as high as 1 in 300 to 1 in 100. Factors increasing the risk include the use of higher than recommended doses, rapid dose escalation and concomitant use of valproate. Most of these problems have developed within 8 weeks of starting lamotrigine and resolved upon withdrawal, but deaths have occurred (Messenheimer *et al.*, 1998; Schlienger *et al.*, 1998).

Pemphigus-like eruptions

Idiopathic pemphigus and bullous pemphigoid are autoimmune disorders. Idiopathic pemphigus typically features superficial flaccid blisters, although sometimes erythema, crusting and scaling are the major clinical signs. Idiopathic bullous pemphigoid is characterised by large tense blisters developing on an erythematous base. The fluid within is often haemorrhagic. A number of drugs, most of which contain a thiol (or sulphydryl) group in their molecular structure, have been implicated in causing a disorder closely resembling these idiopathic conditions (Table 2.8; Vassileva *et al.*, 1998). Cicatricial pemphigoid is a rare variant in which mouth ulcers, eye problems and other complications may develop, with subsequent scarring.

The drug-induced disorder has a broad spectrum of clinical presentation comprising widely scattered large firm bullae, classical but fewer lesions, scarring plaques, an erythema multiforme-like picture and a pemphigus-like picture. In general, affected patients are younger

Table 2.8 Some drugs that may cause pemphigus-like eruptions

Captopril	Interleukin-2
Enalapril	Penicillamine
Flupentixol	Penicillins
Furosemide (frusemide)	Sulfasalazine

than those with idiopathic disease. The drug-induced variant can feature clinical characteristics of both pemphigus and pemphigoid. The mechanism is unknown; both immune and toxic mechanisms have been proposed.

The entire clinical spectrum of pemphigus has been reported in association with penicillamine. As many as 7% of patients taking the drug for more than 6 months develop a pemphigus-like eruption. This is thought to be a cutaneous manifestation of the autoimmunogenic properties of the drug. Evidence suggests that the penicillamine-induced variant of pemphigus is essentially the same as the idiopathic condition (Meyboom and Brodie-Meijer, 1996). The disease usually improves when penicillamine is stopped but may persist for many years and recur on rechallenge.

Photosensitivity

Photosensitivity denotes a reaction occurring when a photosensitising agent in or on the skin reacts to normally harmless doses of ultraviolet or visible light. It may be due to topical or systemic drugs (Table 2.9). Drug-induced photosensitivity is classified as either phototoxic or photoallergic (Ferguson and Katsambas, 1997). Some drugs may induce photosensitivity by precipitating porphyria (e.g. hepatic damage from oral contraceptives) or lupus erythematosus (e.g. hydralazine).

Table 2.9 Some drugs associated with photosensitivity

Frequent	Less frequent
Amiodarone	Antidepressants (tricylic,
Non-steroidal anti-inflammatory drugs	monoamine oxidase inhibitors)
Phenothiazines (particularly	Carbamazepine
chlorpromazine)	Griseofulvin
Retinoids	Quinine
Sulphonamides	Quinolones
Tetracyclines (particularly demeclocycline)	Sulphonylureas
Thiazides	

Phototoxic reactions are common and can be produced in most individuals given a high enough dose of drug and sufficient light exposure. The eruption is usually evident within 5–20 hours of exposure and resembles exaggerated sunburn with erythema, oedema, blistering, weeping and desquamation. The rash is confined to areas exposed to light. Hyperpigmentation may remain after other features have subsided. Patients taking potent photosensitising agents on a long-term basis should be warned of the problem and counselled on the need to avoid direct sunlight and to use sunblocks (Allen, 1993; Ferguson and Katsambas, 1997). Several antibiotic classes are associated with photosensitive reactions, including the sulphonamides, tetracyclines and quinolones (Vassileva *et al.*, 1998).

Amiodarone is associated with a 30–50% incidence of photosensitivity. Symptoms develop within 2 hours of sun exposure as a burning sensation followed by erythema. A small number of affected patients develop slate-grey pigmentation on light-exposed areas. Light sensitivity may persist for up to 4 months after the drug is stopped. Cutaneous pigmentation slowly fades after amiodarone is stopped but may persist for months to years. The problem is related to both the dosage and duration of drug therapy. Skin cells and cells of other organs in affected patients have been found to contain myelin-like lysosomal structures and membrane-bound granules. This generalised derangement of lysosomal storage may be the basis for other adverse effects of amiodarone such as interstitial alveolitis, acute hepatitis and disturbed thyroid function (Chalmers *et al.*, 1982; Zachary *et al.*, 1984).

Chlorpromazine may cause a phototoxic response when given in high doses. The reaction is characterised by a burning, painful erythema within minutes of exposure to sunlight, either directly or through window panes. Erythema may persist for more than 24 hours. Occasionally, a golden-brown or slate-grey pigmentation, predominantly of exposed sites, may be seen.

Photoallergy is less common than phototoxicity and may occur following exposure to chlorpromazine powder (Ferguson and Katsambas, 1997). Photoallergic reactions occur in predisposed individuals who have been previously sensitised. There is a latent period during which sensitisation occurs and the reaction generally develops within 24 hours of re-exposure. Unlike phototoxic reactions, the reaction may spread beyond irradiated areas. Most systemic drugs causing photoallergy also cause phototoxicity. These reactions may occur as a result of local photocontact dermatitis to a topical photoallergen or as a result of systemic drug therapy.

Lichenoid drug eruptions

Lichenoid drug eruptions (LDE) are so called because of their resemblance to idiopathic lichen planus. The first drugs reported to cause lichenoid skin reactions were arsenicals used in the treatment of syphilis. Several causative drugs are now known (Table 2.10), although LDE is quite rare in comparison with other drug-induced skin reactions. The lesions can be described as small, shiny, polygonal, purplish papules, sometimes with a network of white lines known as Wickham's striae. They are usually itchy but they can be asymptomatic. The surrounding skin is completely normal. LDE can rarely affect the buccal mucosa; a characteristic white lace pattern may be present (Highet, 1997).

LDE tend to be extensive and may be linked with, or develop into, an exfoliative dermatitis. LDE can also result from contact dermatitis in photographic workers who handle certain *p*-phenylenediamines (Ellgehausen *et al.*, 1998). The clinical course of LDE has been investigated in many studies. The mechanism is thought to have an immunological basis. The time to onset of the reaction ranges from weeks to months after initiation of therapy. In most patients the symptoms cleared spontaneously within a few weeks of drug withdrawal. In prolonged or severe cases, topical or systemic corticosteroids may be used (Ellgehausen *et al.*, 1998).

Table 2.10 Some drugs that may cause lichenoid eruptions

Antimalarials	Lithium
Beta-blockers	Methyldopa
Captopril	Non-steroidal anti-inflammatory drugs
Gold	Penicillamine
Hydroxycarbamide (hydroxyurea)	Sulphonylureas
Interferon alfa	

Pigmentary disorders

Many skin diseases are followed by changes in skin colour (Table 2.11). In particular, after lichenoid eruptions and fixed drug eruptions there may be residual pigmentation. Drug-induced alteration in skin colour may result from increased (or, more rarely, decreased) melanin synthesis, increased lipofuscin synthesis or cutaneous deposition of drug-related material. Sometimes the exact nature of the pigment is unknown. The pigmentation may be widespread or localized and pigment deposits occasionally occur in internal organs.

Table 2.11 Some drugs that may cause pigmentation

Amiodarone (slate-grey)	Mepacrine (yellow)
Chloroquine (blue-grey or brown)	Minocycline (slate-grey or brown)
Chlorpromazine (blue-grey)	Oral contraceptives (brown)
Gold (blue-grey)	Phenytoin (brown)
Hydroxychloroquine (slate-grey or brown)	

A brown patchy pigmentation on light-exposed areas may be a result of prolonged administration of phenytoin. It occurs in about 10% of patients; women are more likely to be affected. The pigmentation is similar to chloasma, affecting mainly face, neck and arms.

Pigmentary changes develop in about 25% of patients receiving antimalarials for more than 3 or 4 months. The shins and pretibial area are most commonly affected. Irregular patches from grey to blue-black in colour are seen. Patients who develop this pigmentation should undergo an eye examination as corneal depositions and retinal damage frequently coexist. Antimalarials should preferably be discontinued in affected patients, as the retinal damage is irreversible.

Hyperpigmentation has recently been described after long-term use of minocycline and imipramine (Ming *et al.*, 1999).

Alopecia

Many drugs have been reported to cause hair loss (Table 2.12). The human scalp has about 100 000 hairs, 100 of which are shed daily. Human hair follicles undergo three cyclical stages: the actively growing phase of anagen, which lasts about 3 years and features 80–90% of the scalp's follicles; the brief involutionary phase of catagen; and the resting phase of telogen which lasts about 3 months. The telogen phase culminates in the shedding of the hair shaft and at the same time new growth in the hair follicle begins (Tosti *et al.*, 1994; Smith, 1995; Gautam, 1999). Hair follicles produce two types of hair according to the area of the body. Vellus hair is soft and colourless, covering the body surface apart from palms and soles. Terminal hair is the large, coarse, pigmented hair that occurs on the scalp, eyebrows, axillae, etc.

Drugs that induce hair loss may be classified according to the phase of the hair follicle cycle that is affected. In anagen effluvium, drugs induce an abrupt cessation of active anagen growth, and the hairs are shed within days or weeks with tapered and broken roots. Anagen hair loss is an expected pharmacological effect of cytotoxic chemother-

Table 2.12 Some drugs that may cause alopecia

Amfetamines	Hypolipidaemics
Anticoagulants (warfarin, heparin, heparinoids)	Interferons
Antidepressants	Leflunomide
Antithyroid drugs	Lithium
Beta-blockers	Oral contraceptives
Carbamazepine	Retinoids
Cimetidine	Tamoxifen
Cytotoxic agents	Valproate

apy and is often dose-related. The hair loss is almost always reversible but a delay of several weeks is common before regrowth begins. Alopecia is associated with alkylating agents, such as cyclophosphamide, cytotoxic antibiotics, such as bleomycin, vinca alkaloids and platinum compounds. Scalp hypothermia may be useful partially to prevent hair loss in patients undergoing chemotherapy.

Telogen hair loss may be a consequence of drug therapy or events such as severe illness and it can be difficult to establish the cause. It features a conversion in the hair root from the anagen phase to the telogen phase. Drug-induced telogen effluvium usually becomes evident 2–4 months after the treatment is started. Alopecia may or may not be noticeable, depending on the proportion of follicles involved. Hair loss is usually confined to the scalp, although the eyebrows, axillary and pubic regions may be affected. Spontaneous regrowth of hair at the follicle usually occurs within 2–5 months after the causative drug is discontinued. The only way to establish whether or not a particular drug is the cause of the hair loss is to stop the medication, verify improvement and then reinstitute the drug therapy. Alopecia is a well-recognised sign of hypothyroidism and can occur when the disorder is drug-induced (see Chapter 6).

Idiopathic androgenic alopecia (male pattern baldness) presents in several ways but often as a bitemporal recession of the hairline. In women, a diffuse thinning over the top of the scalp with preservation of the anterior hairline occurs. Drugs with androgenic activity may cause this problem, such as danazol, metyrapone and anabolic steroids. It can also occur with the oestrogen receptor antagonist tamoxifen.

Hair gain

There are two patterns of unwanted increase in hair growth, both of which may be associated with drug administration. Hirsutism is an excessive growth of coarse hair with masculine characteristics in a female. This is a consequence of androgenic stimulation of hormone-sensitive hair follicles. Drugs commonly responsible include testosterone, danazol, corticotropin, anabolic steroids and glucocorticoids. Patients with drug-induced hirsutism may also present with other dermatological signs of virilisation such as acne.

Hypertrichosis describes the growth of terminal and/or vellus hair on areas of the body where the hair is usually short, such as the forehead and cheeks. Table 2.13 shows some drugs that have been associated with the development of hypertrichosis. The problem is usually dose-related and reversible after drug withdrawal. Ciclosporin may produce hypertrichosis in 50% of transplant recipients, with the excess growth being most marked on the face and upper back. The problem is less frequent in conditions where lower doses of ciclosporin are used. Minoxidil causes some degree of hypertrichosis in nearly all patients; this effect has led to its theraputic use as a topical treatment for male pattern baldness.

Table 2.13 Some drugs that may cause hypertrichosis

Androgens	Penicillamine
Ciclosporin	Phenytoin
Diazoxide	Psoralens
Minoxidil	Verapamil
Nifedipine	

Nail disorders

A large number of drugs of different classes may be responsible for the development of nail changes (Piraccini and Tosti, 1999). Such changes usually involve several or all of the nails and appear within a few weeks of drug administration. Nail problems can be asymptomatic or associated with pain and impaired digital function. They are usually reversible on drug discontinuation. Nail abnormalities include Beau's lines (horizontal notches in the nail plate), brittle nails, onycholysis (separation of the nail plate from the nail bed), onychomadesis (separation of the nail plate from the matrix area, with progression to shedding) and paronychia (erythematous and tender nail folds).

The nail can be considered to be homologous to hair and the same drugs frequently affect both tissues (Smith, 1995). The pathogenesis of drug-induced nail abnormalities is not well understood but most cases are thought to involve a toxic effect of the drug on the nail epithelia.

Other potential factors may be drug deposition in the nail plate leading to nail discoloration and impaired digital perfusion causing necrosis of the nail apparatus or damage to the nail bed blood vessels. Some drugs that may cause nail disorders are shown in Table 2.14.

Table 2.14 Some drugs that may cause nail disorders

Captopril	8-methoxypsoralen
Chloramphenicol	Penicillamine
Chlorpromazine	Phenytoin
Cytotoxic agents	Retinoids
Fluoroquinolones	Tetracyclines
Gold	Thiazides
Lithium	

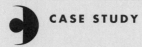

CASE STUDY

A young woman asks for advice about her 14-month-old baby. She explains that 4 days ago she started to give the baby a prescribed course of amoxicillin for a middle-ear infection. Yesterday she noticed that he had developed three or four red blotches on his upper chest and shoulders. She telephoned the local emergency medical service and was advised to use calamine lotion on the blotches, to continue giving the antibiotic and to get back in touch if the rash became worse. Earlier today the baby seemed well but he now seems feverish and the blotches have spread to most parts of the body. On examination the lesions are large, deep red circles which look darker in the centre. There is no sign of blistering or exfoliation. The baby does have a temperature.

What are the most likely possible causes of skin rash in an infant?
There are a number of possible causes, the most obvious of which are viral or bacterial infection (e.g. chickenpox, measles), staphylococcal superinfection of eczema or allergy to a chemical or drug.

What skin disorder does this type of lesion suggest?
The erythematous lesions described are suggestive of the target-like lesions which are characteristic of erythema multiforme. Penicillins are a recognised cause of this sort of reaction but infection is also a common cause. The presence of fever could indicate progression to a more serious skin disorder.

Is there any other information that might be important?
It is important to find out whether the baby has had any other medication recently (e.g. over-the-counter cough mixtures, analgesics, vaccinations). You should check exactly how long the antibiotic has been taken, whether there is any history of eczema or drug allergy, and whether there are any other signs or symptoms, particularly mucous membrane involvement (e.g. lesions in the mouth). It is also worth finding out what brand of amoxicillin was dispensed so that you can check the constituents for artificial colourings, etc.

What advice do you give the child's mother?
You should explain that the rash might be due to an infection or a side-effect of the medication. The baby should not be given any more of the antibiotic in the meantime. Because the rash has spread and the baby has a temperature, medical advice is needed promptly.

References

Allen J E (1993). Drug-induced photosensitivity. *Clin Pharm* 12: 580–587.

Becker D S (1998). Toxic epidermal necrolysis. *Lancet* 351: 1417–1420.

Breathnach S M, Hintner H (1992). *Adverse Drug Reactions and the Skin.* Oxford: Blackwell Scientific Publications.

Cha Y J, Pearson V E (1999). Angioedema due to losartan. *Ann Pharmacother* 33: 936–938.

Chalmers R J, Muston H L, Srinivas V *et al.* (1982). High incidence of amiodarone induced photosensitivity in north-west England. *Br Med J* 285: 341.

Chastain M A, Russo G G, Boh E E *et al.* (1999). Propylthiouracil hypersensitivity: report of two patients with vasculitis and review of the literature. *J Am Acad Dermatol* 41: 757–764.

Chu T C (1997). Acne and other facial eruptions. *Medicine* 25: 30–33.

Committee on Safety of Medicines (1997). Lamotrigine (Lamictal). Increased risk of serious skin reactions in children. *Curr Probl* 23: 8.

DeLeo V A (1998). Skin testing in systemic cutaneous drug reactions. *Lancet* 352: 1488–1490.

Ellgehausen P, Elsner P, Burg G (1998). Drug-induced lichen planus. *Clin Dermatol* 16: 325–332.

Ferguson J, Katsambas A (1997). Photosensitivity disorders. *Medicine* 25: 34–36.

García-Porrúa C, González-Gay M A, López-Lázaro L (1999). Drug associated cutaneous vasculitis in adults in northwestern Spain. *J Rheumatol* 26: 1942–1944.

Gautam M (1999). Alopecia due to psychotropic medications. *Ann Pharmacother* 33: 631–637.

Ghura H S, Carmichael A J, Bairstow D, Finney R (1999). Fatal erythroderma associated with pentostatin. *Br Med J* 319: 549.

Gibbs C R, Lip G Y H, Beevers D G (1999). Angioedema due to ACE inhibitors: increased risk in patients of African origin. *Br J Clin Pharmacol* 48: 861–865.

Golightly L K, Smolinske S S, Bennett M L *et al.* (1988). Pharmaceutical excipients: adverse effects associated with inactive ingredients in drug products (part 1). *Med Toxicol (part 1) 3*: 128–165.

Gupta A K, Lynde C W, Lauzon G J *et al.* (1998). Cutaneous adverse effects associated with terbinafine therapy: 10 case reports and a review of the literature. *Br J Dermatol* 138: 529–532.

Highet A S (1997). Lichen planus and lichenoid eruptions. *Medicine* 25: 75.

Jain K K (1993). Drug-induced cutaneous vasculitis. *Adverse Drug React Toxicol Rev* 12: 263–276.

Jick H, Derby L E (1995). Is co-trimoxazole safe? *Lancet* 345: 1118–1119.

Katugampola G, Katugampola S (1990). Chloroquine and psoriasis. *Int J Dermatol* 29: 153–154.

Kauppinen K, Stubbs S (1985). Fixed eruptions: causative drugs and challenge tests. *Br J Dermatol* 112: 575–578.

Korkij W, Soltani K (1984). Fixed drug eruption. *Arch Dermatol* 120: 520–524.

Kowalzick L (1997). Psoriasis flare caused by recombinant interferon beta injections. *J Am Acad Dermatol* 36: 501.

Kuflik E G (1980). Effects of antimalarial drugs on psoriasis. *Cutis* 26: 153–158.

Mackel S E (1982). Treatment of vasculitis. *Med Clin North Am* 66: 941–954.

Mahboob A, Haroon T S (1998). Drugs causing fixed eruptions: a study of 450 cases. *Int J Dermatol* 37: 833–838.

Malinverni R, Hoigne R, Sonntag R (1996). Sulfonamides, other folic acid antagonists and miscellaneous antibacterial drugs. In: Dukes M N G, ed. *Meyler's Side Effects of Drugs*, 13th edn. Amsterdam: Elsevier Science, chapter 29.

Messenheimer J, Mullens E L, Giorgi L *et al.* (1998). Safety review of adult clinical trial experience with lamotrigine. *Drug Safety* 18: 281–296.

Meyboom R H B, Brodie-Meijer C C E (1996). Metal antagonists. In: Dukes M N G, ed. *Meyler's Side Effects of Drugs,* 13th edn. Amsterdam: Elsevier Science, chapter 23.

Ming M E, Bhawan J, Stefanato C M *et al.* (1999). Imipramine-induced hyperpigmentation: four cases and a review of the literature. *J Am Acad Dermatol* 40: 159–166.

Nowakowski P A, Rumsfield J A, West D P (1997). Drug-induced skin disorders. In: Dipiro J T, Talbert R L, Yee G C *et al.*, eds. *Pharmacotherapy: A Pathophysiologic Approach,* 3rd edn. Connecticut: Appleton & Lange, chapter 91.

Paul C, Janier M, Carlet J *et al.* (1992). Erythroderma induced by teicoplanin. *Ann Dermatol Venereol* 119: 617.

Pauluzzi P, Boccucci N (1999). Inverse psoriasis induced by terbinafine. *Acta Dermato-Venereol* 79: 389.

Piraccini B M, Tosti A (1999). Drug-induced nail disorders. *Drug Safety* 21: 187–201.

Puig L, Goni F J, Roque A M *et al.* (1989). Psoriasis induced by ophthalmic timolol preparations. *Am J Ophthalmol* 108: 455–456.

Pylypchuk G B (1998). ACE inhibitor- versus angiotensin II blocker-induced cough and angioedema. *Ann Pharmacother* 32: 1060–1066.

Rivera J O (1999). Losartan-induced angioedema. *Ann Pharmacother* 33: 933–935.

Roujeau J C (1999). Treatment of severe drug eruptions. *J Dermatol* 26: 718–722.

Roujeau J C, Stern R S (1994). Severe adverse cutaneous reactions to drugs. *N Engl J Med* 331: 1272–1285.

Ryan T J (1995). Diseases of the skin. In: Weatherall D J, Ledingham J G G, Warrell D A, eds. *Oxford Textbook of Medicine,* 3rd edn. Oxford: Oxford University Press, chapter 23.

Sabroe R A, Black A K (1997). Angiotensin-converting enzyme (ACE) inhibitors and angioedema. *Br J Dermatol* 136: 153–158.

Schlienger R G, Shapiro L E, Shear N H (1998). Lamotrigine-induced severe cutaneous adverse reactions. *Epilepsia* 39 (suppl 7): S22–S26.

Smith A G (1994). Important cutaneous adverse drug reactions. *Adverse Drug React Bull* 167: 631–634.

Smith A G (1995). Drug-induced disorders of hair and nails. *Adverse Drug React Bull* 173: 655–658.

Smoot E C (1999). Treatment issues in the care of patients with toxic epidermal necrolysis. *Burns* 25: 439–442.

Tosti A, Misciali C, Piraccini B M *et al.* (1994). Drug-induced hair loss and hair growth. Incidence, management and avoidance. *Drug Safety* 10: 310–317.

Tsankov N, Kazandjieva J, Drenovska K (1998). Drugs in exacerbation and provocation of psoriasis. *Clin Dermatol* 16: 333–351.

Vassileva S (1998). Drug-induced pemphigoid: bullous and cicatricial. *Clin Dermatol* 16: 379–387.

Vassileva S G, Mateev G, Parish L C (1998). Antimicrobial photosensitive reactions. *Arch Intern Med* 158: 1993–2000.

Vervloet D, Durham S (1998). ABC of allergies. Adverse reactions to drugs. *Br Med J* 316: 1511–1513.

Vial T, Descotes J (1996). Drugs acting on the immune system. In: Dukes M N G, ed. *Meyler's Side Effects of Drugs,* 13th edn. Amsterdam: Elsevier Science, chapter 37.

Vleeming W, van Amsterdam J G C, Stricker B H C *et al.* (1998). ACE inhibitor-induced angioedema. *Drug Safety* 18: 171–188.

Webster G (1997). Psoriasis flare caused by recombinant interferon beta injections. *J Am Acad Dermatol* 36: 501.

Wilson N J, Evans S (1998). Severe pustular psoriasis provoked by oral terbinafine. *Br J Dermatol* 139: 168.

Wolfe J T, Singh A, Lessin S R *et al.* (1995). De novo development of psoriatic plaques in patients receiving interferon alfa for treatment of erythrodermic cutaneous T-cell lymphoma. *J Am Acad Dermatol* 32: 887–893.

Wolkenstein P, Revuz J (1995). Drug-induced severe skin reactions. *Drug Safety* 13: 56–68.

Wolkenstein P E, Roujeau J C, Revuz J (1998). Drug-induced toxic epidermal necrolysis. *Clin Dermatol* 16: 399–408.

Wright P (1975). Untoward effects associated with practolol administration: oculo-mucocutaneous syndrome. *Br Med J* i: 595–598.

Zachary C B, Slater D N, Holt D W *et al.* (1984). The pathogenesis of amiodarone-induced pigmentation and photosensitivity. *Br J Dermatol* 110: 451–456.

3

Gastrointestinal disorders

Anne Lee and John Morris

Gastrointestinal (GI) disorders account for about 20% of documented adverse drug reactions (ADRs) (Bates *et al.*, 1995; Smith *et al.*, 1996). Most drugs can affect the gut in some patients and the potential effects vary in severity from dyspepsia to life-threatening GI haemorrhage. The high frequency of reporting of suspected GI ADRs partly reflects the widespread use of aspirin and non-steroidal anti-inflammatory drugs (NSAIDs), whose gastrotoxic properties are renowned. These drugs can cause lesions anywhere in the GI tract, from oesophagus to colon.

Many patients will experience GI complaints related to prescribed or over-the-counter (OTC) medicines and these are an important cause of non-compliance. Healthcare professionals should be familiar with the drugs which frequently cause troublesome GI symptoms, especially where these may be a precursor of more serious toxicity.

The mouth

Taste disorders

The sense of taste (and smell) is mediated by chemosensory nerves that respond to stimulatory chemicals by direct receptor binding, opening ion channels or second messenger systems (Ackerman and Kasbekar, 1997). Taste disturbances may be a feature of acute or chronic disease but drugs can alter taste through an effect on the cellular processes involved. Many drugs can affect the sense of taste, by mechanisms that are unclear. Taste may be blunted (hypogeusia), lost completely (ageusia) or distorted, e.g. sweet things taste sour (dysgeusia) (Seymour, 1998). These problems can lead to non-compliance and occasionally weight loss through poor appetite. Among drug-induced taste disorders, hypogeusia is common but often unrecognised by patients. Dysgeusia is also relatively common; affected patients sense an excessively sweet, bitter, salty or metallic taste while eating. The sensation persists and is incongruous with expected tastes. The problem is thought to be due to a dysfunction of taste buds or ion channels.

Compounds that contain a sulphydryl group, such as penicillamine and captopril, are a common cause of taste disturbance. Penicillamine, the copper chelating agent used in Wilson's disease and as an anti-inflammatory in rheumatoid arthritis, often causes transient taste loss in the first 6 weeks of treatment. Copper depletion is probably the underlying mechanism. Patients with Wilson's disease are less likely to be affected than those with rheumatoid disorders; about a third of rheumatoid patients are affected (Henkin, 1994). Captopril causes taste dysfunction in about 2–4% of patients (Alderman, 1996). It can cause a range of abnormalities from persisting sweetness or saltiness to metallic or bitter tastes. The problem has also occurred with angiotensin-converting enzyme (ACE) inhibitors without a sulphydryl group, although the incidence is much less. The exact mechanism is uncertain, although altered tissue zinc concentrations may be involved.

Terbinafine causes taste disturbance in up to 1% of patients and the problem may persist after treatment is discontinued (Bong *et al.*, 1998); low body weight and old age may be risk factors (Beutler *et al.*, 1993; Stricker *et al.*, 1996).

Metallic taste can occur with gold compounds, metronidazole, metformin and zopiclone (Galan and Grymonpre, 1994). Acetazolamide may cause carbonated drinks to taste bitter (Martinez-Mir *et al.*, 1997). Although ageusia is rare, it has been reported with ACE inhibitors, losartan, etidronate and nifedipine.

Table 3.1 Some drugs that can cause taste disturbance

Taste disturbance	Metallic taste
ACE inhibitors	Allopurinol
Acetazolamide	Gold compounds
Calcium channel blockers	Lithium
Etidronate	Metformin
Griseofulvin	Metronidazole
Isotretinoin	Penicillamine
Levodopa	Zopiclone
Losartan	
Penicillamine	
Propylthiouracil	
Terbinafine	

Many other drugs have been reported to affect taste. Those which are commonly implicated are shown in Table 3.1. Taste disturbances usually resolve when the offending drug is withdrawn, although sometimes this can take many months. Zinc supplements have been used in the treatment of dysgeusia with variable success (Ackerman and Kasbekar, 1997).

Gingival overgrowth

Several drugs can cause an inflammatory gum overgrowth (hypertrophy) that may cover the teeth. Associated symptoms include pain, tenderness or bleeding of the gums. The first drug implicated was phenytoin but ciclosporin and the calcium channel blockers (especially dihydropyridines) are also now a recognised cause (Seymour, 1993; Brunet *et al.*, 1996; Table 3.2). Prevalence studies suggest that about 50% of patients taking phenytoin, 30% of those taking ciclosporin and 10% of those taking nifedipine will experience some degree of gingival overgrowth (Meraw and Sheridan, 1998).

The pathogenesis of this unwanted effect is uncertain. It has been suggested that the causative drug or its metabolites may interfere with the gingival fibroblast, resulting in increased collagen synthesis. Gingival changes usually occur within 3 months of starting the drug. Initially there is enlargement of the gingiva between the teeth which continues until the gingiva appear lobular. The problem seems to be more likely in patients with poor oral hygiene. In some affected patients the gingival changes can be extensive, causing interference with speech and eating, resulting in the need for extensive oral surgery (gingivectomy).

The management of drug-induced gingival overgrowth is unsatisfactory. Stopping the causative drug and changing to an alternative treatment is the preferred approach. However, it is often not practical to stop ciclosporin or phenytoin. Dosage reduction or switching to another drug in the same therapeutic class may be an option. Regression of nifedipine-induced gingival overgrowth has been shown after treatment was changed to isradipine (Meraw and Sheridan, 1998). Patients on

Table 3.2 Some drugs that can cause gingival overgrowth

Calcium channel blockers
Ciclosporin
Phenytoin

chronic therapy with phenytoin, ciclosporin or dihydropyridine calcium channel blockers should be counselled about the importance of good oral hygiene. Where drug-induced gingival overgrowth is suspected, a dentist's opinion may be helpful.

Pigmentation

Tetracyclines, and particularly minocycline, have occasionally caused unusual pigmentation in the mouth in adults (Eisen, 1997; Tanzi and Hecker, 2000).

Dry mouth (xerostomia)

The salivary glands are under the control of the autonomic nervous system and consequently their function can be affected by many drugs (Table 3.3). Most of the drugs that reduce salivary flow do so via anti-cholinergic effects. Dry mouth (xerostomia) is therefore a common problem with the wide range of agents with anticholinergic properties. It can cause problems with speech, eating and swallowing and patients become more susceptible to oral infections, particularly candidiasis. It may also predispose to dental caries. Caries has been a particular problem in patients treated with tricyclic antidepressants (DeVries and Peeters, 1995). It is important to advise patients starting treatment with anticholinergic agents, tricyclic antidepressants, phenothiazines or central nervous system stimulants that they may experience a dry mouth. Saliva substitutes or sugar-free chewing gum may provide some relief.

Table 3.3 Some drugs that commonly cause xerostomia

Amfebutamone
Anticholinergic agents
Antihistamines
Central nervous system stimulants (e.g. phentermine)
Phenothiazines
Tricyclic antidepressants

Ptyalism

Salivary secretion is increased by drugs that have a cholinergic effect (e.g. pilocarpine). Clozapine-induced nocturnal sialorrhoea is a well-recognised unwanted effect that can cause choking (Pearlman, 1994).

This problem is particularly troublesome in patients with Parkinson's disease as their swallowing is often impaired.

Stomatitis and mouth ulcers

Inflammation of the mouth (stomatitis) and tongue (glossitis) may be drug-induced. Contact stomatitis is a hypersensitivity reaction of the oral mucosa which occurs after repeated contact with an allergen. Hypersensitivity can develop at any time – from days to years – after exposure to the allergen. Common causes include toothpastes, mouthwashes, antiseptic lozenges, lipsticks and lipsalves, food additives and chewing gum (Seymour, 1998).

Mouth ulcers may occur during treatment with many cytotoxic drugs, NSAIDs, proguanil, gold compounds and sulfasalazine. They usually resolve quickly after the drug is stopped (Galan and Grymonpre, 1994). The oral mucous membranes are commonly involved in erythema multiforme and, in the severe form – Stevens–Johnson syndrome – massive mucous membrane ulceration can occur throughout the gut (see Chapter 2). Drugs causing this potentially life-threatening effect include penicillins, sulphonamides and phenytoin. Intensive supportive therapy is the mainstay of management.

Nicorandil, a potassium channel activator used in the management of angina, has been linked with recurrent aphthous ulcers (Agbo-Godeau *et al.*, 1998; Cribier *et al.*, 1998; Desruelles *et al.*, 1998; Shotts *et al.*, 1999). Large, painful mouth ulcers affecting the tongue, the inside of the cheeks and the gingiva have been described. Often the ulcers persisted despite symptomatic treatment or relapsed soon afterwards. Affected patients were treated for 1–36 months before developing the ulcers, although in most cases the onset was noted within 1 year. In general the ulcers healed completely within several weeks of stopping nicorandil. It has been suggested that the problem is dose-related, occur-

Table 3.4 Some drugs that may cause mouth ulcers/stomatitis

Aspirin	Leflunomide
Auranofin	Nicorandil
Barbiturates	Non-steroidal anti-inflammatory
Captopril	drugs
Cytotoxics	Penicillamine
Griseofulvin	Proguanil
Interferon alfa	Sulfasalazine
Isoniazid	

ring more often with doses above 30 mg daily. The underlying mechanism for this adverse effect remains unclear. Table 3.4 shows some drugs that commonly cause mouth ulcers/stomatitis.

The oesophagus

Drugs that relax the lower oesophageal sphincter may cause symptoms secondary to acid reflux or heartburn. This has been described with calcium channel blockers (Ganginella and Maxfield, 1988), opioids and anticholinergic drugs.

Drug-induced oesophageal injury is a common cause of oesophageal complaints. Major oesophageal symptoms are dysphagia (difficulty in swallowing), heartburn and painful swallowing (odynophagia). Oesophageal ulceration, which can lead to stricture, has occurred secondary to drug therapy. Patients with oesophageal injury typically present with sudden onset of odynophagia or substernal chest pain within a period of hours to days after taking the medication. Occasionally the pain is severe enough to be misdiagnosed as angina or myocardial infarction. Other features include dysphagia or a persistent foreign body sensation in the oesophagus. The diagnosis of drug-induced oesophageal injury is confirmed by radiography or endoscopy (Levine, 1999; Jaspersen, 2000). Other conditions associated with the development of ulcers in the upper or mid oesophagus include herpes oesophagitis, reflux oesophagitis and Crohn's disease. Drug-induced mucosal injury is an essential part of the differential diagnosis of oesophageal ulceration.

Patients with drug-induced oesophagitis typically have a history of ingesting their medication with little or no water immediately before going to bed. The tablet or capsule then tends to become lodged in the upper or mid oesophagus where it can produce a contact oesophagitis. Several pharmaceutical factors are important, including the chemical formula, the molecular concentration, the duration of contact with the mucosa, the pH of the drug and the size of the tablet/capsule. Most injured patients have no predisposing factors but mechanical obstruction of the oesophagus, for example by compression of the oesophagus by an enlarged left atrium or dilated aorta, can contribute to this problem. Mechanical obstruction is thought to be important in cases of oesophagitis that have occurred with potassium chloride tablets and with quinidine in patients with cardiac problems (Jaspersen, 2000).

Antibiotics such as tetracyline and doxycycline are the most frequently offending agents, accounting for about half of all reported cases of drug-induced oesophagitis (Keller, 1992; Jaspersen, 2000). Both tetracycline and doxycycline capsules are relatively acidic and prolonged contact with the oesophageal wall can cause ulceration. There is a strong association between aspirin and oesophagitis (Shallcross and Heatley, 1990). Oesophagitis and oesophageal strictures have also been documented with a variety of NSAIDs. Chronic NSAID therapy may also aggravate pre-existing oesophageal disease (Semble *et al.*, 1989; Jaspersen, 2000).

Bisphosphonates are a recognised cause of oesophageal reactions. Alendronate has been reported to cause reflux, oesophagitis and ulceration (Committee on Safety of Medicines, 1996). To reduce the risk, patients prescribed alendronate must be carefully counselled about how to take the drug. In addition, it should be used with caution in patients with upper GI problems and in those taking NSAIDs or aspirin. If oesophagitis occurs, alendronate should be discontinued; it is not sufficient to prescribe a concomitant acid-suppressing drug.

Most uncomplicated cases of drug-induced oesophageal disorder heal spontaneously, resolving within days or weeks. Management generally comprises stopping the offending drug and supportive care. Parenteral or liquid analgesics may be required for the acute erosive stages of damage and sucralfate may also help. To minimise this problem, patients should be aware of the importance of swallowing their medicines while sitting or standing and to drink at least 100 ml of water immediately afterwards.

Drugs which may cause oesophageal reactions are shown in Table 3.5.

Table 3.5 Some drugs that may cause oesophageal disorders

Ascorbic acid	Lincomycin
Aspirin	Non-steroidal anti-inflammatory drugs
Bisphosphonates	Potassium chloride
Clindamycin	Quinidine
Doxycycline	Tetracycline
Ferrous sulphate	Theophylline

Nausea and vomiting

Nausea and/or vomiting are listed as potential side-effects in the prescribing information for many drugs. In practice, it is important to know which drugs frequently cause these symptoms (e.g. most cytotoxics, levodopa, opioids). With many drugs these symptoms will often resolve with continued use, although concurrent antiemetics may be required. If nausea and vomiting are severe, treatment may need to be stopped. For some drugs (e.g. digoxin, theophylline), nausea and vomiting may be an indicator of toxicity.

The pathophysiology of nausea and vomiting is poorly understood, but most drugs are thought to cause the problem through effects on the chemoreceptor trigger zone. Some drugs cause nausea through direct gastric irritation (e.g. iron salts, potassium). The mechanism by which antibiotics cause nausea is unclear. Drugs that are a common cause of nausea and vomiting are shown in Table 3.6.

Table 3.6 Some drugs that commonly cause nausea and/or vomiting

Bromocriptine	Levodopa
Cytotoxics	Oestrogens (high-dose)
Digoxin	Opioids
Ergot alkaloids	Selective serotonin reuptake inhibitors
Erythromycin	Theophylline
Iron salts	

Stomach and duodenum

NSAID gastrotoxicity

NSAIDs, including aspirin, are the most widely used class of medicines in the world. In the UK, more than 20 million prescriptions a year are issued for them. Their potential to damage the GI tract is their biggest disadvantage and such damage is the most prevalent category of ADR. Aspirin-induced gastric bleeding was confirmed by gastroscopy in 1938 (Douthwaite and Lintott, 1938) and cases of melaena and GI haemorrhage were first described in the 1950s. NSAID-related GI side-effects range in severity to include asymptomatic mucosal damage revealed on endoscopy, symptoms such as abdominal pain, heartburn and dyspepsia, and serious GI complications such as ulcers or bleeding requiring hospitalisation. All these side-effects involve various degrees of damage to the gastric mucosa resulting from prostaglandin inhibition. All NSAIDs inhibit the enzyme cyclooxygenase and so reduce the synthesis of prostaglandins which, among their many actions, mediate aspects of inflammation (Vane, 1971). Prostaglandins also have a physiological role in protecting the gastric mucosa. Inhibition of prostaglandin synthesis and, to a lesser extent, topical irritant effects on the gastric epithelium are responsible for NSAID gastrotoxicity (Wallace, 1997). All

NSAIDs have been found to cause gastric toxicity and severe toxicity is not prevented by parenteral or rectal administration (Anon, 1994). Although NSAID use is primarily associated with upper GI problems, such as GI bleeding, gastric ulcers and perforations, they also cause lower GI problems such as inflammation, haemorrhage, perforation and stricture formation.

Epidemiology

Estimates of the prevalence of NSAID-induced GI complications vary widely. In general, at least 10–20% of patients have dyspepsia while taking an NSAID, although the reported prevalence ranges from 5 to 50%. The overall prevalence of endoscopically confirmed gastric lesions arising during treatment is about 15–30%. Within a 6-month treatment period, 5–15% of patients with rheumatoid arthritis can be expected to discontinue NSAID therapy because of dyspepsia (Singh *et al.*, 1996).

In the US, the Food and Drug Administration estimates that symptomatic GI ulcers, bleeding and perforation occur in about 2–5% of patients using NSAIDs for 1 year.

Studies have used odds ratios, relative risks and risk ratios to express the risk of NSAID-related events relative to that in a control population (Langman *et al.*, 1985, 1994; Garcia-Rodriguez and Jick, 1994; Rees Willett *et al.*, 1994; Tannenbaum *et al.*, 1996). Langman *et al.* reported an odds ratio of 4.5 for peptic ulceration and bleeding due to NSAIDs (Langman *et al.*, 1994). Garcia-Rodriguez and Jick found a risk ratio of 3.9 for hospitalisation (Garcia-Rodriguez and Jick, 1994). In a meta-analysis of 40 studies published between 1975 and 1990, Gabriel and colleagues found that the overall odds ratio for serious NSAID-induced GI complications was 2.74 and the odds ratio for GI surgery was 7.75 (Gabriel *et al.*, 1991).

Prospective data from the US Arthritis, Rheumatism and Aging Medical Information System (ARAMIS) indicate that 15 of every 1000 rheumatoid arthritis patients who take NSAIDs for 1 year have a serious GI complication. This equates to a relative risk of 5.49 compared with that in patients not taking NSAIDs. The corresponding figure for serious complications in osteoarthritis patients is 7.3 per 1000 patients per year (relative risk versus patients not taking NSAIDs = 2.51).

The rate of serious GI complications requiring hospitalisation appears to be declining, presumably due to increased awareness as a result of efforts to educate prescribers about the magnitude of the problem. The mortality rate among patients who are hospitalised for NSAID-induced upper GI bleeding is about 5–10% (Armstrong and Blower, 1987). ARAMIS data suggest that the relative risk of death due to GI toxicity in rheumatoid arthritis patients taking NSAIDs is 4.21 times that in patients not using NSAIDs. Although the annual mortality rate (0.22%) in these patients may not seem high, the lifetime risk for patients with chronic arthritis is substantial.

US data suggest that there are at least 107 000 hospital admissions each year due to serious GI complications of NSAIDs, with associated costs in excess of US$1 billion (Singh and Rosen Ramey, 1998). The total number of deaths is believed to be similar to the number of deaths from human immunodeficiency virus (HIV) complications. Further-more, these data do not take into account usage of OTC NSAIDs.

Another cause for concern is the evidence that many regular NSAID users are unaware or unconcerned about possible GI complica-tions. In a recent survey of 4799 Americans, 807 had taken NSAIDs (prescribed or OTC) at least twice in the past year for 5 or more consec-utive days (Singh and Triadofilopoulos, 1999). About 45% of NSAID users reporting taking them for 5 or more consecutive days at least once a month and 40% took both OTC and prescribed NSAIDs. Nearly 75% of regular users were either unaware or unconcerned about possible GI complications. A large proportion of users indicated that they would expect warning signs before the development of a serious GI problem. This contrasts with the available evidence showing that only a minority of patients who develop such problems (<20%) report any antecedent dyspepsia.

Pathophysiology

Gastroduodenal mucosal injury develops when the deleterious effect of gastric acid overwhelms the normal defensive properties of the mucosa. Inhibition of prostaglandin synthesis by NSAIDs leads to decreases in epithelial mucus, bicarbonate secretion, mucosal blood flow, epithelial perforation and mucosal resistance to injury. The impairment in mucosal resistance permits injury by endogenous factors, including acid, pepsin and bile salts, as well as exogenous factors such as NSAIDs. Topical injury caused by NSAIDs contributes to the development of gas-troduodenal mucosal injury but systemic effects appear to have the pre-dominant role. The use of enteric-coated aspirin preparations and parenteral or rectal administration of NSAIDs in order to prevent topical damage has failed to prevent the development of ulcers.

The metabolism of arachidonic acid to prostaglandins is catalysed by the cyclooxygenase pathway. Two related but unique isoforms of cyclooxygenase, designated cyclooxygenase 1 (COX-1) and cyclooxygenase 2 (COX-2) have been demonstrated (Appleton *et al.*, 1994; Lipsky *et al.*, 1998). COX-1 appears to function as a 'housekeeping' enzyme in most tissues, including the gastric mucosa, the kidneys and the platelets. The expression of COX-2 can be induced by inflammatory stimuli in many tissues. It has been suggested that the anti-inflammatory properties of NSAIDs are mediated through the inhibition of COX-2 and that adverse effects, such as gastroduodenal ulceration, occur via effects on COX-1. NSAIDs have been developed which have less effect on COX-1; those described as 'COX-2 preferential' include nabumetone and etodolac. These may confer a slightly lower risk for serious GI toxicity than traditional drugs. A new generation of COX-2 selective compounds has now been developed (Lipsky *et al.*, 1998). Designed to cause little, if any, inhibition of COX-1 function at therapeutic doses, these agents are expected to exert anti-inflammatory and analgesic effects without the gastrotoxicity or platelet dysfunction that is characteristic of traditional NSAIDs. It has been suggested that COX-2 (like COX-1) is present in normal gastric mucosa (although not every study has found this) and, if so, it could play a physiological role there. Animal studies suggest that COX-2-derived prostaglandins may have a role in gastric ulcer healing but the relevance of this to humans is uncertain.

NSAID-induced GI damage can be categorised into three groups:

1   superficial damage such as mucosal haemorrhages and erosions which may cause symptoms but not ulcer formation
2   endoscopically diagnosed non-symptomatic ('silent') ulcers
3   symptomatic ulcers, including complications such as GI haemorrhage

Currently there are no definitive data that correlate findings on endoscopy with resultant GI haemorrhage, perforation or obstruction. However, it appears likely that all agents that increase the frequency of endoscopically defined ulcers will impose an increased risk of GI haemorrhage. Outcome data documenting a significant reduction in the incidence of GI bleeding, ulceration and perforation will be necessary to show conclusively that a compound has no clinically meaningful effect on gastric COX-1 function. Preliminary data suggest that celecoxib and rofecoxib are associated with fewer clinically symptomatic ulcers and ulcer complications than traditional NSAIDs (Langman *et al.*, 1999; Feldman and McMahon, 2000). The actual risk for serious GI complications will only become apparent during wider clinical use.

In the majority of patients, NSAID-induced gastroduodenal mucosal injury is superficial and self-limiting. However, peptic ulcers do develop in some patients and they may lead to gastroduodenal haemorrhage, perforation and death. The spectrum of NSAID-related gastroduodenal injury includes subepithelial haemorrhages, erosions and ulcerations and this is often referred to as NSAID gastropathy. No area of the stomach is resistant to mucosal injury; the most frequent and severely affected site is the gastric antrum. Duodenal mucosal injury is less common than gastric damage; however, the incidence of bleeding and perforation from the two sites is similar (Langman *et al.*, 1985).

Risk factors

Because serious GI events occur frequently in patients taking NSAIDs who have not experienced any warning symptoms, it is important to identify factors that increase the risk of serious GI complications and to consider how the risk can be reduced. Advanced age has been consistently found to be a primary risk factor; the risk increases linearly with age (Henry *et al.*, 1993; Wolfe *et al.*, 1999). It was previously thought that the risk of problems was greatest early in the course of treatment, but a recent study suggests that the risk of GI haemorrhage remains constant over an extended period of observation (Singh and Triadafilopoulus, 1999). The identification of *Helicobacter pylori* infection as a factor in the development of peptic ulcer has raised the question of a possible synergistic relationship between *H. pylori* infection and NSAID use. However, recent data suggest that any associated increase in risk is minimal. Recognised risk factors for NSAID-induced gastrotoxicity are shown in Table 3.7.

Relative safety

All traditional NSAIDs have been shown to cause the full spectrum of GI side-effects, but there are differences among NSAIDs with respect to the frequency of side-effects, mucosal damage and serious GI complica-

Table 3.7 Risk factors for NSAID-induced ulcer

Age over 60 years	Concomitant corticosteroids
Previous history of gastrointestinal problems (e.g. peptic ulcer, gastrointestinal bleeding)	Concomitant warfarin
	Serious systemic disorder
High NSAID dosage	Cigarette smoking (possible)
Hepatorenal dysfunction	Alcohol consumption (possible)

tions. The rate of reporting of serious upper GI effects to the Committee on Safety of Medicines (corrected for annual reporting trends) was used in 1994 to group the drugs in order of increasing frequency of their GI side-effects (Committee on Safety of Medicines, 1994). Ibuprofen was associated with the lowest risk. Diclofenac, naproxen and indometacin all had similar GI risk, greater than ibuprofen. Ketoprofen and piroxicam were associated with a greater risk. The rate was highest for azapropazone. This ranking is consistent with the findings of two large case-control studies and several epidemiological studies (Garcia-Rodriguez and Jick, 1994; Langman *et al.*, 1994).

Aspirin causes significant GI toxicity, even in the low doses used for cardiovascular prophylaxis (Weil *et al.*, 1995). Patients should be prescribed the lowest effective dose (usually 75 mg daily) in an attempt to reduce the incidence of GI complications (Anon, 1997). There is no evidence that at these doses the risk of clinically significant GI bleeding is reduced by using enteric-coated or modified-release formulations (Kelly *et al.*, 1996).

Treatment of NSAID-related dyspepsia

Symptoms associated with NSAIDs such as dyspepsia or heartburn are common and can generally be treated empirically with a histamine H_2-receptor antagonist (H_2A) or a proton pump inhibitor. However, the risk of serious GI complications was found to be higher in rheumatoid arthritis patients with no GI symptoms who were taking antacids or H_2As than in those taking no prophylaxis (Singh and Rosen Ramey, 1998). The reason for this finding is unknown but it may be explained by the masking of dyspeptic symptoms associated with mucosal injury.

In general, if a gastroduodenal ulcer develops in a patient taking an NSAID, the most prudent approach is to discontinue the NSAID and switch to a simple analgesic such as paracetamol. If treatment with the NSAID must be continued, a proton pump inhibitor should be prescribed concurrently, since these drugs have been shown to heal ulcers at the same rate, whether or not NSAID therapy is continued.

Prevention of GI complications

Because of the prevalance and severity of GI complications, recent efforts have been directed at the prevention of gastrotoxicity. However, there are no clear published guidelines on which patients should receive prophylaxis.

A recent endoscopic study compared omeprazole and ranitidine in the prevention of recurrent gastroduodenal ulcers in a large number of patients with arthritis in whom NSAID therapy could not be discontinued (Yeomans *et al.*, 1998). After 6 months of treatment 16.3% of patients treated with ranitidine had gastric ulcers and 4.2% had duodenal ulcers. In the omeprazole group 5.2% of patients had gastric ulcers and 0.5% had duodenal ulcers. H_2A are effective only in the prevention of NSAID-induced duodenal ulcers and are less effective than proton pump inhibitors, so their use cannot be recommended.

Misoprostol can be used for the prevention of NSAID-induced ulcers (gastric and duodenal) and has been shown to protect against clinically important complications (Maiden and Madhok, 1995; Silverstein *et al.*, 1995). It must be taken at least three times a day to provide adequate prophylaxis. In the Misoprostol Ulcer Complications Outcomes Safety Assessment (MUCOSA) study, concomitant treatment with misoprostol achieved a 40% reduction in the overall rate of NSAID-induced complications compared with placebo. Patients at particular risk of complications who require continued NSAID administration may benefit from prophylaxis with misoprostol or a proton pump inhibitor.

NSAID-induced GI complications account for a considerable number of hospital admissions and deaths and it has been estimated that 2000 UK hospital admissions each year could be prevented if simple guidelines on NSAID use were followed. Healthcare professionals have an important role in minimising the occurrence of these problems (Table 3.8).

Table 3.8 Minimising the risk of non-steroidal anti-inflammatory drug (NSAID)-induced gastrotoxicity

---

- No more than one NSAID should be taken at any one time
- If an NSAID is indicated, one of the less toxic agents should be first choice
- The lowest effective dose should be used
- The maximum recommended dose should not be exceeded
- Patients at particular risk of gastrointestinal complications (including those over 65 years old) should receive prophylaxis with misoprostol or a proton pump inhibitor
- Patients on long-term repeat prescription should be reviewed regularly, to avoid unnecessarily prolonged treatment, especially the elderly
- Patients should receive appropriate counselling. They should be advised not to take more than the recommended dose, and to consult their doctor immediately if they have any blood-stained vomit, black tarry stools or other signs of internal bleeding

---

Other drugs

Corticosteroids

There has been much debate about whether oral corticosteroids cause peptic ulcer. Several studies have suggested such a link, but most have weaknesses in the methodology. A large case-control study confirmed that patients taking steroids had twice the risk of developing a peptic ulcer, but the increased risk was confined to patients on concurrent NSAIDs (Piper *et al.*, 1991).

Calcium channel blockers

A study assessing the incidence of GI haemorrhage in a cohort of elderly patients with hypertension concluded that calcium channel blocker therapy was associated with an increased risk (Pahor *et al.*, 1996). However, subsequent research indicates that an increased risk is unlikely (Desboeuf *et al.*, 1998; Smalley *et al.*, 1998; Suissa *et al.*, 1998; Kelly *et al.*, 1999).

Selective serotonin reuptake inhibitors (SSRIs)

Published case reports have suggested an association between SSRIs and bleeding disorders. Most of the patients had mild bleeding disorders, for example, ecchymoses, purpura or prolonged bleeding time, but several had more serious conditions, including GI haemorrhage (De Abajo *et al.*, 1999). A case-control study investigating the potential link using the UK General Practice Research Database concluded that SSRIs increase the risk of upper GI bleeding by a factor of three. The increased risk appeared similar for all antidepressants that inhibit serotonin, suggesting that it is a class effect. The absolute effect was equivalent to the risk associated with low-dose ibuprofen. The results also suggested that concurrent use of SSRIs with NSAIDs greatly increased the risk of upper GI bleeding. Further research on this association is needed. In the meantime caution is needed in patients taking SSRIs together with other drugs known to affect platelet function and in those with a history of bleeding disorders (Li Wan Po, 1999).

Clopidogrel

Clopidogrel is an antiplatelet drug indicated for the prevention of ischaemic events in patients with a history of symptomatic ischaemic disease. It acts by irreversible inhibition of adenosine diphosphate (ADP) receptor function. In the pivotal study comparing the safety and efficacy of clopidogrel and low-dose aspirin (Harker *et al.*, 1999), there were significantly fewer GI adverse events with clopidogrel than aspirin overall (27.1% vs 29.8%; $P<0.001$) although the incidence of severe events did not differ significantly between groups (3% vs 3.6%). Clopidogrel is a possible cause of GI side-effects and should not be regarded as a safe alternative to aspirin.

Small intestine

Ulceration and perforation

The healthy small intestine, from the duodenum to the caecum, facilitates the absorption of nutrients, electrolytes and vitamins and acts as an effective barrier against the permeation of macromolecules, bacteria and luminal toxins (Tibble *et al.*, 1999). Adverse effects of drugs on the small intestine are rarely considered in clinical practice, although the small bowel mucosa is often affected, as high drug concentrations occur there. Poor recognition of intestinal ADRs may be explained by the fact that there are often few symptoms of small intestinal disease until substantial damage has occurred. In addition, the small bowel is not easily accessible to clinical investigation.

NSAID enteropathy

It is now clear that NSAIDs also damage the small intestine, causing a small bowel inflammation (enteropathy), perforation, ulceration and stricture (Lanas *et al.*, 1992; Bjorkman, 1998; Lanza, 1998; Tibble *et al.*, 1999). The overall incidence of NSAID-related injury to the GI tract distal to the duodenum is much less than that seen in the stomach and proximal duodenum. Nevertheless, it occurs frequently enough to warrant serious consideration. Several diagnostic techniques are used to detect NSAID enteropathy. Depending on the method used, the prevalence of small intestinal inflammation found in long-term NSAID users is 20–65% (Morris *et al.*, 1991; Tibble *et al.*, 1999). The enteropathy is seen with all commonly used NSAIDs. The vast majority of patients have no symptoms from this inflammation, but clinical problems arise from the associated complications, including blood loss, protein loss, ulceration and stricture formation.

- Blood loss (2–10 ml per day) may contribute to an iron-deficiency anaemia in patients receiving these drugs long-term. Because this level of blood loss may not be sufficient to produce a positive faecal occult blood test, patients are frequently subjected to upper GI endoscopy and colonoscopy before NSAID enteropathy is considered.

- Protein loss (equivalent to 30–300 ml serum per day) from the damaged intestinal mucosa can lead to severe hypoalbuminaemia with peripheral oedema and other signs of fluid retention.

- Ulcers can be demonstrated at enteroscopy in many patients taking NSAIDs, but small ulcers are unlikely to be associated with complications. Most patients with larger ulcers present clinically with substantial small intestinal haemorrhage or obstruction.

- Strictures, termed 'diaphragm' strictures, which appear as thin, concentric narrowings are highly characteristic of NSAID injury to the small bowel. Affected patients present with intermittent postprandial colicky abdominal pain (subacute intestinal obstruction) and often have a history of iron deficiency and hypoalbuminaemia. These strictures are very difficult to diagnose.

In 1983 a novel osmotic pump delivery system of indometacin (Osmosin) was withdrawn from the UK market because of reports of perforation and ulceration (Committee on Safety of Medicines, 1983). Small intestinal ulceration and perforation have also been described with slow-release potassium preparations, cocaine misuse and arsenic.

Paralytic ileus and pseudo-obstruction

Intestinal obstruction is a common surgical emergency. Drug-induced intestinal obstruction, or pseudointestinal obstruction, although rare, is important to recognise because its management is usually conservative (Iredale and George, 1993). Early recognition can therefore prevent unnecessary surgical intervention. The mechanisms by which this problem can occur include: physical obstruction within the small bowel lumen; physical obstruction from within the gut wall (e.g. intramural haematomas induced by anticoagulants); bowel dysmotility via drug effects on smooth muscle or autonomic nerve transmission; and obstruction from outside the gut wall as a result of vascular occlusion or peritoneal fibrosis (Iredale and George, 1993). Several patient groups may be at greater risk of these problems such as those with a predisposing lesion (e.g. Crohn's disease, carcinoma) and patients with cystic fibrosis or gastroparesis. Neural control of the gut occurs via the sympathetic and parasympathetic nervous systems. A large number of drugs can decrease intestinal motility and prolong transit time, including opioids and calcium channel blockers (Mantzoros *et al.*, 1994).

Atropine and related cholinergic muscarinic receptor antagonists block parasympathetic transmission to the postganglionic muscarinic receptors. This results in reduced forward propulsion of intestinal contents. Tricyclic antidepressants have potent anticholinergic effects and commonly produce constipation and intestinal obstruction. Phenothiazines also cause constipation and obstruction and the problem can be made worse by anticholinergic drugs if required for parkinsonian side-effects. Patients taking such combinations are at particular risk of developing severe paralytic ileus, which is associated with a high mortality. Clozapine has been reported to cause severe GI complications, including bowel obstruction, faecal impaction and paralytic ileus (Schwartz and Frisolone, 1993; Erickson, 1995; Anon, 1999); some of the reactions have been fatal. The mechanism is thought to relate to clozapine's anticholinergic effects and the risk is increased when it is given together with other anticholinergic medications. Patients with a history of colonic disease or previous bowel surgery may be at greater risk of this problem.

Drug-induced neuropathy can also affect the nerve supply to the gut, producing a syndrome similar to paralytic ileus. This has been reported with vincristine. Table 3.9 shows some drugs that may cause intestinal obstruction and pseudo-obstruction.

The vascular supply of the bowel may be damaged in a number of ways. Mesenteric vein thrombosis has been associated with oral contraceptive use but current low-dose formulations do not incur this risk.

Other drug effects on the small bowel

Neomycin is used in patients with hepatic encephalopathy to reduce bacterial colonisation of the intestine. In doses greater than 4 g daily it has a direct toxic effect on the enterocytes, causing villous atrophy resembling that seen in coeliac disease (Longstreth and Newcomer,

Table 3.9 Some drugs that may cause intestinal obstruction and pseudo-obstruction

Acarbose	Opioids
Calcium channel blockers	Phenothiazines
Clozapine	Potassium salts
Colestyramine	Tricyclic antidepressants
Laxatives (bulk-forming)	Vincristine
Loperamide	Vinorelbine

1975). This results in reduced hydrolysis of disaccharidases and consequent carbohydrate malabsorption.

Colchicine is a notorious cause of nausea, vomiting, colicky abdominal pain and diarrhoea. The underlying mechanism is unclear but appears to be local as symptoms are not seen after intravenous administration. These symptoms usually resolve within 24 hours of stopping the drug.

Malabsorption

Malabsorption of drugs or nutrients can occur as a result of an interaction between these agents in the small bowel. The anion exchange resins, colestyramine and colestipol, and the faecal softener liquid paraffin can interfere with the absorption of fat-soluble vitamins (A, D and K), calcium and other nutrients. Orlistat is an intestinal lipase inhibitor which has been shown to assist weight reduction by increasing faecal fat excretion. When fat excretion exceeds 20% of ingested fat, bulky, pale steatorrhoeic stools may become a problem. This agent too can interfere with the absorption of fat-soluble vitamins. Metformin can interfere with the absorption of vitamin B_{12} in a third of patients on long-term therapy, occasionally leading to megaloblastic anaemia (Adams *et al.*, 1983). Serum B_{12} levels should be checked annually in patients taking metformin.

Colon

Although adverse drug effects on the colon are rare, it is important that problems are recognised because the offending medication usually needs to be withdrawn (Cappell and Simon, 1993). Pseudo-obstruction of the colon can occur secondary to treatment with the agents discussed above.

Diarrhoea

Diarrhoea is a common ADR that has been reported with many drugs (Chassany *et al.*, 2000). Antimicrobials are the most frequent cause, accounting for about 25% of drug-induced diarrhoea. The drugs most commonly implicated are shown in Table 3.10. The high frequency of drug-induced diarrhoea is not surprising, since the intestinal mucosa is the first absorption site of orally administered drugs. The mechanism of these reactions is often multifactorial and sometimes remains unclear.

The most important pathophysiological mechanisms are:

- osmotic diarrhoea: ingestion of unusual amounts of poorly absorbed and osmotically active solutes such as mannitol, sorbitol
- secretory diarrhoea: increased small intestinal ion secretion or inhibition of normal active ion absorption, leading to an excess of water and electrolytes in the intestinal lumen and stools
- impairment of fluid absorption by activation of adenylate cyclase within the small intestinal enterocyte, which increases the level of cyclic adenosine monophosphate
- disturbance of intestinal motility, i.e. shortened transit time
- exudative diarrhoea: exudation of blood, mucus and proteins into the bowel lumen because of disruption of the integrity of the intestinal mucosa through inflammatory and ulcerated lesions
- malabsorption or maldigestion of fat and carbohydrates

Often more than one of these mechanisms is present simultaneously. In most cases of drug-induced diarrhoea there is no detectable organic lesion, except for in antibiotic-associated pseudomembranous colitis and rare observations of enteropathy and colitis. In practice, the two main types of diarrhoea seen are acute diarrhoea, which usually appears during the first few days of treatment, and chronic diarrhoea, lasting several weeks and which can appear a long time after the start of drug treatment. Both can be severe and poorly tolerated.

Antimicrobials

Diarrhoea occurs in up to 30% of individuals treated with antimicrobial agents (Bateman and Aziz, 1998). Most cases can be classified into two categories: diarrhoea associated with *Clostridium difficile* infection and cases in which no pathophysiological mechanism is identified. Most

Table 3.10 Some drugs that commonly cause diarrhoea

Acarbose	Iron preparations
Antibiotics	Laxatives
Biguanides	Leflunomide
Bile salts	Magnesium-containing antacids
Colchicine	Misoprostol
Cytotoxics (docetaxel, idarubicin, irinotecan, epirubicin, mitoxantrone (mitozantrone))	Non-steroidal anti-inflammatory drugs (especially mefenamic acid)
	Olsalazine
Dipyridamole	Orlistat
Gold compounds	Ticlopidine

antimicrobial-induced diarrhoea is benign, appearing during the first few days of treatment and resolving after treatment stops. The cause is generally thought to be disruption of the normal intestinal microflora which can lead to proliferation of pathogenic micro-organisms and impairment of the metabolic function of the microflora. Usually, changes in the composition of the gut microflora are of no clinical significance and the normal microflora is re-established shortly after antimicrobial treatment is complete. In some patients, however, modification of the microflora and the loss of normal colonisation resistance can lead to proliferation of opportunistic pathogens such as *C. difficile*, which is responsible for more than 20% of cases of antimicrobial-associated diarrhoea and almost all cases of pseudomembranous colitis. This organism can release specific toxins (A and B) which may cause mucosal damage and inflammation. Changes in the normal intestinal microflora can also lead to osmotic or secretory diarrhoea.

Pseudomembranous colitis

Pseudomembranous colitis is a rare but potentially severe complication of antimicrobial treatment, which is characterised by the proliferation of *C. difficile* in the colon. Symptoms generally begin 5–10 days after the start of therapy, but both shorter and longer times to onset are possible. The acute colitis can be severe with profuse watery diarrhoea (rarely with blood), abdominal pain, fever and bloating (Anon, 1995; Chassany *et al.*, 2000). Endoscopy reveals raised plaques or membranes ('pseudomembranes') covering the colonic mucosa. The membranes consist of fragments of fibrin, leukocytes and epithelial cells. The diagnosis of *C. difficile* infection depends on the detection of its toxins in the stools. Outbreaks of *C. difficile* diarrhoea are common in hospitals and long-term care establishments.

C. *difficile*-associated diarrhoea is more likely to occur with broad-spectrum antibiotics, such as amoxicillin, second- and third-generation cephalosporins and clindamycin, and those that achieve high concentrations in the intestinal lumen (e.g. agents that are poorly or incompletely absorbed or secreted into the bile) lead to greater changes in gut commensals (Gorbach, 1999). For example, the third-generation cephalosporin ceftriaxone, which is mainly eliminated by biliary secretion, is associated with a 10–40% frequency of diarrhoea (Thompson and Jacobs, 1993).

Other risk factors are the duration of antimicrobial therapy, multiple or repeated antibiotic regimens, severe underlying illness, advanced age, immunodeficiency, use of a nasogastric tube, intensive care and prolonged hospital stay. The dose of the antimicrobial and the route of administration are not risk factors.

C. *difficile* colitis may have a fatal outcome due to local complications (e.g. toxic megacolon, haemorrhage, perforation) or general complications (e.g. sepsis).

Other antimicrobial agents occasionally associated with pseudomembranous colitis include aminoglycosides, tetracyclines, macrolides, quinolones, sulphonamides, imidazoles and chloramphenicol. Antibiotic therapy should be stopped as soon as possible in a patient who develops severe diarrhoea. Patients with proven or suspected C. *difficile* infection will require treatment with oral metronidazole or vancomycin. If an antimicrobial must be continued for the primary infection it should be one that is less likely to cause C. *difficile* diarrhoea, such as a quinolone or a parenteral aminoglycoside. Because of the magnitude of the problem of antibiotic-associated colitis, care should be taken to ensure that an antibiotic appropriate for the infecting pathogen is prescribed. Broad-spectrum antimicrobials should generally be reserved for severe infections. Loperamide, which controls diarrhoea by inhibiting GI peristalsis, has caused paralytic ileus that progressed to necrotising enterocolitis in adults and in children (Chow *et al.*, 1986; Motala *et al.*, 1990; Olm *et al.*, 1990). It should not be used where ileus or abdominal distension is present, or in patients with pseudomembranous colitis associated with broad-spectrum antibiotics.

Other causes of diarrhoea

Laxative abuse, possibly linked with an eating disorder, is a possible cause of chronic diarrhoea (Eastwood, 1995; Chassany *et al.*, 2000). A rare complication is cathartic colon with severe diarrhoea and hypokalaemia. This has been linked to prolonged and surreptitious laxative consumption.

Gold therapy is associated with frequent diarrhoea in about 40–50% of patients, usually within the first 3 months of treatment (Marcuard *et al.*, 1987). The problem usually resolves on dosage reduction or with the use of antidiarrhoeal agents but some patients may need to discontinue treatment. Occasionally, severe enterocolitis has also occurred, with rectal bleeding and vomiting, usually within the first 3 months of treatment. Septicaemia is a common complication (Marcuard *et al.*, 1987).

Ischaemic colitis

Ischaemic colitis has been reported as a complication of treatment with various drugs. It commonly presents with sudden onset of severe abdominal pain, nausea, vomiting, diarrhoea and abdominal distension. Tachycardia, pyrexia, leukocytosis (raised white cell count) and bloody stools are often present. Other conditions associated with colonic ischaemia include atherosclerosis, arrhythmias, valvular heart disease and recent myocardial infarction. Examination of the colon may show erythematous, ulcerated, haemorrhagic mucosa. Drugs that are recognised causes of ischaemic colitis include ergotamine, oestrogens, amphetamines, digoxin and cocaine. Ergotamine, although now seldom used in migraine, can cause local ischaemia due to vasospasm (Jost *et al.*, 1991). Colitis has been described after oral administration and the suppositories can cause proctitis.

Ischaemic colitis has recently been reported in association with sumatriptan (Knudsen *et al.*, 1998) and with docetaxel and vinorelbine combination therapy (de Matteis *et al.*, 2000; Ibrahim *et al.*, 2000). NSAIDs, particularly mefenamic acid, have been reported to cause or exacerbate colitis (Cappell and Simon, 1993; Evans *et al.*, 1997). Proctocolitis was described in a patient taking isotretinoin; the symptoms resolved after medication withdrawal.

Drugs that may cause colitis are shown in Table 3.11.

Table 3.11 Some drugs that may cause colitis

Amfetamines	Non-steroidal anti-inflammatory drugs
Cocaine	Oestrogens
Digoxin	Salicylates
Docetaxel	Sulfasalazine
Ergotamine	Sumatriptan
Methotrexate	Vasopressin
Methyldopa	Vinorelbine
Methysergide	

Constipation

The fact that many drugs cause constipation is often overlooked. The drugs most frequently implicated include anticholinergic agents, opioids, iron salts and verapamil. Common drug causes of constipation are shown in Table 3.12.

Table 3.12 Some drugs that commonly cause constipation

Anion exchange resins	Opioids
Anticholinergics	Peppermint oil
Antihistamines	Phenothiazines
Clozapine	Sucralfate
Diuretics	Tricyclic antidepressants
Iron preparations	Verapamil
Mebeverine	Vincristine
Monoamine oxidase inhibitors	

Pancreatitis

Although drug-induced pancreatic dysfunction is rarer than many other GI adverse reactions, it is increasingly recognised as a complication of treatment with a wide range of drugs (Doucette, 1998; Eland *et al.*, 1999). Acute pancreatitis is a severe disease associated with considerable morbidity and mortality and the incidence in western countries seems to be rising. Despite advanced critical care, the mortality rate remains about 5–10%. Gallstones and alcohol consumption are the most important risk factors for acute pancreatitis. Other risk factors include hyperlipidaemia, hypercalcaemia, endoscopic retrograde cholangiopancreatography and trauma. In 10–25% of patients with acute pancreatitis no obvious risk factors are present.

The incidence of drug-induced pancreatitis is not known. A recent review estimated that about 2% of cases are caused by drugs, with much higher proportions in specific populations, such as children and HIV-positive patients (Wilmink and Frick, 1996). Acute pancreatitis typically presents with sudden onset of upper abdominal pain and vomiting. Symptoms include tachycardia, fever, jaundice and a rigid, tender abdomen. The most useful biochemical marker is a serum amylase level over four times the upper limit of normal.

Most cases of drug-induced pancreatitis are mild. The management consists of immediate withdrawal of the suspected drug and standard supportive treatment. Published literature contains many anecdotal case reports; drugs which have been consistently implicated with positive rechallenge include the aminosalicylates, azathioprine, cimetidine, interferon alfa, sodium valproate, oestrogen and didanosine. When reports of pancreatitis first appeared with sulfasalazine, the sulphonamide component was thought to be responsible. However, the problem has since occurred with mesalazine and olsalazine, suggesting that the salicylate component is the most likely cause.

There is a strong association between sodium valproate and pancreatitis, most cases occurring in the first year of treatment. There is no obvious relation to dose or serum concentration of valproate, suggesting that it is an idiosyncratic reaction. Pancreatitis has been reported as part of the azathioprine or mercaptopurine hypersensitivity reaction and required withdrawal of treatment in 1.3% of patients with Crohn's disease (Pearson *et al.*, 1995; Lamers *et al.*, 1999). An association with drug-induced pancreatitis is likely but not proven for thiazide diuretics, ACE inhibitors, vinca alkaloids, pentamidine and clozapine. Corticosteroids are frequently suspected to cause pancreatitis (Steinberg and Lewis, 1981), but the data are contradictory and the association is difficult to support.

Table 3.13 shows some drugs that may cause pancreatitis.

Table 3.13 Some drugs that may cause pancreatitis

Aminosalicylates (olsalazine, mesalazine, sulfasalazine)	Interferon alfa
	Metronidazole
Angiotensin-converting enzyme (ACE) inhibitors	Oestrogens
	Pentamidine
Azathioprine	Propofol
Didanosine	Sodium valproate
Furosemide (frusemide)	Sulindac
Gemfibrozil	Thiazide diuretics
Histamine H_2-receptor antagonists	

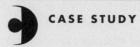 **CASE STUDY**

Mrs B is a 62-year-old woman with rheumatoid arthritis and osteoporosis. Her regular medication consists of transdermal oestradiol, calcium and vitamin D tablets, ibuprofen (400 mg three times a day) and, for the last 2 months, alendronic acid 10 mg daily. She is currently taking a 10-day course of amoxicillin (250 mg three times a day) for acute sinusitis. While collecting her repeat prescription, Mrs B tells the community pharmacist that she has had a peculiar sensation of something caught in her throat for the last few days.

Could this be anything to worry about?
Early medical referral is essential in any patient with dysphagia.

Could this be a drug-induced problem?
A sensation of something being stuck in the throat is suggestive of oesophagitis, which has been described with alendronic acid. To minimise the risk of oesophageal adverse reactions, patients should be carefully counselled about how to take this medicine.

Alendronic acid should be swallowed on rising for the day with a full glass of water (not less than 200 ml). Patients should not lie down for at least 30 minutes after taking it, and not until after eating, which should be at least 30 minutes after taking the tablet. The drug should not be taken at bedtime.

What questions would you ask the patient to help clarify the problem?
Other symptoms signalling a possible oesophageal reaction include painful or difficult swallowing, retrosternal pain and new or worsening heartburn. Mrs B should be asked whether she has noticed any of these symptoms. She should also be questioned carefully about whether she has been complying with the guidance for administration and whether she has any history of upper GI problems (dysphagia, oesophageal disease, gastritis, duodenitis and peptic ulceration). The frequency of upper GI adverse reactions with alendronic acid appears to be increased by concurrent NSAIDs or aspirin.

Mrs B has been able to swallow her food and medication without difficulty but she has had some heartburn recently, which she thought was caused by the antibiotic. She was given some quite complicated instructions on how to take the alendronic acid when it was first prescribed. She has generally been very strict in following these, but since she has been poorly with sinusitis, she has gone straight back to bed most mornings after taking her medicines. She had a course of cimetidine about 10 years ago for a peptic ulcer, but no problems since.

What advice do you give Mrs B?
Mrs B should be advised to stop her alendronic acid and visit her GP as soon as possible as her symptoms may be related to her drug therapy. Although she appears to be only mildly inconvenienced by the problem at present, there could be serious sequelae if she continues to take the drug.

References

Ackerman B H, Kasbekar N (1997). Disturbances of taste and smell induced by drugs. *Pharmacotherapy* 17: 482–496.

Adams J F, Clark J S, Ireland J T *et al.* (1983). Malabsorption of vitamin B_{12} and intrinsic factor secretion during biguanide therapy. *Diabetologica* 24: 16–18.

Agbo-Godeau S, Joly P, Lauret P *et al.* (1988). Association of major aphthous ulcers and nicorandil. *Lancet* 352: 1598–1599.

Alderman C P (1996). Adverse effects of the angiotensin-converting enzyme inhibitors. *Ann Pharmacother* 30: 55–61.

Anon. (1994). Rational use of NSAIDs for musculoskeletal disorders. *Drug Ther Bull* 32: 91–95.

Anon. (1995). Antibiotic-induced diarrhoea. *Drug Ther Bull* 33: 23–24.

Anon. (1997). Which prophylactic aspirin? *Drug Ther Bull* 35: 7–8.

Anon. (1999). Clozapine and gastrointestinal obstruction. *WHO Drug Inf* 13: 92.

Appleton I, Tomlinson A, Willoughby D A (1994). Inducible cyclo-oxygenase (COX-2): a safer therapeutic target? *Br J Rheumatol* 33: 410–412.

Armstrong C P, Blower A L (1987). Non-steroidal anti-inflammatory drugs and life threatening complications of peptic ulceration. *Gut* 28: 527–532.

Bateman D N, Aziz E E (1998). Gastrointestinal disorders. In: Davies D M, Ferner R E, de Glanville H, eds. *Textbook of Adverse Drug Reactions*, 5th edn. London: Chapman and Hall Medical, 259–274.

Bates D W, Cullen D J, Laird N *et al.* (1995). Incidence of adverse drug events and potential adverse drug events. Implications for prevention. *JAMA* 274: 29–34.

Beutler M, Hartmann K, Kluhn M, Gartmann J (1993). Taste disorders and terbinafine. *Br Med J* 307: 26.

Bjorkman D (1998). Nonsteroidal anti-inflammatory drug-associated toxicity of the liver, lower gastrointestinal tract, and oesophagus. *Am J Med* 105: 17S–21S.

Bong J L, Lucke T W, Evans C D (1998). Persistent impairment of taste resulting from terbinafine. *Br J Dermatol* 139: 747–748.

Brunet L, Miranda J, Farre M *et al.* (1996). Gingival enlargement induced by drugs. *Drug Safety* 15: 219–231.

Cappell M S, Simon T (1993). Colonic toxicity of administered medications and chemicals. *Am J Gastroenterol* 88: 1684–1699.

Chassany O, Michaux A, Bergmann J F (2000). Drug-induced diarrhoea. *Drug Safety* 1: 53–72.

Chow C B, Li S H, Leung N K (1986). Loperamide associated necrotising enterocolitis. *Arch Pediatr Scand* 75: 1034.

Committee on Safety of Medicines (1983). Osmosin (controlled release indomethacin). *Curr Probl Pharmacovigilance* 11: 1–2.

Committee on Safety of Medicines (1994). Relative safety of oral non-aspirin NSAIDs. *Curr Probl Pharmacovigilance* 20: 9–11.

Committee on Safety of Medicines (1996). Oesophageal reactions with alendronate sodium. *Curr Probl Pharmacovigilance* 22: 5–6.

Cribier B, Marquart-Elbaz C, Lipsker D *et al.* (1998). Chronic buccal ulceration induced by nicorandil. *Br J Dermatol* 138: 372–373.

De Abajo F, Garcia Rodriguez L A, Montero D (1999). Association between selective serotonin reuptake inhibitors and upper gastrointestinal bleeding: population based case-control study. *Br Med J* 319: 1106–1109.

de Matteis A, Nuzzo F, Rossi E *et al.* (2000). Intestinal side-effects of docetaxel/vinorelbine combination. *Lancet* 355: 1098–1099.

Desboeuf K, Lapeyre-Mestre M, and Montastruc J L (1998). Risk of gastrointestinal haemorrhage with calcium antagonists. *Br J Clin Pharmacol* 46: 87–89.

Desruelles F, Bahadoran P, Lacour J P *et al.* (1998). Giant oral aphthous ulcers induced by nicorandil. *Br J Dermatol* 138: 712–713.

DeVries M W, Peeters F (1995). Dental caries with longterm use of antidepressants. *Lancet* 346: 1640.

Doucette D (1998). Drug-induced acute pancreatitis. *Can Pharm J* 131: 26–32.

Douthwaite A H, Lintott S A M (1938). Gastroscopic observation of the effect of aspirin and certain other substances on the gut. *Lancet* 2: 1222–1225.

Eastwood M (1995). The dilemma of laxative abuse. *Lancet* 346: 1115.

Eisen D (1997). Minocycline-induced oral pigmentation. *Lancet* 349: 400.

Eland I A, van Puijenbroek E P, Sturkenboom J C M *et al.* (1999). Drug-associated acute pancreatitis: twenty-one years of spontaneous reporting in the Netherlands. *Am J Gastroenterol* 94: 2417–2422.

Erickson B (1995). Clozapine-associated postoperative ileus: case report and review of the literature. *Arch Gen Psychiatry* 52: 508–509.

Evans J M M, McMahon A D, Murray F E *et al.* (1997). Non-steroidal anti-inflammatory drugs are associated with emergency admission to hospital for colitis due to inflammatory bowel disease. *Gut* 40: 619–622.

Feldman M, McMahon A T (2000). Do cyclooxygenase-2 inhibitors provide benefits similar to those of traditional nonsteroidal anti-inflammatory drugs, with less gastrointestinal toxicity? *Ann Intern Med* 132: 134–143.

Gabriel S E, Jaakkimainen L, Bombardier C (1991). Risk for serious gastrointestinal complications related to use of nonsteroidal anti-inflammatory drugs. A meta-analysis. *Ann Intern Med* 115: 787–796.

Galan D, Grymonpre R (1994). Adverse oral effects of systemic drug use. *Can J Hosp Pharm* 47: 155–164.

Ganginella T S, Maxfield D L (1988). Calcium channel blocking agents and chest pain. *Drug Intell Clin Pharm* 22: 623.

Garcia-Rodriguez L A, Jick H (1994). Risk of upper gastrointestinal bleeding and perforation associated with individual non-steroidal anti-inflammatory drugs. *Lancet* 343: 769–772.

Gorbach S L (1999). Antibiotics and *Clostridium difficile*. *N Engl J Med* 341: 1690–1691.

Harker L A, Boissel J P, Pilgrim A J *et al.* (1999). Comparative safety and tolerability of clopidogrel and aspirin. *Drug Safety* 4: 325–335.

Henkin R I (1994). Drug-induced taste and smell disorders. Incidence, mechanisms, and management related primarily to treatment of sensory receptor dysfunction. *Drug Safety* 11: 318–377.

Henry D, Dobson A, Turner C (1993). Variability in the risk of major gastro-intestinal complications from nonaspirin non-steroidal anti-inflammatory drugs. *Gastroenterology* 105: 1078–1088.

Ibrahim N K, Sahin A A, Dubrow R A et al. (2000). Colitis associated with docetaxel-based chemotherapy in patients with metastatic breast cancer. *Lancet* 355: 281–283.

Iredale J P, George C F (1993). Drugs causing gastrointestinal obstruction. *Adverse Drug React* 12: 163–175.

Jaspersen D (2000). Drug-induced oesophageal disorders. *Drug Safety* 22: 237–249.

Jost W H, Raulf F, Muller-Lobeck H (1991). Anorectal ergotism: induced by migraine therapy. *Acta Neurol Scand* 84: 73–74.

Keller H (1992). Chapter 27. In: Dukes M N G, ed. *Meyler's Side Effects of Drugs*, 12th edn. Amsterdam: Elsevier, 637–671.

Kelly J P, Kaufman D W, Jurgelon J M et al. (1996). Risk of aspirin-associated major upper-gastrointestinal bleeding with enteric-coated or buffered product. *Lancet* 348: 1413–1416.

Kelly J P, L'aszio A, Kaufman D W et al. (1999). Major upper gastrointestinal bleeding and the use of calcium channel blockers. *Lancet* 353: 559.

Knudsen J F, Friedman B, Goldwasser J E (1998). Ischemic colitis and sumatriptan use. *Arch Intern Med* 158: 1946–1948.

Lamers C B H, Griffioen G, van Hogezand R A et al. (1999). Azathioprine: an update on clinical efficacy and safety in inflammatory bowel disease. *Scand J Gastroenterol* 34: 111–115.

Lanas A, Sekar M C, Hirschowitz B I (1992). Objective evidence of aspirin use in both ulcer and nonulcer upper and lower gastrointestinal bleeding. *Gastroenterology* 103: 862–869.

Langman M J S, Morgan L, Worrall A (1985). Use of anti-inflammatory drugs by patients admitted with small or large bowel perforations and haemorrhage. *Br Med J* 290: 347–349.

Langman M J S, Weil J, Wainwright P et al. (1994). Risks of bleeding peptic ulcer associated with individual non-steroidal anti-inflammatory drugs. *Lancet* 343: 1075–1078.

Langman M J, Jensen D M, Watson D J et al. (1999). Adverse upper gastrointestinal effects of rofecoxib compared with NSAIDs. *JAMA* 282: 1929–1933.

Lanza F L (1998). A guideline for the treatment and prevention of NSAID-induced ulcers. *Am J Gastroenterol* 93: 2037–2046.

Levine M S (1999). Drug-induced disorders of the esophagus. *Abdom Imaging* 24: 3–8.

Li Wan Po A (1999). Antidepressants and upper gastrointestinal bleeding. *Br Med J* 319: 1081–1082.

Lipsky P E, Abramson S B, Crofford L et al. (1998). The international COX-II study group. The classification of cyclooxygenase inhibitors. *J Rheumatol* 25: 2298–2303.

Longstreth G F, Newcomer A D (1975). Drug-induced malabsorption. *Mayo Clin Proc* 50: 284–293.

Maiden N, Madhok R (1995). Misoprostol in patients taking non-steroidal anti-inflammatory drugs. *Br Med J* 311: 1518–1519.

Mantzoros C S, Prabhu A S, Sowers J R (1994). Paralytic ileus as a result of diltiazem treatment. *J Intern Med* 235: 613–614.

Marcuard S P, Ehrinpreis M N, Fitter W F (1987). Gold-induced ulcerative proctitis: report and review of the literature. *J Rheumatol* 14: 142–144.

Martinez-Mir I, Badenes J N, Larrea V P (1997). Taste disturbance with acetazolamide. *Ann Pharmacother* 31: 373.

Meraw S J, Sheridan P J (1998). Medically induced gingival hyperplasia. *Mayo Clin Proc* 73: 1196–1199.

Morris A J, Madhok R, Sturrock R D *et al.* (1991). Enteroscopic diagnosis of small bowel ulceration in patients receiving non-steroidal anti-inflammatory drugs. *Lancet* 337: 520.

Motala C, Hill I D, Mann M D, Bowie M D (1990). Effect of loperamide on stool output and duration of acute infectious diarrhoea in infants. *J Pediatr* 117: 467–471.

Olm M, Gonzalez F J, Garcia-Valdecasas J C *et al.* (1990). Necrotising enterocolitis with perforation in diarrhoeic patients treated with loperamide. *Eur J Clin Pharmacol* 40: 415–416.

Pahor M, Gurainik J M, Furberg C D *et al.* (1996). Risk of gastrointestinal haemorrhage with calcium antagonists in hypertensive persons over 67 years old. *Lancet* 347: 1061–1065.

Pearlman C (1994). Clozapine, nocturnal sialorrhea and choking. *J Clin Psychopharmacol* 14: 283.

Pearson D, May G, Fick G *et al.* (1995). Azathioprine and 6-mercaptopurine in Crohn disease. A meta-analysis. *Ann Intern Med* 123: 132–142.

Piper J M, Ray W A, Daugherty J R, Griffin M R (1991). Corticosteroid use and peptic ulcer disease: role of non-steroidal anti-inflammatory drugs. *Ann Intern Med* 114: 735–740.

Rees Willett L, Carson J L, Strom B L (1994). Epidemiology of gastrointestinal damage associated with nonsteroidal anti-inflammatory drugs. *Drug Safety* 10: 170–181.

Schwartz B J, Frisolone J A (1993). A case report of clozapine-induced gastric outlet obstruction. *Am J Psychiatry* 150: 1563.

Semble E L, Wu W C, Castell D O (1989). Nonsteroidal anti-inflammatory drugs and oesophageal injury. *Semin Arth Rheum* 19: 99.

Seymour R (1993). Drug-induced gingival overgrowth. *Adverse Drug React Toxicol Rev* 12: 215–232.

Seymour R A (1998). Oral and dental disorders. In: Davies D M, Ferner R E, de Glanville H, eds. *Textbook of Adverse Drug Reactions*, 5th edn. London: Chapman and Hall, chapter 11.

Shallcross T M, Heatley R V (1990). Effect of non-steroidal anti-inflammatory drugs on dyspeptic symptoms. *Br Med J* 300: 368–369.

Shotts R H, Scully C, Avery C M *et al.* (1999). Nicorandil-induced severe oral ulceration. *Oral Surg Oral Med Oral Pathol Oral Radiol Endod* 87: 706–707.

Silverstein F E, Graham D Y, Senior J R *et al.* (1995). Misoprostol reduces serious gastrointestinal complications in patients with rheumatoid arthritis receiving nonsteroidal anti-inflammatory drugs: a randomised, double-blind, placebo-controlled trial. *Ann Intern Med* 123: 241–249.

Singh G, Rosen Ramey D (1998). NSAID induced gastrointestinal complications: the ARAMIS perspective – 1997. *J Rheumatol* 25 (suppl 51): 8–16.

Singh G, Triadafilopoulus G (1999). Epidermiology of NSAID-induced GI complications. *J Rheumatol* 26 (suppl 26): 18–24.

Singh G, Rosen Ramey D, Morfeld D *et al.* (1996). Gastrointestinal tract complications of nonsteroidal anti-inflammatory drug treatment in rheumatoid arthritis: a prospective observational cohort study. *Arch Intern Med* 156: 153–156.

Smalley W E, Ray W A, Daugherty J R *et al.* (1998). No association between calcium channel blocker use and confirmed bleeding peptic ulcer disease. *Am J Epidemiol* 148: 350–354.

Smith C C, Bennett P M, Pearce H M *et al.* (1996). Adverse drug reactions in a hospital general medical unit meriting notification to the Committee on Safety of Medicines. *Br J Clin Pharmacol* 42: 423–429.

Steinberg W, Lewis J (1981). Steroid-induced pancreatitis: does it really exist? *Gastroenterology* 81: 799–808.

Stricker B H Ch, van Riemsdijk M M, Sturkenboom M C J M, Ottervanger J P (1996). Taste loss to terbinafine: a case control study of potential risk factors. *Br J Clin Pharmacol* 42: 313–318.

Suissa S, Bourgault C, Barkun A *et al.* (1998). Antihypertensive drugs and the risk of gastrointestinal bleeding. *Am J Med* 105: 230–235.

Tannenbaum H, Davis P, Russell A S *et al.* (1996). An evidence-based approach to prescribing NSAIDs in musculoskeletal disease: a Canadian consensus. *Can Med Assoc J* 155: 77–88.

Tanzi E L, Hecker M S (2000). Minocycline-induced hyperpigmentation of the tongue. *Arch Dermatol* 136: 427–428.

Thompson J W, Jacobs R F (1993). Adverse effects of newer cephalosporins. *Drug Safety* 9: 132–142.

Tibble J, Smale S, Bjarnason I (1999). Adverse effects of drugs on the small bowel. *Adverse Drug React Bull* 198: 755–758.

Vane J R (1971). Inhibition of prostaglandin synthesis as a mechanism of action for aspirin-like drugs. *Nature* 231: 232–235.

Wallace J L (1997). Nonsteroidal anti-inflammatory drugs and gastroenteropathy: the second hundred years. *Gastroenterology* 112: 1000–1016.

Weil J, Colin-Jones D, Langman M *et al.* (1995). Prophylactic aspirin and risk of peptic ulcer bleeding. *Br Med J* 310: 827–830.

Wilmink T, Frick T W (1996). Drug-induced pancreatitis. *Drug Safety* 14: 406–423.

Wolfe M M, Lichtenstein D R, Singh G (1999). Gastrointestinal toxicity of nonsteroidal anti-inflammatory drugs. *N Engl J Med* 340: 1888–1899.

Yeomans N D, Tulassay Z, Juhasz L *et al.* (1998). A comparison of omeprazole with ranitidine for ulcers associated with nonsteroidal anti-inflammatory drugs. *N Engl J Med* 338: 719–726.

4

Hepatic disorders

Fiona Ward and Mike Daly

Drug-induced hepatotoxicity accounts for approximately 2% of cases of inpatient jaundice and the liver is involved in 3–10% of all adverse drug reactions (ADRs). Between 20 and 30% of all cases of acute liver failure (which is associated with a 90% mortality rate) are thought to be drug-related (O'Grady *et al.*, 1989; Dossing and Sonne, 1993; Farrell, 1997). This chapter discusses the different types of hepatotoxic reaction that can be produced and the main drugs implicated.

The liver is central to the metabolism of virtually all foreign substances ingested. If these substances are potentially toxic, they can damage the liver either directly or as a consequence of the metabolic changes that occur in the organ. Most drugs have been implicated as a cause of liver injury, if all published case reports are taken into account. However, if only drugs where there is reasonable evidence of a causal relationship are considered, several hundred can be classed as hepatotoxic (Dossing and Sonne, 1993).

The spectrum of drug hepatotoxicity is wide, ranging from asymptomatic reversible alterations in liver function tests (LFTs) to fatal acute hepatic necrosis.

Classification and mechanism

Adverse effects of drugs on the liver can be classified into two main types, namely, predictable (type A) and unpredictable (type B) reactions. Predictable hepatic reactions are dose-dependent and affect the majority of individuals who ingest a sufficient amount of the drug. Examples of dose-dependent hepatotoxins are paracetamol (acetaminophen), salicylates, tetracycline and methotrexate. Idiosyncratic or unpredictable liver reactions (type B) are generally less frequent, typically occurring in fewer than 1% of exposed individuals (Farrell, 1994). Examples of drugs involved are chlorpromazine, halothane and isoniazid. Both types of reaction can cause similar patterns of liver damage and several drugs can cause more than one type of damage (Jim and Gee, 1995).

The time between starting treatment and the appearance of liver injury (the latent period) varies greatly. The latency period for type A reactions generally ranges between days and weeks, while for type B reactions this period may be months or even years (Dossing and Sonne, 1993). Although drug-induced liver damage is relatively rare in comparison with some other types of ADR, healthcare professionals should have some knowledge of the problem. In particular, they should be familiar with the drugs most frequently implicated, the most susceptible patients, the types of damage which can occur and the situations in which monitoring liver function is advisable.

Signs and symptoms of liver disorders

There may be few clinical signs on physical examination of a patient with liver disease other than fever and the general appearance of being unwell. The liver is often tender and may be slightly enlarged, while a skin rash may indicate a drug hypersensitivity reaction. Less frequent signs of hypersensitivity reactions include lymphadenopathy, splenomegaly and arthritis (Farrell, 1994).

Anorexia, nausea and vomiting are the usual presenting symptoms in patients with hepatitis. Abdominal discomfort is common, particularly in the right upper quadrant, while dark urine, pale stools and jaundice tend to become evident after the first few days of illness. If these symptoms are associated with pruritus, they indicate possible obstruction of the common bile duct, causing cholestasis. In the absence of cholestasis, however, the presence of jaundice may indicate that the liver injury is severe. Fatalities from drug-induced hepatitis occur in between 5 and 30% of jaundiced patients, but are rare in those without jaundice (Farrell, 1994).

Risk factors

Pre-existing liver disease

Patients with liver disease may be at increased risk of ADRs because of a reduced drug-metabolising capacity of the affected liver (Bass and Williams, 1988). The risk of terfenadine-induced ventricular arrhythmias, for example, is greater in patients with significant liver disease (Committee on Safety of Medicines, 1992). Care should be taken with drug dosing in patients with cirrhosis, ascites or encephalopathy.

Gender

Women appear to be more susceptible to drug-induced liver disease than men. For example, halothane-induced hepatitis occurs more often in women (Benjamin *et al.*, 1985) and the rate of isoniazid hepatotoxicity appears to be higher in women (Nolan *et al.*, 1999).

Age

Older patients have a higher incidence of drug-induced liver disease and reactions tend to be more severe (James, 1985). In general, drug-induced liver disease is rare in children, except in those receiving sodium valproate. Children under the age of two on multiple enzyme-inducing antiepileptics and with developmental delay seem to be particularly susceptible to idiosyncratic hepatotoxicity with sodium valproate (Pirmohamed *et al.*, 1994). The mechanism is not fully understood but is thought to involve a toxic metabolite (Anderson *et al.*, 1992).

The other drug causing hepatotoxicity specifically in children is aspirin. The use of salicylates in children with a viral infection results in a greater risk of developing Reye's syndrome. The condition is characterised by coma, hypoglycaemia, seizures and hepatic steatosis leading to fulminant liver failure. Once the association with aspirin was confirmed by epidemiological studies (Starko *et al.*, 1980; Hall *et al.*, 1988) aspirin became contraindicated in children under 12 years except for use in juvenile arthritis. The mechanism of the toxicity remains unknown. Data from the USA suggest that cases of aspirin-induced Reye's syndrome in children still occur (Poss *et al.*, 1994). Healthcare professionals should ensure that children are not inadvertently treated with aspirin.

Children appear to be less susceptible than adults to the hepatotoxic effects of paracetamol in overdose; severe or fatal reactions are rare in this age group (Penna and Buchanan, 1991). This may be because children have an enhanced capacity for sulphate conjugation and a relative immaturity of microsomal enzymes catalysing formation of the active metabolite (Choonara *et al.*, 1996; Davis, 1998).

Genetic factors

Genetic factors are increasingly recognised as potentially important determinants of drug-induced liver disease. The composition of the cytochrome P450 isoenzymes in the liver is genetically determined, and the relative concentrations of these can determine the extent to which an individual may produce toxic metabolites or have reduced protective mechanisms when exposed to a particular drug (Finlayson, 1994).

Epidemiological studies have not led to a definitive conclusion on whether acetylator status is an important determinant of isoniazid-induced liver damage. Rapid acetylators of isoniazid were originally believed to be more susceptible to hepatotoxicity, but further studies have refuted this and some have suggested that the risk is in fact higher in slow acetylators (Farrell, 1994).

Enzyme inducers

Enhancement of drug-metabolising enzymes via the induction of cytochrome P450 isoenzymes may lead to an increased risk of liver damage when an individual is subsequently exposed to drugs which can produce toxic metabolites. For example, the incidence of hepatotoxicity due to sodium valproate is increased in patients on enzyme-inducing anticonvulsants (Pirmohamed et al., 1994).

Alcohol

Chronic ethanol consumption induces the cytochrome P450 system and, as a result, can potentiate toxicity induced by certain drugs. Doses of paracetamol smaller than those which are usually hepatotoxic may cause liver damage in chronic alcohol abusers. In addition, toxicity caused by isoniazid and methotrexate is more likely in alcoholics (Farrell, 1994).

Multidrug regimens

There are some circumstances in which drug combinations are associated with an increased risk of toxic reactions. In these cases one drug commonly causes induction of cytochrome P450 which then increases the quantity of the toxic metabolite formed by the other drug. For example, the risk of hepatotoxicity with isoniazid is substantially greater when rifampicin is given concomitantly (Steele et al., 1991).

Other diseases

Certain pre-existing conditions can increase the risk of drug-induced hepatic injury. For example, patients with insulin-dependent diabetes mellitus are at increased risk of hepatic fibrosis caused by methotrexate.

The risk of liver injury caused by tetracycline is increased in patients with renal failure (Lee, 1995).

Nutritional status

Obesity increases the risk of liver injury caused by methotrexate and halothane. Fasting patients are more likely to be predisposed to hepato-toxicity caused by paracetamol as hepatic glutathione, which is needed for normal paracetamol metabolism, is depleted (Lee, 1995).

Diagnosis of drug-induced liver damage

To assess the likelihood that a particular drug or compound is responsible for causing liver disease, several factors must be considered. These include: drug exposure, time to onset of abnormalities, time to resolution of abnormalities, clinical features, exclusion of other causes of liver disease, LFTs and biopsy results.

Routine LFTs involve measurement of total bilirubin, alanine aminotransferase and alkaline phosphatase. Impairment of the synthetic function of the liver is detected by total protein, albumin and the pro-thrombin time. The gamma-glutamyltransferase level may also be elevated in drug-induced liver disease. Conjugated bilirubin may be measured to establish whether there is biliary obstruction. Liver biopsy and histological evaluation are useful in the diagnosis of acute hepato-cellular dysfunction where a drug-induced cause is suspected.

Drug exposure

It is essential that a detailed and thorough medication history is obtained from any patient in whom liver disease is suspected. This history should include all drugs (current and past), with specific questions about the use of over-the-counter medicines, herbal remedies, oral contraceptives and any drugs of abuse. Some drugs, including digoxin and theophylline, are seldom implicated as causes of liver injury, whereas drugs such as the non-steroidal anti-inflammatory agents and some antibiotics (e.g. flu-cloxacillin) are commonly implicated (Farrell, 1997).

Onset of abnormalities

The most effective way to identify the drug causing a reaction is to consider carefully when drugs were ingested in relation to the onset of signs and symptoms. Healthcare professionals should be particularly suspicious of any potentially hepatotoxic drug begun during the 3 months before the onset of symptoms (Farrell, 1997). There is usually a latent period between the first administration of a drug and the onset of an adverse reaction on the liver. The interval may vary from a few hours (in the case of a drug causing potent dose-dependent hepatotoxicity), to several weeks (for most forms of drug-induced acute hepatitis or cholestasis), to more than 6 months (in cases of chronic liver disease). Although there is some variability, the latent period for many drugs is sufficiently reproducible to be of some diagnostic value (Farrell, 1994).

Resolution of abnormalities

A striking improvement in symptoms of liver impairment on discontinuing a drug strongly suggests that it may be implicated as a hepatotoxin. Time to resolution of abnormalities will depend very much on the individual drug and the type of disease it has induced. The recovery period can take many months. Confirmation of drug-induced hepatotoxicity can sometimes be sought by performing a rechallenge with the suspected drug, but as this is potentially dangerous for the patient it is usually unacceptable in practice (Farrell, 1997). In some cases, such as when a patient with tuberculosis develops abnormal liver function while taking isoniazid or rifampicin, therapy is often reintroduced sequentially, with careful monitoring, as the potential benefits of therapy generally outweigh the risks associated with not giving the most effective antituberculous regimen (Ormerod et al., 1996). If the patient develops further liver abnormalities, an alternative drug may then need to be substituted.

Clinical features

The clinical features which guide causality assessment in drug-induced hepatotoxicity include an evaluation of the signs and symptoms at diagnosis, the systemic features of the reaction and the availability of a specific diagnostic test. If drug-induced hepatotoxicity is suspected and the liver injury is accompanied by fever, rash and eosinophilia, for example, it is possible that the patient is suffering from an immunologically mediated (type B) ADR (Farrell, 1994).

There are very few specific diagnostic tests that can confirm drug-induced liver disease other than routine determinations of liver function. One possible exception relates to halothane hepatotoxicity, which involves both direct hepatotoxicity and immune mechanisms.

The major metabolite of halothane is trifluoroacetic acid (TFA). TFA–liver protein complexes are formed in all individuals exposed to halothane, yet only those who develop severe halothane hepatitis have antibodies to them (Kenna *et al.*, 1988; Howard Fee and Thompson, 1997).

Exclusion of other possible causes

It is essential to exclude other possible causes of liver disease, in case the hepatic changes are unrelated to drug exposure. Viral and autoimmune causes of hepatitis can be identified by serological tests, and in cases of cholestasis the common bile duct can be investigated radiologically to exclude physical obstruction by gallstones, other masses or strictures.

Liver function tests

Abnormalities in LFTs may indicate the presence of liver disease, although some are crude and non-specific. In general, markers of liver function (such as serum gamma-glutamyltransferase, alanine aminotransferase, aspartate aminotransferase, alkaline phosphatase or the conjugated bilirubin concentration) are defined as abnormal when they are increased to more than twice the upper limit of the normal reference range (Danan and Benichou, 1993). Elevations in LFTs are common with certain drugs but only in a minority of cases does significant hepatic injury follow (Davis, 1989). For example, serum aminotransferases rise in up to 40% of patients taking isoniazid, but symptomatic hepatotoxicity occurs in fewer than 5% (Ormerod *et al.*, 1996).

Patterns of changes in LFTs may distinguish the type of liver disease present, which in turn may help to determine whether a particular drug is implicated. Marked increases in LFTs together with signs and symptoms associated with liver disease (nausea, vomiting, abdominal pain, ascites, pruritus, jaundice) suggest that liver injury has occurred.

When potentially hepatotoxic drugs are prescribed, it is important to measure LFTs before the start of treatment, so that baseline values are available to compare with subsequent measurements. Monitoring LFTs in the first few weeks of therapy with drugs known to cause hepatic damage by metabolic idiosyncrasy (e.g. isoniazid, pyrazinamide) can give early warning of an impending severe reaction.

Liver biopsy

Data on the histological and ultrastructural features of hepatic lesions may be necessary to confirm a suspected diagnosis. This is generally achieved by taking a needle biospy of the liver through the abdomen under local anaesthetic. Certain drugs cause characteristic lesions, for example, amiodarone therapy can lead to infiltration of the hepatocytes with phospholipid droplets (Richer and Robert, 1995). Liver biopsy is not a risk-free procedure, and is generally only performed routinely in specialist centres. The value of liver biopsy in patients taking low-dose methotrexate is controversial (Neuberger, 1995) but it may be recommended if liver dysfunction is suspected (American College of Rheumatology Guidelines, 1996; Boffa and Chalmers, 1996).

Types of drug-induced liver disease

Dose-dependent hepatotoxicity

Paracetamol is safe when taken in the recommended therapeutic dose of 1–4 g daily but in excessive doses it is hepatotoxic. It is the most common cause of drug-induced liver disease, leading to about 200 deaths each year in the UK (Fagan and Wannan, 1996). In therapeutic doses, paracetamol is mainly metabolised by conjugation to the glucuronide and sulphate compounds, which are then excreted in the urine. A small proportion (5–10%) is oxidised by mixed-function oxidase enzymes to form the highly reactive N-acetyl-p-benzoquinoneimine (NAPQI). In overdose, the conjugation pathway becomes saturated, and a greater proportion of paracetamol is oxidised. As a result, liver glutathione stores become depleted and the liver is unable to deactivate the toxic metabolite NAPQI. This compound can bind directly to liver cells, leading to necrosis.

Replenishment of glutathione stores is of value in paracetamol poisoning. Intravenous N-acetylcysteine and oral methionine are effective antidotes, provided they are administered within 8–10 hours of the ingestion of the overdose (Vale and Proudfoot, 1995). For this reason, all patients should be referred to hospital immediately if there is a suspicion that they have taken an overdose of paracetamol.

After an overdose of paracetamol patients usually remain asymptomatic for the first 24 hours, although anorexia, nausea and vomiting are sometimes present. The absence of symptoms can lead to a delay in seeking medical advice, and thus increase the risk of potentially fatal liver failure. Liver damage is not usually detectable by routine LFTs until at least 18 hours after ingestion of the drug. Hepatic tenderness and abdominal pain are seldom seen before the second day after ingestion. Maximum liver damage, as assessed by plasma alanine aminotransferase or aspartate aminotransferase activities or prothrombin time, occurs 72–96 hours after ingestion. Hepatic failure (manifest by jaundice and encephalopathy) may then develop between the third and fifth day; the rate of clinical deterioration reflects the severity of the overdose. Hepatic coma, metabolic acidosis, high peak prothrombin time and renal failure are all indicators of poor outcome. Death can occur between 4 and 18 days after the overdose, usually from cerebral oedema, sepsis and multiorgan failure. The overall mortality from paracetamol poisoning in untreated patients is about 5%.

Any patient who ingests more than 150 mg per kg body weight of paracetamol, or more than 12 g in total, should be considered at risk of severe liver damage. Patients who present 12 hours or more after ingestion are at greater risk of serious liver damage as the antidotes are less effective after this time. Patients taking enzyme-inducing drugs, those with eating disorders and chronic alcohol abusers are at greater risk of hepatotoxic damage. In patients with a high alcohol intake paracetamol doses of 2–6 g have been associated with fatal hepatotoxicity. Treatment with N-acetylcysteine or methionine should be initiated at lower plasma paracetamol concentrations in these high-risk patients.

Points to remember about paracetamol include the following:

- There is evidence that the public has a poor knowledge of paracetamol's toxicity in overdose. There is a tendency to misjudge the potentially lethal dose
- Accidental deaths have occurred after self-medication with multiple paracetamol- containing preparations at the same time
- Healthcare professionals have an active role to play in educating the public about the dangers of paracetamol overdose. Patients should be counselled about the importance of not exceeding the maximum daily dose of 4 g
- Any patient who reports having taken a paracetamol overdose, either accidentally or deliberately, should be advised to seek medical advice immediately

Dose-independent hepatotoxicity

Hepatocellular damage from dose-independent reactions can present with a wide spectrum of changes, from mild, asymptomatic elevations in serum transaminases to a severe hepatic illness with jaundice. Minor abnormalities in LFTs are sometimes self-limiting and resolve with continued drug administration, while in other cases they progress to symptomatic hepatitis. Hepatitis from some drugs often occurs in the context of a hypersensitivity reaction, with prominent skin rashes, arthralgia and eosinophilia, while for other agents such features are rarely, if ever, seen. Tables 4.1–4.7 illustrate the diversity of drugs which have the potential to have adverse effects on the liver. They are not exhaustive summaries of all the drugs implicated in liver injury but select those most frequently documented in the literature.

Acute hepatocellular necrosis (Table 4.1)

In hepatic necrosis there are LFT abnormalities with a modestly increased alkaline phosphatase level and a markedly increased alanine aminotransferase level up to 200 times the upper limit of normal. In severe cases jaundice is present and the prothrombin time is greatly increased. Microscopy reveals necrosis of the hepatocytes in a characteristic pattern.

This type of liver disease is frequently thought to be a manifestation of drug hypersensitivity or due to metabolic idiosyncrasy. Halothane, for example, can produce severe hepatocellular necrosis leading to fulminant hepatic failure. Halothane hepatitis has a low incidence (estimated at between 1 in 22 000 and 1 in 35 000 halothane anaesthetics) but a high mortality. Severe hepatic damage is more common in patients who have been exposed to halothane on more than one occasion, particularly if the interval between exposures is short (Lee, 1995; Davis, 1998). For this reason it is recommended that repeat exposure within 3 months should be avoided (Committee on Safety of Medicines, 1986, 1997). In practice, the use of halothane has been superseded by newer and safer anaesthetic agents.

Table 4.1 Some drugs that may cause acute hepatocellular necrosis

Allopurinol	Labetalol
Aspirin	Methyldopa
Carbamazepine	Minocycline
Cocaine	Monoamine oxidase inhibitors
Cyclophosphamide	Non-steroidal anti-inflammatory drugs
Dantrolene	(NSAIDs), e.g. indometacin, diclofenac
Didanosine	Paracetamol
Ecstasy (MDMA; methylene	Pennyroyal (herbal)
dioxymethamfetamine)	Sodium valproate
Halothane	Sulphonamides
Isoniazid	Troglitazone

Acute hepatitis (Table 4.2)

Acute hepatitis is usually a self-limiting episode of hepatocyte inflam-mation or damage that normally resolves completely. In rare cases the hepatocyte damage is so severe that it affects the whole liver, causing hepatic coma and death (fulminant hepatic failure). The best indica-tor of severity is the prothrombin time. Acute hepatitis can occur in response to a variety of drugs (Table 4.2). The injury produced may be characterised by cytotoxic cellular breakdown (hepatocellular destruction), arrested bile flow (cholestasis) or a mixed presentation of both.

Table 4.2 Some drugs causing acute hepatitis

Angiotensin-converting enzyme (ACE) inhibitors	Nicotinamide
	Nifedipine
Chinese herbs	Nitrofurantoin
Co-trimoxazole	Phenytoin
Cyproterone	Pyrazinamide
Dantrolene	Rifampicin
Isoniazid	Sulfasalazine
Ketoconazole	Sulphonamides
Methoxyflurane	Tizanidine
Methyldopa	Tolcapone
Monoamine oxidase inhibitors (MAOIs)	Tricyclic antidepressants

Steatosis

Steatosis or fatty liver can be characterised into two categories: an acute form and a subacute or chronic form that resembles alcoholic hepatitis, usually termed steatohepatitis. Blood glucose may be low and blood ammonia levels high. Acute microvesicular fatty changes of the liver are associated with the hepatocytes becoming filled with small droplets of lipid, and can be caused by drugs such as tetracy-cline, sodium valproate and L-asparaginase. Occasionally, the lipid droplets are much larger, leading to macrovesicular fatty liver, which can be caused by corticosteroids, methotrexate and also by alcohol (Farrell, 1994; Lee, 1995). Steatohepatitis differs from diffuse fatty change as the clinical symptoms and biochemistry resemble those of chronic parenchymal disease. Amiodarone can complex with phos-pholipids causing chronic steatohepatitis. This may progress to cirrhosis.

Cholestasis (Tables 4.3 and 4.4)

Partial or complete obstruction of the common bile duct, with resulting retention of bile acids, leads to the condition known as cholestasis. This may occur with or without associated hepatitis and bile duct injury or destruction. Long-standing obstruction of the bile outflow from the liver can cause inflammation, scarring and eventually cirrhosis.

Table 4.3 Some drugs causing cholestasis with hepatitis

Angiotensin-converting enzyme (ACE) inhibitors	Nitrofurantoin
Azathioprine	Non-steroidal anti-inflammatory drugs, e.g. sulindac
Carbimazole	Penicillamine
Chlorpropamide	Phenindione
Cimetidine	Phenothiazines, e.g. chlorpromazine
Clavulanic acid	Phenytoin
Co-trimoxazole	Ranitidine
Dextropropoxyphene	Sulphonamides
Erythromycin	Sulphonylureas
Flucloxacillin	Thiouracils
Flutamide	Ticlopidine
Fusidic acid	Tricylic antidepressants
Gold salts	Troglitazone
Ketoconazole	

Table 4.4 Some drugs causing cholestasis without hepatitis

Ciclosporin	Oral contraceptives
Flucloxacillin	Tamoxifen
Glibenclamide	Warfarin
Griseofulvin	

Cholestasis without hepatitis is associated with a raised bilirubin and a normal or minimally raised alanine aminotransferase level. No inflammation or hepatocellular necrosis is seen. In contrast, in cholestasis associated with hepatitis the laboratory picture is normally one of elevated levels of alkaline phosphatase, alanine aminotransferase and conjugated bilirubin.

Chlorpromazine is a common cause of cholestasis with an estimated incidence of 0.5–1% in patients taking the drug for more than 2 weeks. The median latent period is 2–3 weeks, with symptoms usually resolving within 4 weeks of discontinuation in the majority of cases.

Abnormal LFTs without jaundice are much more common and may be seen in a quarter or more of patients treated with phenothiazines (Davis, 1998).

Chronic active hepatitis (Table 4.5)

Drug-induced chronic active hepatitis has mixed characteristics, with features of both acute and chronic hepatic injury. Serum transaminases are usually raised and serum albumin low. The disease is defined as chronic when it is present for more than 3 months, as determined by histological and laboratory results. The histology resembles that of autoimmune chronic active hepatitis and is associated with circulating antibodies. The condition usually resolves on drug withdrawal.

Table 4.5 Some drugs causing chronic active hepatitis

Cimetidine	Minocycline
Dantrolene	Nitrofurantoin
Diclofenac	Paracetamol
Etretinate	Phenytoin
Herbal medicines (e.g. germander, chaparral)	Sulphonamides
Isoniazid	Tricyclic antidepressants

Fibrosis and cirrhosis

Fibrosis may occur without cirrhosis and is partially reversible, whereas cirrhosis is characterised by dense fibrosis and hepatocellular degeneration which is irreversible. In fibrosis, serum transaminases may be only transiently raised and are not good predictors of hepatic damage. Microscopy shows deposition of fibrous tissue. Cirrhosis results from continued injury to hepatocytes, which may occur in chronic cholestasis, steatohepatitis and chronic active hepatitis, although it may also develop despite discontinuation of a causal drug (Cadman, 1996). Methotrexate and vitamin A have both been implicated in causing a gradual progression to cirrhosis without any symptoms or abnormalities in LFTs.

Methotrexate-induced liver damage is dose-related. The high incidence of hepatic fibrosis and cirrhosis reported in early studies reflected the use of high daily doses of the drug. There is also good evidence that daily dosing is more hepatotoxic than giving the same cumulative amount in weekly doses. With the doses currently used in psoriasis and rheumatoid arthritis the incidence of liver damage is minimal. Other factors that increase susceptibility to liver injury from methotrexate include underlying liver disease, alcohol abuse and the combination of obesity and diabetes mellitus. The incidence of liver toxicity also seems to be higher in patients with psoriasis than in those with rheumatoid arthritis. This is probably related both to dose and the higher prevalence of alcohol abuse in psoriasis patients. Regular monitoring of LFTs is required in patients taking methotrexate.

Chronic cholestasis (Table 4.6)

A syndrome that clinically and histologically resembles primary biliary cirrhosis occurs in association with a number of drugs, all of which have been shown to produce acute cholestasis. Histologically there is disappearance of small intrahepatic bile ducts (vanishing bile duct syndrome). The syndrome may be manifested as chronic cholestatic jaundice with its attendant complications or, just as persistently, abnormal LFTs (predominantly alkaline phosphatase) with no symptoms or signs. Even when the offending agent is stopped, there is usually chronic cholestasis, often with jaundice, and high alkaline phosphatase and gamma-glutamyltransferase activities for several years (McCarthy and Wilkinson, 1999). In some cases abnormalities may be permanent. Some drugs reported to cause chronic cholestasis are shown in Table 4.6.

Table 4.6 Some drugs causing chronic cholestasis

Carbamazepine
Chlorpromazine
Co-amoxiclav
Co-trimoxazole
Erythromycin
Flucloxacillin
Phenytoin
Prochlorperazine

Granulomatous hepatitis (Table 4.7)

Granulomatous hepatitis is characterised by proliferative inflammatory lesions and is often the result of an immunoallergic reaction. Resolution of the clinical, laboratory and histological abnormalities usually occurs promptly after discontinuation of the responsible drug.

Table 4.7 Some drugs causing granulomatous hepatitis

Allopurinol	Phenytoin
Carbamazepine	Procainamide
Chlorpromazine	Quinidine
Gold	Quinine
Hydralazine	Sulfasalazine
Methyldopa	Sulphonamides
Nitrofurantoin	Sulphonylureas
Penicillin	Tacrine
Phenylbutazone	

Vascular disorders

A variety of drugs can cause veno-occlusive disease and Budd–Chiari syndrome. Veno-occlusive disease is characterised by non-thrombotic concentric narrowing of the central hepatic veins by connective tissue. Severe centrilobular congestion and necrosis reflect the venous blockage. Presentation may be acute with right upper quadrant pain, ascites and, in the most severe cases, hepatic failure. This progresses to cirrhosis in those who survive. Alternatively, cirrhosis may develop insidiously over a number of years and present with its complications, including hepatocellular carcinoma. Veno-occlusive disease may be caused by azathioprine, dactinomycin, dacarbazine and high-dose busulfan or cyclophosphamide. High-dose chemotherapy with busulfan or cyclophosphamide for bone marrow transplantation is complicated by veno-occlusive disease of the liver in about 25% of patients (Styler *et al.*, 1996). The risk of this complication may be reduced by careful dose adjustment and heparin prophylaxis. Herbal remedies containing pyrrolizidine alkaloids, for example comfrey and heliotropium, have also been reported to cause veno-occlusive disease.

Budd–Chiari syndrome is characterised by the obstruction of large hepatic veins, and has been reported in association with oral contraceptives and cytotoxic agents (Maddrey, 1987; Valla and Benhamou, 1988).

Hepatic tumours

Hepatocellular adenoma and carcinoma, although rare, have been associated with the use of steroidal compounds such as the oral contraceptives, danazol and anabolic steroids (Davis, 1998; Farrell, 1994).

Management of patients with drug-induced hepatic disease

Stopping the administration of a suspected hepatotoxic drug is the most important action in the management of drug-induced liver disease. In some circumstances attempts to remove a drug from the body can be made, i.e. with dose-dependent acute hepatotoxins, such as paracetamol or heavy metal poisoning, where the unabsorbed drug may be removed by emptying the stomach. If available, a suitable antidote, such as N-acetylcysteine or methionine, may be used as a cytoprotectant in the management of paracetamol overdose.

There are conflicting views on the value of corticosteroids as anti-inflammatory agents to treat drug-induced liver disease. It is generally considered reasonable to give corticosteroids to patients with a hepato-cellular drug-induced injury if improvement is not apparent within 3 months of discontinuing the drug, or possibly as early as 6 weeks where deterioration persists after the causative agent has been stopped (Lee, 1995).

Additional supportive therapy may be needed, ranging from the symptomatic management of pruritus with systemic antihistamines or colestyramine, to liver transplantation for cases where hepatic encephalopathy or fulminant hepatic failure has developed.

Liver dysfunction of any kind is classed as a serious reaction, so any suspicion that a drug has had an adverse effect on the liver should be reported to the appropriate regulatory authority.

Prevention of drug-induced hepatic damage

Regular monitoring of LFTs should be carried out for all patients treated with certain drugs that are common causes of hepatotoxicity (Table 4.8). Baseline liver function tests should be carried out before treatment starts. There is uncertainty about the level of abnormality at which drugs should be discontinued. In general, an increase in any one parameter to two to three times the baseline measurement may indicate drug-induced hepatotoxicity and the drug should be withdrawn. However, where drugs are commonly known to cause elevations in certain liver enzymes, then the threshold for discontinuing the drug may be higher.

Patient education is essential in the prevention of drug-induced hepatotoxicity. Many drug reactions can develop within days, so monitoring of LFTs is not a complete safeguard against toxicity. Patients who do not realise that drug-induced injury is possible, and those who con-

Table 4.8 Some drugs for which regular monitoring of liver function tests (LFTs) is recommended

Drug	LFT monitoring recommended (in UK)
Amiodarone	Monitor LFTs (particularly transaminases) at baseline and then every 6 months
Cyproterone	Check baseline LFTs and then recheck if symptoms develop
Dantrolene	Check baseline LFTs and repeat 6 weeks after starting therapy
Leflunomide	Check baseline LFTs and repeat periodically thereafter
Methotrexate	Check baseline LFTs, then every 2–3 months
Methyldopa	Check baseline LFTs, then at intervals during first 6–12 weeks of treatment
Nevirapine	Check baseline LFTs then every 2 weeks during first 3 months of treatment, after dose increases and periodically thereafter
Rifampicin	In patients with pre-existing liver disease or if pretreatment LFTs are abnormal, LFTs should be checked weekly for the first 2 weeks then at 2–4 week intervals
Rosiglitazone	Check baseline LFTs then repeat every 2 months for the first 12 months and periodically thereafter
Sodium valproate	Check baseline LFTs and repeat periodically during first 6 months of therapy
Statins	Check baseline LFTs and check periodically after that (e.g. every 6–12 months)
Sulfasalazine	Check baseline LFTs, then every 2–3 months

tinue to take a drug despite initial signs of toxicity, are at highest risk of fatal reactions. For example, patients taking antituberculous medication should be encouraged to report to their doctor any gastrointestinal symptoms, which may indicate drug-induced hepatitis, such as anorexia, nausea, vomiting or abdominal pain.

One area where healthcare professionals can have a valuable educational role is with over-the-counter preparations, which members of the public widely assume to be safer than drugs available only on prescription. Health food products ('nutraceuticals') and herbal remedies may also be judged to be innocuous but toxic reactions, including liver damage, may occur.

Finally, the latency period of many hepatotoxic reactions may lead to diagnostic difficulties when patients present with the non-specific signs of actual or impending hepatic damage. Ensuring adequate monitoring of patients, and providing information to prescribers about drugs that are potentially hepatotoxic, is therefore an essential educational role.

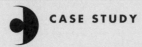

CASE STUDY

Mrs A is a 72-year-old woman with a history of chronic obstructive airways disease. She was recently prescribed a 1-week course of amoxicillin for a chest infection. The infection did not resolve, so she was then given a prescription for a 10-day course of co-amoxiclav. Two weeks later Mrs A felt that her chest infection had improved but she felt generally unwell. She complained of several recent episodes of vomiting and the development of an itch all over her body, and particularly on her arms and legs.

What symptoms are indicative of liver disease and what is the possible cause?
General malaise, tiredness and gastrointestinal symptoms of nausea and vomiting are common signs of drug-induced liver disease. Pruritus in particular is associated with liver dysfunction of cholestatic origin, where it is thought that bile salts are deposited either in or under the skin, with associated itching.

Co-amoxiclav contains amoxicillin and clavulanic acid. Clavulanic acid can cause hepatotoxic reactions which are usually reversible on discontinuation.

What other questions would you ask the patient to help confirm your suspicions?
It is important to obtain details of time of symptom onset in relation to drug ingestion. Onset of illness associated with co-amoxiclav is usually within 1–6 weeks of starting the drug, but has been reported up to 6 weeks after completing a course (Farrell, 1994). While it may be likely that co-amoxiclav is the causative agent, a full drug history should still be taken to exclude other drugs or other causes of potential illness. The patient may have a history of liver disease which might confuse the picture, and this should be clarified.

The patient was admitted to hospital 2 days later. LFTs on admission (with normal level in brackets) were:

Albumin 35 g/l (normal 35–55 g/l)
Aspartate aminotransferase 123 u/l (< 35 u/l)
Alkaline phosphatase 642 u/l (30–130 u/l)
Bilirubin 84 μmol/l (3–17 μmol/l)

What type of liver dysfunction is indicated by these results?
The liver function tests reveal a cholestatic picture of injury. Significant elevations in serum bilirubin and alkaline phosphatase commonly occur in cases of cholestatic jaundice, whereas elevations in the hepatocellular enzymes aspartate and alanine transaminase tend to be less significant in this respect. The albumin is in the normal reference range, which indicates that the liver injury is acute rather than chronic. LFTs can only provide a crude guide to the type of liver disease, and changes do not always accurately indicate the extent of liver damage.

→

> ● **CASE STUDY** (continued)
>
> **How would you recommend that this patient is managed?**
> Cholestatic jaundice associated with co-amoxiclav is usually relatively mild and patients normally recover within 1–4 months of stopping therapy. Liver function should be monitored regularly to detect any deterioration.
>
> Pruritus is a common and debilitating effect of cholestatic injury, and will probably be the main symptomatic complaint. Once the patient has been assessed, treatment with antihistamines, colestyramine and/or topical therapy with menthol in aqueous cream may be considered. In general, sedating antihistamines, such as chlorphenamine (chlorpheniramine), are used because of their longer-term safety record and because lack of sleep is a debilitating feature of pruritus. However, they should only be used in patients with stable liver disease. Non-sedating antihistamines, such as loratadine or cetirizine, may also be of some benefit. Resolution of the underlying condition will provide the most effective relief from the pruritus.
>
> Probably the most important aspect of the patient's long-term management is that she should not be prescribed any products containing clavulanic acid in the future. The appropriate regulatory authority should be notified of the adverse reaction.

References

American College of Rheumatology Ad Hoc Committee on Clinical Guidelines (1996). Guidelines for monitoring drug therapy in rheumatoid arthritis. *Arth Rheum* 39: 723–731.

Anderson G D, Acheampong A A, Wilensky A J et al. (1992). Effect of valproate dose on formation of hepatotoxic metabolites. *Epilepsia* 33: 736.

Bass N M, Williams R L (1988). Guide to drug dosage in hepatic disease. *Clin Pharmacokinet* 15: 396–420.

Benjamin S B, Goodman Z D, Ishak K G et al. (1985). The morphologic spectrum of halothane-induced hepatic injury: analysis of 77 cases. *Hepatology* 5: 1163–1171.

Boffa M J, Chalmers R J G (1996). Methotrexate for psoriasis. *Clin Exp Dermatol* 21: 399–408.

Cadman B (1996). Drug induced liver disease. *Hosp Pharm* 3: 31–35.

Choonara I, Gill A, Nunn A (1996). Drug toxicity and surveillance in children. *Br J Clin Pharmacol* 42: 407–410.

Committee on Safety of Medicines (1986). Halothane hepatotoxicity. *Curr Probl Pharmacovigilance* 18: 1–2.

Committee on Safety of Medicines (1992). Ventricular arrhythmias due to terfenadine and astemizole. *Curr Probl* 35: 1–2.

Committee on Safety of Medicines (1997). Reminder: halothane hepatotoxicity. *Curr Probl Pharmacovigilance* 23: 7.

Danan G, Benichou C (1993). Causality assessment of adverse reactions to drugs. I. A novel method based on the conclusions of international consensus meetings: application to drug-induced liver injuries. *J Clin Epidemiol* 46: 1323–1330.

Davis M (1989). Drugs and abnormal liver function tests. *Adverse Drug React Bull* 139: 520–523.

Davis M (1998). Hepatic disorders. In: Davies D M, Ferner R E, de Glanville H, eds. *Textbook of Adverse Drug Reactions,* 5th edn. London: Chapman and Hall Medical, 275–338.

Dossing M, Sonne J (1993). Drug-induced hepatic disorders. Incidence, management and avoidance. *Drug Safety* 9: 441–449.

Fagan E, Wannan G (1996). Reducing paracetamol overdoses. *Br Med J* 313: 1417–1418.

Farrell G C (1994). *Drug-induced Liver Disease,* 1st edn. Melbourne: Churchill-Livingstone.

Farrell G C (1997). Drug-induced hepatic injury. *J Gastroenterol Hepatol* 12: S242–S250.

Finlayson N D C (1994). Drugs and the liver. *Med Int* 22: 455–458.

Hall S M, Plaster P A, Glasgow J F T *et al.* (1988). Preadmission antipyretics in Reye's syndrome. *Arch Dis Child* 63: 857–866.

Howard Fee J P, Thompson G H (1997). Comparative tolerability profiles of the inhaled anaesthetics. *Drug Safety* 16: 157–170.

James O F W (1985). Drugs and the aging liver. *J Hepatol* 1: 431–435.

Jim L K, Gee J P (1995). Applied therapeutics: the clinical use of drugs. In: Koda Kimble M A, Young L Y, eds. *Adverse Effects of Drugs on the Liver,* 6th edn. Vancouver: Applied Therapeutics, chapter 26.

Kenna J G, Neuberger J, Williams R (1988). Evidence for expression in human liver of halothane-induced neoantigens recognised by antibodies in sera from patients with halothane hepatitis. *Hepatology* 8: 1635–1641.

Lee W M (1995). Drug-induced hepatotoxicity. *N Engl J Med* 333: 1118–1127.

Maddrey W C (1987). Hepatic vein thrombosis (Budd–Chiari syndrome): possible association with the use of oral contraceptives. *Semin Liver Dis* 7: 32–39.

McCarthy M, Wilkinson M L (1999). Hepatology. *Br Med J* 318: 1256–1259.

Neuberger J (1995). Selected side-effects: 16. Methotrexate and liver disorders. *Prescribers' J* 35: 158–163.

Nolan C M, Goldberg S V, Buskin S E (1999). Hepatotoxicity associated with isoniazid preventive therapy. *JAMA* 281: 1014–1018.

O'Grady J G, Alexander G J M, Hayllar K M *et al.* (1989). Early indicators of prognosis in fulminant hepatic failure. *Gastroenterology* 97: 439–445.

Ormerod L P, Skinner C, Wales J (1996). Hepatotoxicity of antituberculous drugs. *Thorax* 51: 111–113.

Penna A, Buchanan N (1991). Paracetamol poisoning in children and hepatotoxicity. *Br J Clin Pharmacol* 32: 143–149.

Pirmohamed M, Kitteringham N R, Park B K (1994). The role of active metabolites in drug toxicity. *Drug Safety* 11: 114–144.

Poss W B, Vernon D D, Dean J M. (1994). A re-emergence of Reye's syndrome. *Arch Pediatr Adolesc Med* 148: 879–882.

Richer M, Robert S (1995). Fatal hepatotoxicity following oral administration of amiodarone. *Ann Pharmacother* 29: 582–586.

Starko K M, Ray G C, Dominguez L B *et al.* (1980). Reye's syndrome and salicylate use. *Pediatrics* 66: 859–864.

Steele M A, Burke R F, Des Prez R M (1991). Toxic hepatitis with isoniazid and rifampicin. A meta-analysis. *Chest* 99: 465–471.

Styler M J, Crilley P, Biggs J *et al.* (1996). Hepatic dysfunction following busulfan and cyclophosphamide myeloablation: a retrospective, multicenter analysis. *Bone Marrow Transplant* 18: 171–176.

Vale J A, Proudfoot A T (1995). Paracetamol (acetaminophen) poisoning. *Lancet* 346: 547–552.

Valla D, Benhamou J P (1988). Drug-induced vascular and sinusoidal lesions of the liver. *Baillieres Clin Gastroenterol* 2: 481–500.

5

Renal disorders

Sharon Hems

Drug-induced renal disease is an important clinical problem. Studies suggest that up to 30% of cases of acute renal failure are secondary to drugs and chemicals and that 2–5% of hospitalised patients develop drug-induced acute renal impairment (Hoitsma *et al.*, 1991; Davidman *et al.*, 1991; Cove-Smith, 1995). In one analysis, drugs contributed to 29% of all cases of acute renal failure in hospital patients, with antibiotics, non-steroidal anti-inflammatory drugs (NSAIDs), angiotensin-converting enzyme (ACE) inhibitors and diuretics most commonly implicated (Davidman *et al.*, 1991). Hospital-acquired acute renal failure is often due to a combination of factors, such as the use of aminoglycosides in patients with sepsis or the use of radiocontrast media in patients on ACE inhibitors. Herbal medicines also have the potential to cause renal impairment; recent case reports have described nephropathy associated with the use of Chinese herbal medicines containing *Aristolochia* (Committee on Safety of Medicines, 1999; Yang *et al.*, 2000).

The kidneys together weigh less than 500 g, but receive 25% of cardiac output. They have an essential role in the elimination of many substances, control of fluid and electrolyte balance and hormonal homoeostasis. They are particularly susceptible to the toxic effects of drugs. Drug toxicity may occur through a variety of mechanisms, including direct and indirect biochemical effects as well as immunological effects. The spectrum of drug-induced renal disease is wide; many drugs can cause several types of defect. For example, NSAIDs can cause functional renal insufficiency, interstitial nephritis, glomerulonephritis, oedema, hyponatraemia and hyperkalaemia.

Loss of renal function is often reversible on discontinuation of therapy, but may occasionally lead to end-stage renal failure. Renal dysfunction of any kind is considered a serious reaction and, if suspected to be drug-related, should always be reported to the appropriate regulatory authority.

Risk factors

Patients at particular risk of nephrotoxicity include those with pre-existing renal impairment, dehydration, sodium-retaining states such as cirrhosis or heart failure and specific clinical conditions such as diabetes. Seriously ill patients with sepsis, shock or failure of multiple body systems are also at increased risk. The elderly appear to be more susceptible to renal toxicity than younger people, possibly because of reduced renal reserve.

Diagnosis of drug-induced renal dysfunction

Several criteria are important in determining whether renal dysfunction has occurred. There is a fall in glomerular filtration rate (GFR), manifest as a rise in blood urea or creatinine. A change in the volume of urine output may also be significant; output may be reduced to less than 400 ml/day (oliguria) or it may be increased (polyuria).

Healthy adults may excrete up to 200 mg of protein daily in urine. Heavy proteinuria is usually due to an abnormally permeable glomerular membrane and suggests glomerular disease (Gaskin, 1999). Other causes of proteinuria include reduced tubular reabsorption due to tubular damage or overflow of proteins present in the plasma at high concentrations.

Routine dipstick testing of the urine for blood, protein and sugar is carried out in all patients suspected of having renal disease. Microscopy of urine may reveal casts, which are cylindrical bodies moulded in the shape of the distal tubular lumen (Cattell *et al.*, 1994). Casts are composed of glycoprotein, cells, cell debris and other proteins. The characteristics of the casts may be helpful; pigmented granular casts are typically found in acute tubular necrosis, white cell casts in interstitial nephritis and red cell casts in glomerulonephritis.

Imaging techniques such as ultrasonography may be useful in the diagnosis of obstruction or the estimation of renal size. Renal biopsy is of value where a knowledge of the histology will influence management. Tissue should be examined by conventional histochemical staining, electron microscopy and immunofluorescence.

Acute renal failure

In acute renal failure (ARF), kidney function deteriorates rapidly over days or weeks. It is a medical emergency characterised by a rapid rise in serum creatinine and usually accompanied by oliguria, although this is less common in drug-induced acute renal failure (Cattell *et al.*, 1994). Symptoms are often non-specific and renal failure is commonly diagnosed after incidental observation of elevated creatinine or urea. Hyperkalaemia, hypocalcaemia or hyperphosphataemia may also be present (Swan and Bennett, 1993; Harper, 1994).

In the later stages of failure, an accumulation of excess urea and other substances in the blood leads to uraemia and associated symptoms. These include nausea, vomiting, gastrointestinal haemorrhage, muscle cramps, predisposition to infection and decreased consciousness. The overall mortality due to acute renal failure depends on the cause but averages about 50%; septicaemia is the most common cause of death.

As shown in Figure 5.1, acute renal failure is generally categorised as prerenal, intrarenal and postrenal failure.

Prerenal failure

Prerenal failure is precipitated by a fall in renal perfusion (Becker *et al.*, 1992). Usually renal function returns to normal once the offending drug is withdrawn and perfusion restored. However, if it persists, acute tubular necrosis may develop (see intrarenal failure, below). Renal perfusion may decline for a number of reasons, such as volume depletion secondary to excessive use of diuretics or laxatives (Wang and Lai, 1994). Volume depletion may manifest as fatigue, hypotension and muscle cramps. Patients especially at risk include the elderly, those with renal impairment and those receiving other nephrotoxic agents (Burnett, 1993).

Intrarenal failure

This condition arises from changes to the renal infrastructure. It can be subdivided into effects on the GFR, acute interstitial nephritis (AIN), acute tubular necrosis and glomerulonephritis.

Effects on the glomerular filtration rate

The GFR is largely controlled by the relative tone of the afferent and efferent arterioles. In the afferent arteriole, tone is mainly mediated by vasodilatory prostaglandins, while in the efferent arteriole the renin–angiotensin–aldosterone system is mainly involved. When renal perfusion falls, activation of these systems will help to control the filtration pressure across an individual glomerulus (Hoitsma *et al.*, 1991).

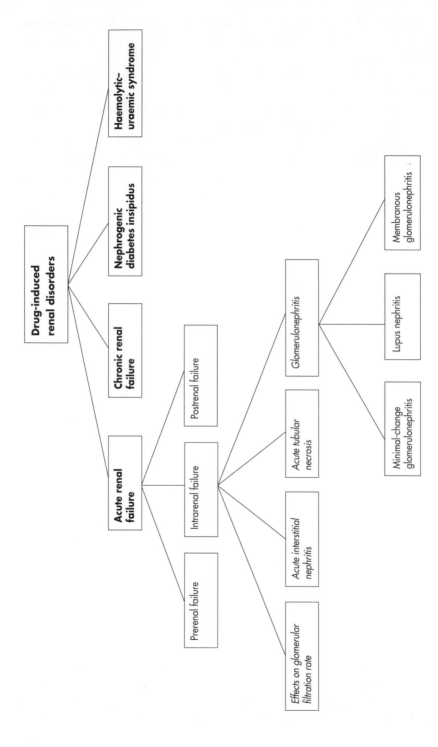

Figure 5.1 Classification of drug-induced renal disorders.

Angiotensin II does this via vasoconstriction of the efferent glomerular arteriole while prostaglandins stimulate vasodilation of the afferent glomerular arteriole.

ACE inhibitors prevent the conversion of angiotensin I to angiotensin II in the renin–angiotensin–aldosterone system. Angiotensin II is a potent vasoconstrictor of the systemic and the renal vascular bed. Consequently, ACE inhibitors produce systemic and renal vasodilation, resulting in decreased blood pressure and increased renal blood flow. As renal vasodilation is mainly mediated by the efferent arteriole, filtration pressure is reduced by ACE inhibition. The lower filtration pressure does not automatically lead to a reduction in GFR, but this may occur in some situations (Navis *et al.*, 1996). Patients at risk include those with renal artery stenosis, particularly bilateral stenoses, those with severe cardiac failure and those receiving NSAIDs or diuretics. The overall incidence of acute renal failure in patients taking ACE inhibitors is less than 1%. However, it increases to 25% in those with bilateral renal disease; it is therefore essential to monitor renal function regularly before and during therapy in at-risk patients.

NSAIDs can cause renal damage by inhibiting prostaglandin production in the kidney, particularly the vasodilatory prostaglandins E_2, D_2 and I_2 (prostacyclin). Where renal blood flow is decreased, these prostaglandins protect against renal ischaemia by antagonising vasoconstrictor substances. In some circumstances, when renal blood flow is already compromised, as in congestive cardiac failure or cirrhosis, NSAID therapy can precipitate an acute fall in GFR. Mild cases are manifest only as increased serum creatinine or hypertension due to salt and water retention, but acute renal failure can occur. NSAIDs have been associated with 7% of all cases of ARF and 36% of drug-related cases of ARF (Porile *et al.*, 1990). Functional renal insufficiency is the most common adverse renal effect of NSAIDs. Patients who are volume-depleted or those with pre-existing renal impairment are also particularly susceptible (Henrich *et al.*, 1996).

Acute interstitial nephritis

AIN is a hypersensitivity reaction characterised by interstitial inflammation and tubular damage. It is often drug-induced. The incidence of AIN is difficult to assess because the presenting symptoms are not specific and diagnosis requires biopsy. Acute renal failure normally occurs within 2 weeks of drug exposure (Mathew, 1992). The signs and symptoms are fever, skin rash, arthralgias, gross haematuria, blood eosinophilia and a variable degree of acute renal failure (Hoitsma *et al.*, 1991; Davison *et al.*, 1997). Mild proteinuria and microscopic haematuria are always present, with urinary white and red cell casts. Proteinuria within the nephrotic range is almost exclusively found in NSAID-related AIN. The renal failure is often non-oliguric and dialysis is required in about a third of patients.

Most patients recover fully following withdrawal of the nephrotoxin but this may take several months. The recovery of renal function depends on how long there had been renal failure before the discovery of AIN. Although evidence for their use is limited, corticosteroids may be prescribed to shorten recovery time if spontaneous recovery does not occur within 10 days of drug withdrawal (Murray and Keane, 1992; Hoitsma *et al.*, 1991). Steroids should be discontinued if no response is obtained after up to 4 weeks of treatment. More than 70 drugs have been implicated in AIN, of which the most common are beta-lactam antibiotics and NSAIDs (Table 5.1).

Table 5.1 Some drugs associated with acute interstitial nephritis

Allopurinol	Minocycline
Azathioprine	Non-steroidal anti-inflammatory drugs
Captopril	Omeprazole
Cephalosporins	Penicillins
Cimetidine	Phenobarbital
Co-trimoxazole	Phenytoin
Erythromycin	Pyrazinamide
Fluoroquinolones	Rifampicin
Furosemide (frusemide)	Sulphonamides
Isoniazid	Thiazides
Methyldopa	Vancomycin

Beta-lactam antibiotics Beta-lactams give the most characteristic picture of drug-induced AIN (Davison *et al.*, 1997). Many cases of methicillin-induced AIN were reported during the 1970s. The incidence of renal dysfunction ranged from 12 to 20% of patients treated. Symptoms of AIN appeared between 2 and 60 days after the start of treatment. Fever often occurred and about half of affected adults had an increased blood urea. Macroscopic haematuria, skin rash, blood eosinophilia and eosinophiluria were present in one-third of patients. More than 90% of affected patients recovered. Other penicillin derivatives linked to AIN are ampicillin, amoxicillin, penicillin G and piperacillin, although the problem is comparatively rare with these agents. Renal and extrarenal symptoms may recur if the patient is rechallenged with the same or chemically related drugs. All beta-lactam antibiotics are best avoided in anyone who has developed AIN during treatment with a penicillin or cephalosporin. Cephalosporins are a rare cause of AIN.

NSAIDs   NSAIDs are a recognised cause of AIN, but the clinical picture is different to that seen with beta-lactam antibiotics. There may be no symptoms or signs of hypersensitivity and renal insufficiency has a progressive onset, discovered several months or years after the start of treatment. Extrarenal signs are rare. More than 80% of patients with NSAID-induced AIN develop a nephrotic syndrome; with beta-lactams this occurs in fewer than 1% of patients (Grunfeld *et al.*, 1993). In biopsies the glomeruli show minimal change. Minimal-change nephrotic syndrome without AIN has also been reported with many NSAIDs (see below).

Other drugs   AIN has also been described in association with the allopurinol hypersensitivity syndrome, where additional symptoms include rash, hepatotoxicity, fever, eosinophilia and leukocytosis (Arellano and Sacristan, 1993; Elasy *et al.*, 1995). The syndrome usually develops within 6 weeks of starting therapy, although this is variable and overall mortality is about 25%. Fortunately, the syndrome is rare, although it has been described in patients with renal impairment in whom the drug dose has not been reduced appropriately. This results in accumulation of allopurinol and its metabolite, oxypurinol, to which and a hypersensitivity reaction develops (Arellano and Sacristan, 1993).

Rifampicin-induced AIN usually occurs following intermittent therapy and is a dose-dependent effect (Murray and Keane, 1992). It is thought that anti-rifampicin antibodies, still detectable weeks to months after rifampicin withdrawal, stimulate an immunological reaction when the drug is reintroduced (Bennett *et al.*, 1991; Murray and Keane, 1992). Initial symptoms often include an influenza-like illness (fever, malaise, chills, myalgia, headache), typically following 3–6 months of intermittent therapy (Levine *et al.*, 1991). These symptoms generally develop within 2 hours of rifampicin administration and resolve within 8 hours. Intermittent rifampicin therapy should therefore be avoided and patients previously exposed to rifampicin should be closely monitored on re-exposure.

Acute tubular necrosis

Acute tubular necrosis is the most common drug-induced renal disease. The most important causes are aminoglycosides, amphotericin, cisplatin, ciclosporin and radiocontrast agents (Table 5.2; Wang and Lai, 1994). These drugs produce a direct toxic effect on the renal tubule resulting in necrosis of the tubular cells. However, acute tubular necrosis may also result from persistent renal hypoperfusion which causes ischaemic tubular cell damage and necrosis (Hoitsma *et al.*, 1991; Harper, 1994).

Table 5.2 Some drugs associated with acute tubular necrosis

Amphotericin	Gentamicin
Ciclosporin	Methotrexate
Ciprofloxacin	Radiocontrast agents
Cisplatin	Rifampicin

Aminoglycoside antibiotics Aminoglycoside antibiotics cause transient renal failure in 10–30% of patients and are the cause of half of all cases of drug-induced acute renal failure in hospital (Bennett and Porter, 1990). Clinical features include mild elevation of creatinine accompanied by normal urine output (non-oliguric renal failure). Serum creatinine levels typically increase after 3–5 days of treatment but occasionally, acute renal failure may only become apparent after treatment is stopped.

The major site of aminoglycoside damage is the proximal renal tubule. The exact mechanism of nephrotoxicity is unclear, but accumulation of drug and phospholipids within lysosomes is involved. The lysosomes become overloaded with phospholipid, destabilise and rupture, releasing acid hydrolases and high concentrations of aminoglycoside into the cytoplasm where they disrupt cell structure and function (Begg and Barclay, 1995). The toxic potential of individual aminoglycosides is directly related to their capacity to disrupt lysosomal membrane function. It has been suggested that the aminoglycosides may be ranked in decreasing order of nephrotoxicity as follows: gentamicin > tobramycin > amikacin > netilmicin, although the differences may only be marginal.

It is essential that plasma drug concentrations and renal function are monitored throughout aminoglycoside therapy and doses adjusted as appropriate. Gentamicin is the most frequently implicated, with

6–26% of recipients developing renal impairment within 10 days of treatment (Humes, 1988). Development of renal failure is dependent on the dose and duration of therapy, as well as the presence of risk factors such as renal or hepatic disease or concurrent administration of other nephrotoxic agents (Appel, 1990; Swan, 1997; Table 5.3). Renal function usually recovers completely when aminoglycosides are withdrawn, although this may take several weeks.

Table 5.3 Risk factors for aminoglycoside nephrotoxicity

Choice of aminoglycoside	High peak or trough serum concentrations
High total dose of aminoglycoside	Concurrent liver disease
Hypotension	Concurrent use of other nephrotoxic
Volume depletion	drugs

The approach to aminoglycoside dosing has changed recently, with a move towards giving larger doses less frequently. It is believed that once-daily dosing will lead to reduced tissue accumulation and so decrease the incidence of nephrotoxicity. However, there is no agreed way of monitoring aminoglycoside concentrations to ensure optimum efficacy and safety with once-daily dosing (Anon, 1997).

Amphotericin   Parenteral amphotericin still has an important role in the management of systemic fungal infections, but dose-dependent nephrotoxicity occurs to some degree in almost all patients receiving the drug (Hoeprich, 1992). Toxicity may be manifest as a decrease in renal blood flow and GFR with increased serum creatinine, distal renal tubular acidosis and renal tubular potassium, sodium and magnesium wasting into urine. Toxicity may occur with doses as low as 300 mg and reaches a prevalence of 80% with cumulative doses approaching 4 g. Risk factors include high mean daily doses, diuretic use and volume depletion and abnormal baseline renal function (Fisher *et al.*, 1989; Sabra and Branch, 1990).

The risk of nephrotoxicity may be minimised by volume repletion and administration with an intravenous saline load. New preparations of amphotericin in which the drug is encapsulated in or available as a complex with, liposomes may be less toxic (Tollemar and Ringden, 1995). If nephrotoxicity occurs, the drug should be stopped. Renal tubular dysfunction and glomerular filtration will improve in most patients, although in some cases damage may be irreversible.

Contrast media The incidence of nephrotoxicity associated with contrast agents varies from 0.6% in patients with normal renal function to almost 100% in renally impaired diabetics. The pathogenesis of contrast nephropathy includes both direct tubular nephropathy and renal ischaemia. Pre-existing renal impairment is the major risk factor, present in 60% of cases, but other factors may be implicated, such as congestive heart failure, myeloma and dehydration (Swan and Bennet, 1993). Renal failure usually develops within 24 hours of administration of the contrast agent, with serum creatinine concentrations reaching a maximum within 4 days, followed by gradual recovery within 10 days.

Contrast nephropathy can be prevented by using alternative imaging procedures in high-risk patients. If contrast media must be used, the smallest adequate dose, preferably of a low-osmolality agent, should be administered. In addition, it has been recommended that patients at risk should receive intravenous fluids (0.45% saline) before and after administration of these agents to protect against acute renal failure (Barrett, 1994; Barrett and Parfrey, 1994; Oliveira, 1999).

Glomerulonephritis

Glomerulonephritis describes a disorder in which there is immunologically mediated damage to the glomeruli of both kidneys. There are several forms of glomerulonephritis, including membranous glomerulonephritis, minimal-change glomerulonephritis and lupus nephritis (Becker *et al.*, 1992). Drug-induced glomerulonephritis may present as proteinuria which, if prolonged and severe (usually more than 3.5 g/day), leads to oedema and hypoalbuminaemia; this is known as the nephrotic syndrome (Becker *et al.*, 1992; Critchley *et al.*, 1997).

Membranous glomerulonephritis In membranous glomerulonephritis, antigens stimulate the production of antibodies and then combine with them to form an immune complex. The immune complex deposits in the kidney to produce thickening of the capillary basement membrane. This form of glomerulonephritis has been described in association with gold and penicillamine therapy (Cattell *et al.*, 1994). Genetic factors appear to be important in conferring susceptibility.

With gold therapy, proteinuria has been described in 2–19% of patients (Collins, 1987). Onset is usually within the first 6 months of treatment but appears to be unrelated to the daily or cumulative dose. It is more common with parenteral than with oral gold therapy. Usually renal function remains normal and proteinuria resolves 6–12 months following drug withdrawal (Collins, 1987; Mathew, 1992). However, about 10–30% of patients affected develop the nephrotic syndrome, usually with membranous glomerulonephritis as the underlying pathology (Collins, 1987; Hall *et al.*, 1987). To minimise the risk of complications, urinalysis must be carried out regularly during gold therapy and treatment discontinued if severe proteinuria develops.

Penicillamine causes proteinuria in up to 30% of patients, usually within the first 12 months of therapy. The incidence is dose-related. The problem usually resolves within 6–12 months of drug withdrawal (Hoitsma *et al.*, 1991; Critchley *et al.*, 1997). However, since proteinuria often remits with continued treatment, therapy may be continued as long as renal function remains normal, oedema is absent and urinary protein excretion does not exceed 2 g/24 hours.

Membranous glomerulonephritis is found in 12% of patients treated with penicillamine and 85% of those with penicillamine-induced nephrotic syndrome (Cassidy and Kerr, 1991; Critchley *et al.*, 1997). Urinalysis should be conducted regularly throughout therapy.

Minimal-change glomerulonephritis   In minimal-change glomerulonephritis, light microscopy of biopsy tissue shows normal glomeruli but electron microscopy reveals abnormal epithelial cells (Cattell *et al.*, 1994). It is most commonly observed with NSAIDs, especially in patients with renal failure and elderly patients on diuretics (Hoitsma *et al.*, 1991; Critchley *et al.*, 1997). The nephrotic syndrome develops following 2 weeks to 2 years of therapy and usually disappears following drug withdrawal, although this may take several weeks (Murray and Keane, 1992). Steroids may assist recovery but progression to chronic renal failure has been described despite their administration.

Lupus nephritis   More than 50 drugs have been associated with a syndrome resembling the autoimmune disease systemic lupus erythematosus (Cassidy and Kerr, 1991; see Chapter 8). In the US, about 10% of cases of systemic lupus erythematosus are estimated to be drug-related and symptoms resemble those of the spontaneously occurring disease: antinuclear antibodies are present and there may be fever, arthralgia, rashes, pleurisy, pleural effusions and pericarditis. Renal involvement in drug-induced systemic lupus erythematosus (lupus nephritis) is rare (about 5%) and the disease usually resolves following drug withdrawal

(Cassidy and Kerr, 1991; Wang and Lai, 1994; McLaughlin *et al.*, 1998).

Lupus erythematosus was recognised with hydralazine in the 1950s and has been reported in 10–20% of patients, of whom 2–20% have renal involvement (Cove-Smith, 1995; Stratton, 1985). Risk is increased in women, patients who are slow acetylators or possess the HLA-DR4 genotype and following prolonged therapy, particularly if doses exceed 100 mg daily (Cove-Smith, 1995). Acetylator status should be determined if the dose is to be increased beyond 100 mg daily. Initial symptoms of lupus nephritis may include microhaematuria, proteinuria and positive titres of antinuclear factors. Regular urinalysis is therefore important during long-term therapy.

Procainamide is the commonest cause of drug-induced systemic lupus erythematosus, with antinuclear antibodies appearing in 50–100% of patients, of whom 5–30% develop signs and symptoms of systemic lupus erythematosus (Stratton, 1985). Usually the lupus-like syndrome appears within 2–6 months of therapy, more commonly in slow acetylators. There have been several reports of lupus nephritis associated with procainamide, but this appears to occur less frequently than with hydralazine (Stratton, 1985; McLaughlin *et al.*, 1998).

Postrenal failure

Postrenal failure results from urinary tract obstruction. It may develop during chemotherapy, when the breakdown of tumour cells leads to overproduction of uric acid which precipitates and blocks the renal tubules. This can be prevented by prior administration of allopurinol which inhibits uric acid production and by ensuring adequate hydration and alkalinisation of the urine.

Obstruction may also occur from precipitation of the drug itself. For example, aciclovir crystals may precipitate in the renal collecting tubules following intravenous administration, because of the drug's low solubility (Cassidy and Kerr, 1991; Krieble *et al.*, 1993). Risk factors include bolus administration, pre-existing renal impairment, hypovolaemia and high dosage. It resolves following drug withdrawal. With high-dose intravenous aciclovir, adequate hydration is essential to prevent crystallisation.

Similarly, methotrexate or its metabolites may precipitate in the renal tubules when administered in high doses. Adequate hydration and alkalinisation of the urine are recommended to avoid this problem.

Sulphonamides have, rarely, been implicated in obstructive

nephropathy due to formation of crystals which obstruct the urinary tract, leading to haematuria, renal colic and anuria (Cribb *et al.*, 1996). The risk of nephrotoxicity depends on the solubility of the sulphonamide, the dose, the presence of pre-existing renal impairment, dehydration or low urinary pH. Older agents such as sulfadiazine and sulfapyridine are more likely to cause crystalluria and obstructive nephropathy than newer, more soluble sulphonamides such as sulfamethoxazole. However, there have been two reports of sulfamethoxazole-induced crystalluria as a result of hypoalbuminaemia leading to increased free concentrations of sulfamethoxazole (Buchanan, 1978).

Obstructive nephropathy has been reported in acquired immune deficiency syndrome (AIDS) patients treated with high doses of sulphonamides for *Pneumocystis carinii* pneumonia infection or *Toxoplasma* encephalitis (Simon *et al.*, 1990). More recently, indinavir has been associated with renal stones in approximately 4% of patients, and this may be complicated by renal failure and urinary tract obstruction (Anon, 1998).

In rhabdomyolysis acute muscle damage occurs, causing release of cell contents, such as myoglobin, enzymes and electrolytes into the circulation (Molnar and Shearer, 1996). Several mechanisms have been suggested to explain the ensuing acute renal failure, such as impaired renal vascular flow or tubular obstruction by myoglobin casts or urate crystals (Prendergast and George, 1993). At urinary pH less than 5.6, myoglobin is converted to ferrihaem which may act as a direct tubular cell toxin or may precipitate and obstruct the tubules. Alternatively, it may be that by scavenging vasodilatory nitric oxide, myoglobin produces intrarenal vasoconstriction and acute renal failure.

It has been estimated that about 30% of patients with rhabdomyolysis develop acute renal failure (Molnar and Shearer, 1996). Drugs have been implicated in about 80% of cases of rhabdomyolysis, with alcohol accounting for at least 20% (Table 5.4; Prendergast and George, 1993). The risk of rhabdomyolysis in association with lipid-lowering agents (fibrates and statins) is recognised (Committee on Safety of Medicines, 1995) (see Chapter 8). The presenting symptom is muscle pain, with elevated creatine phosphokinase and myoglobinuria. The risk may be increased in renal impairment, hypothyroidism, combined therapy with a fibrate and a statin or concomitant ciclosporin. Patients who develop muscle pain, tenderness or weakness while taking these drugs should be referred to their GP.

Table 5.4 Some drugs associated with rhabdomyolysis

Amphotericin B	Monoamine oxidase inhibitors
Barbiturates	Opioids
Benzodiazepines	Phenothiazines
Cimetidine	Retinoids
Colchicine	Statins
Co-trimoxazole	Theophylline
Fibrates	
Lithium	

Bromocriptine, methysergide and other ergot derivatives and beta-blockers have been implicated in retroperitoneal fibrosis (Lim and Devane, 1988; Hely *et al.*, 1991). This is characterised by fibrosis over the posterior abdominal wall and retroperitoneum (Cattell *et al.*, 1994). The ureters become embedded in the fibrous tissue, resulting in an obstructive uropathy. Symptoms of retroperitoneal fibrosis may include malaise, fatigue, back pain, weight loss, abdominal pain, flank pain and dysuria (Lim and Devane, 1988). Because of the hazards, continuous therapy with methysergide should not exceed 6 months without a drug-free period of at least 1 month. Although retroperitoneal fibrosis usually recedes following drug withdrawal, it may progress and require corticosteroid therapy or surgery (Cassidy and Kerr, 1991).

Chronic renal failure

Chronic renal failure is defined as a gradual deterioration in renal function developing over months or years. Typical signs and symptoms are shown in Table 5.5 (Gaskin, 1999). Analgesic nephropathy is the commonest drug cause. Long-term abuse or use of analgesics for chronic pain disorders, such as rheumatoid arthritis, can lead to chronic interstitial nephritis and renal papillary necrosis (Henrich *et al.*, 1996). The problem was identified in the early 1950s and phenacetin was the first drug to be incriminated. However, the problem has not resolved with phenacetin's withdrawal. Studies have shown that analgesic nephropathy is usually associated with combinations of paracetamol with salicylates, codeine or caffeine. The mechanism involved is not clear but is thought to involve the generation of reactive metabolites. Stopping analgesic use generally results in stabilisation or improvement of renal function, while continued use leads to progressive renal damage (Cove-Smith, 1995).

Table 5.5 Signs and symptoms associated with chronic renal failure

Anaemia	Oedema
Breathlessness	Paraesthesia
Drowsiness	Polyuria
Electrolyte disturbances (e.g. hyper-kalaemia, hypocalcaemia)	Pruritus
	Renal bone disease
Hypertension	Restless legs syndrome
Malaise	Seizures
Muscle cramps	Tiredness
Nausea/vomiting	

Abuse of compound analgesics is more common in women and has been attributed to the presence of addictive substances, such as caffeine. In contrast, abuse of single-component analgesics (paracetamol, aspirin, codeine, NSAIDs) and nephropathy secondary to their chronic use, is rare (Wang and Lai, 1994; Elseviers and de Broe, 1996). Paracetamol has been implicated more often than NSAIDs or aspirin. The low doses of aspirin used for its antiplatelet effect are unlikely to affect the kidneys in this way (Patrono, 1994).

The prevalence of analgesic nephropathy varies widely throughout the world. Surveys have shown that the percentage of patients with end-stage renal disease associated with analgesic abuse is as high as 36% in Belgium and as low as 0.07–0.4% in the UK (McGoldrick and Bailie, 1997). In Australia, in the 1970s, a quarter of all patients commencing dialysis had developed renal failure secondary to analgesic nephropathy (Wang and Lai, 1994). In Australia, Sweden and Canada, the withdrawal of over-the-counter sales of compound analgesics significantly reduced the incidence of analgesic nephropathy (Henrich *et al.*, 1996). This led to an ad hoc committee of the US National Kidney Foundation recommending that compound analgesics should be available only on prescription and that all NSAIDs and compound analgesics should be clearly labelled with a warning about the risk of nephrotoxicity.

Nephrogenic diabetes insipidus

In nephrogenic diabetes insipidus, the renal tubules are partially or totally resistant to the effects of antidiuretic hormone (vasopressin), resulting in polyuria and polydipsia (Burke *et al.*, 1995). Unlike central diabetes insipidus, it does not respond to desmopressin.

Lithium reduces the responsiveness of the kidney to antidiuretic hormone, thus impairing its ability to concentrate urine and causing polyuria in up to one-third of patients. The decline in urine-concentrating ability is probably progressive over the first 10 years of therapy (Gitlin, 1999). However, although initially functional and reversible, renal dysfunction may become structural and irreversible during long-term treatment (Waller, 1997). Recommendations to reduce the risk of renal dysfunction include monitoring serum lithium levels to achieve optimal efficacy at the lowest possible concentration. In addition, serum creatinine levels should be monitored regularly during therapy.

Demeclocycline also produces a reversible, dose-dependent nephrogenic diabetes insipidus. In this case, however, the 'adverse effect' has been put to therapeutic use in the management of hyponatraemia caused by the syndrome of inappropriate antidiuretic hormone secretion.

Haemolytic–uraemic syndrome

The haemolytic–uraemic syndrome (HUS) is associated with the production of microthrombi in the renal arterioles and glomeruli, with symptoms including haemolytic anaemia, thrombocytopenia and acute renal failure (Becker *et al.*, 1992; Abuelo, 1995). The syndrome has been associated with ciclosporin, mitomycin C, oral contraceptives and, in children, metronidazole (Cassidy and Kerr, 1991).

The first reports of quinine-induced HUS appeared in 1991 (McDonald *et al.*, 1997). Since quinine is widely consumed, either as a treatment for muscle cramps or in drinks such as tonic water and bitter lemon, careful questioning of the patient is vital. Unlike HUS due to other drugs, with quinine the problem is immune-mediated. Quinine-dependent antibodies directed against red cells, granulocytes and platelets have been demonstrated (Anon, 1996). Treatment with corticosteroids and plasma exchange has been suggested. The prognosis is favourable, with most reports documenting normal renal function at follow-up.

Conclusion

Many drugs can cause renal failure, from mild reversible to severe irreversible. Some drugs for which renal function monitoring is recommended are shown in Table 5.6. There is a wide spectrum of renal lesions and many drugs can produce more than one type. A knowledge and understanding of the pathogenesis assist early diagnosis and prevent unnecessary interventions.

Table 5.6 Some drugs for which regular renal function monitoring is recommended

Amphotericin	Cyclophosphamide
Aminoglycoside antibiotics (systemic)	Gold (injectable and oral)
Carboplatin	Methotrexate
Chlorambucil	Penicillamine
Ciclosporin	Tacrolimus
Cisplatin	Vancomycin

 CASE STUDY

Mrs L is a 53-year-old woman who requests advice on the management of cystitis. Although she has never suffered from cystitis before, she recognises the symptoms. Mrs L has been passing a lot of urine, sometimes blood-stained, and she describes severe loin pain.

Are these symptoms suggestive of cystitis?
Cystitis is characterised by a burning pain on passing urine (dysuria), urinary frequency, urgency and loin pain. The urine may be cloudy with an offensive odour, suggesting bacterial infection and blood may be present due to inflammation of the lining of the bladder and urethra. Any patient who presents with loin pain or haematuria needs further investigation to confirm the diagnosis.

On further questioning Mrs L reports no pain on urination and she has not noticed that her urine is cloudy or has an offensive smell. She is otherwise healthy and not on any prescribed medication. When asked about medicines bought without a prescription, however, she tells you that she buys a painkiller from the supermarket for persistent headaches. She says she has probably taken this on most days for the past 15 years. The analgesic contains aspirin, paracetamol and caffeine.

What could be causing Mrs L's symptoms?
These symptoms and the drug history suggest a possible diagnosis of analgesic nephropathy, although further investigation is necessary to confirm this and to eliminate other causes. Compound analgesics containing caffeine, such as that taken by Mrs L, are particularly prone to abuse since they produce a psychological lift and rebound headache on withdrawal (Becker *et al.*, 1992).

References

Abuelo J G (1995). Diagnosing vascular causes of renal failure. *Ann Intern Med* 123: 601–614.

Anon. (1996). Quinine and haemolytic uraemic syndrome. *Aust Adverse Drug React Bull* 15: 2.

Anon. (1997). Aminoglycosides once daily? *Drug Ther Bull* 35: 36–37.

Anon. (1998). Renal and urinary reactions. *HIV ADR Reporting Scheme News* 1: 2.

Appel G B (1990). Aminoglycoside nephrotoxicity. *Am J Med* 88 (suppl 3C): 16–20.

Arellano F, Sacristan J (1993). Allopurinol hypersensitivity syndrome: a review. *Ann Pharmacother* 27: 337–343.

Barrett B J (1994). Contrast nephrotoxicity. *J Am Soc Nephrol* 5: 125–137.

Barrett B J, Parfrey P S (1994). Prevention of nephrotoxicity induced by radiocontrast agents. *N Engl J Med* 331: 1449–1450.

Becker G J, Whitworth J A, Kincaid-Smith P (1992). *Clinical Nephrology in Medical Practice*. London: Blackwell Scientific Publications.

Begg E J, Barclay M L (1995). Aminoglycosides – 50 years on. *Br J Clin Pharmacol* 39: 597–603.

Bennett W M, Porter G A (1990). Nephrotoxicity of common drugs used by urologists. *Urol Clin North Am* 17: 145–156.

Bennett W M, Elzinga L W, Porter G A (1991). Tubulointerstitial disease and toxic nephropathy. In: Brenner B M, Rector F C, eds. *The Kidney*, 4th edn. London: WB Saunders, chapter 29.

Buchanan N (1978). Sulphamethoxazole, hypoalbuminaemia, crystalluria and renal failure. *Br Med J* ii: 172.

Burke C, Fulda G J, Castellano J (1995). Lithium-induced nephrogenic diabetes insipidus treated with intravenous ketorolac. *Crit Care Med* 23: 1924–1927.

Burnett J C (1993). Acute renal failure associated with cardiac failure and hypovolaemia. In: Lazarus J M, Brenner B M, eds. *Acute Renal Failure*, 3rd edn. London: Churchill Livingstone, chapter 7.

Cassidy M J D, Kerr D N S (1991). Renal disorders. In: Davies D M, ed. *Textbook of Adverse Drug Reactions*, 4th edn. Oxford: Oxford University Press, chapter 12.

Cattell W R, Baker L R I, Greenwood R N (1994). Renal disease. In: Kumar P J, Clark M L, eds. *Clinical Medicine*, 3rd edn. London: Baillière Tindall, chapter 9.

Collins A J (1987). Gold treatment for rheumatoid arthritis: reassurance on proteinuria. *Br Med J* 295: 739–740.

Committee on Safety of Medicines (1995). Rhabdomyolysis associated with lipid-lowering drugs. *Curr Probl Pharmacovigilance* 21: 3.

Committee on Safety of Medicines (1999). Renal failure associated with Chinese herbal medicines. *Curr Probl Pharmacovigilance* 25: 18.

Cove-Smith R (1995). Drugs and the kidney. *Medicine* 23: 165–173.

Cribb A E, Lee B L, Trepanier L A *et al.* (1996). Adverse reactions to sulphonamide and sulphonamide–trimethoprim antimicrobials: clinical syndromes and pathogenesis. *Adverse Drug React Toxicol Rev* 15: 9–50.

Critchley J A J H, Chan T Y K, Cumming A D (1997). Renal diseases. In: Speight T M, Holford N H G, eds. *Avery's Drug Treatment,* 4th edn. New Zealand: Adis International, chapter 24.

Davidman M, Olson P, Kohen J *et al.* (1991). Iatrogenic renal disease. *Arch Intern Med* 151: 1809–1812.

Davison A E, Stewart Cameron A E, Grunfeld J P *et al.* (1997). *Oxford Textbook of Clinical Nephrology.* Oxford: Oxford University Press.

Elasy T, Kaminsky D, Tracy M *et al.* (1995). Allopurinol hypersensitivity syndrome revisited. *West J Med* 162: 360–361.

Elseviers M M, de Broe M E (1996). Combination analgesic involvement in the pathogenesis of analgesic nephropathy: the European perspective. *Am J Kidney Dis* 28 (suppl 1): S48–S55.

Fisher M A, Talbot G H, Maislin G *et al.* (1989). Risk factors for amphotericin B-associated nephrotoxicity. *Am J Med* 87: 547–552.

Gaskin G (1999). Signs and symptoms of renal disease. *Medicine* 27: 1–4.

Gitlin M (1999). Lithium and the kidney. *Drug Safety* 20: 231–243.

Grunfeld J P, Kleinknecht D, Droz D (1993). Acute interstitial nephritis. In: Schrier R W, Gottschalk C W, eds. *Diseases of the Kidney,* vol. 2, 5th edn. Boston: Little Brown, 1331–1353.

Hall C L, Fothergill N J, Blackwell M M *et al.* (1987). The natural course of gold nephropathy: long term study of 21 patients. *Br Med J* 295: 745–748.

Harper A (1994). Acute renal failure. In: Walker R, Edwards C, eds. *Clinical Pharmacy and Therapeutics.* London: Churchill Livingstone, chapter 14.

Hely M A, Morris J G L, Lawrence S *et al.* (1991). Retroperitoneal fibrosis, skin and pleuropulmonary changes associated with bromocriptine therapy. *Aust NZ J Med* 21: 82–84.

Henrich W, Agodoa L, Barrett B *et al.* (1996). Analgesics and the kidney: summary and recommendations to the scientific advisory board of the National Kidney Foundation from an Ad Hoc Committee of the National Kidney Foundation. *Am J Kidney Dis* 27: 162–165.

Hoeprich P D (1992). Clinical use of amphotericin B and derivatives: lore, mystique, and fact. *Clin Infect Dis* 14 (suppl 1): S114–S119.

Hoitsma A J, Wetzels J F M, Koene R A P (1991). Drug-induced nephrotoxicity. Aetiology, clinical features and management. *Drug Safety* 6: 131–147.

Humes H D (1988). Aminoglycoside nephrotoxicity. *Kidney Int* 33: 900–911.

Krieble B F, Rudy D W, Glick M R, Clayman M D (1993). Case-report: acyclovir neurotoxicity and nephrotoxicity – the role for hemodialysis. *Am J Med Sci* 305: 36–39.

Levine M, Collin K, Kassen B O (1991). Acute hemolysis and renal failure following discontinuous use of rifampin. *Drug Intell Clin Pharm* 25: 743–744.

Lim C, Devane C L (1988). Retroperitoneal fibrosis and migraine therapy. *Drug Intell Clin Pharm* 22: 405–406.

Mathew T H (1992). Drug-induced renal disease. *Med J Aust* 156: 724–729.

McDonald S P, Shanahan E M, Thomas A C *et al.* (1997). Quinine-induced hemolytic uremic syndrome. *Clin Nephrol* 47: 397–400.

McGoldrick M D, Bailie G R (1997). Non-narcotic analgesics: prevalence and estimated economic impact of toxicities. *Ann Pharmacother* 31: 221–227.

McLaughlin K, Gholoum B, Guiraudon C *et al.* (1998). Rapid development of drug-induced lupus nephritis in the absence of extrarenal disease in a patient receiving procainamide. *Am J Kidney Dis* 32: 698–702.

Molnar Z L, Shearer E S (1996). Rhabdomyolysis on the intensive care unit – an under diagnosed condition. *Care Crit Ill* 12: 165–168.

Murray K M, Keane W R (1992). Review of drug-induced acute interstitial nephritis. *Pharmacotherapy* 12: 462–467.

Navis G, Faber H J, de Zeeuw D *et al.* (1996). ACE inhibitors and the kidney. *Drug Safety* 15: 200–211.

Oliveira D B G (1999). Prophylaxis against contrast-induced nephropathy. *Lancet* 353: 1638–1639.

Patrono C (1994). Aspirin as an antiplatelet agent. *N Engl J Med* 330: 1287–1294.

Porile J L, Bakris G L, Garella S (1990). Acute interstitial nephritis with glomerulopathy due to nonsteroidal anti-inflammatory agents: a review of its clinical spectrum and effects of steroid therapy. *J Clin Pharmacol* 30: 468–475.

Prendergast B D, George C F (1993). Drug-induced rhabdomyolysis – mechanisms and management. *Postgrad Med J* 69: 333–336.

Sabra R, Branch R A (1990). Amphotericin B nephrotoxicity. *Drug Safety* 5: 94–108.

Simon D I, Brosius F C, Rothstein D M (1990). Sulphadiazine crystalluria revisited. The treatment of toxoplasma encephalitis in patients with acquired immunodeficiency syndrome. *Arch Intern Med* 150: 2379.

Stratton M A (1985). Drug-induced systemic lupus erythematosus. *Clin Pharm* 4: 657–663.

Swan S K (1997). Aminoglycoside nephrotoxicity. *Semin Nephrol* 17: 27–33.

Swan S K, Bennett W M (1993). Nephrotoxic acute renal failure. In: Lazarus J M, Brenner B M, eds. *Acute Renal Failure*, 3rd edn. London: Churchill Livingstone.

Tollemar J, Ringden O (1995). Lipid formulations of amphotericin B. Less toxicity but at what economic cost? *Drug Safety* 13: 207–218.

Waller D (1997). Lithium-induced polyuria. *Prescribers' J* 37: 24–28.

Wang A, Lai K N (1994). Drug-induced renal diseases. *Adverse Drug React Bull* 168: 635–638.

Yang C S, Lin C H, Chang S H *et al.* (2000). Rapidly progressive fibrosing interstitial nephritis associated with Chinese herbal drugs. *Am J Kidney Dis* 35: 313–318.

6

Endocrine disorders

Janice Watt

Endocrine disease affects a wide range of body systems. It may be characterised as congenital or acquired; the majority is idiopathic, has an autoimmune cause or is secondary to an endocrine tumour (most commonly of the pituitary, thyroid or parathyroid). Autoimmune diseases are characterised by the presence of specific antibodies in the serum that may be present for many years before symptoms occur. Autoimmune disease has been observed involving every endocrine organ (Drury, 1994). A wide range of drugs affects the functions of the endocrine glands. Drugs may act on the synthesis and release of endocrine hormones or may interfere with the tests used to identify endocrine disease. Some knowledge of drugs that interfere with tests for endocrine disease is particularly important as, if this is not considered, misdiagnosis may result in inappropriate treatment. This chapter gives an overview of drugs that affect the endocrine system, highlighting those commonly implicated.

Drugs affecting thyroid function

Thyroid hormone is synthesised from dietary iodine. The minimum daily requirement of iodine is 50 μg. There is an autoregulatory mechanism within the thyroid gland that protects against iodine deficiency and excess. Iodine is reduced to iodide in the gastrointestinal tract and, following its absorption, is 'organified' (i.e. combines with tyrosyl residues of thyroglobulin) to form mono-iodotyrosines and di-iodotyrosines. Release of thyroid-stimulating hormone (TSH) from the pituitary results in these compounds being coupled to form levothyroxine (thyroxine) (T_4) and tri-iodothyronine (T_3) which are then released from the thyroid. T_3 and T_4 are transported throughout the body via carrier proteins, including thyroxine-binding globulin (TBG). Most thyroid disease is secondary to autoimmune processes but some drugs cause thyroid dysfunction by interacting with aspects of thyroid hormone synthesis and release (Table 6.1).

Table 6.1 Some drugs that can affect thyroid function

Drugs associated with hyperthyroidism	Drugs associated with hypothyroidism
Amiodarone	Amiodarone
Interferon alfa	Interferon alfa
Lithium	Lithium
Radiographic contrast media (transient)	

Iodine and the thyroid gland

Iodine has complex effects on the thyroid gland and thyroid status and is recognised as causing both hypothyroidism and thyrotoxicosis (hyperthyroidism) (Gittoes and Franklyn, 1995). However, in iodine-replete areas, such as the UK and US, the effects of iodine and iodine-containing preparations on thyroid function are seldom clinically relevant.

Amiodarone

Amiodarone contains 37% by weight of iodine; a daily dose of 200–400 mg provides 6–12 mg of free iodine, which is about 100 times that consumed in an average diet (Quin and Thomson, 1994). Thyroid hormone dynamics change in almost all patients receiving amiodarone. This results in the following typical abnormal thyroid function tests in most patients: elevated T_4 (free and total), elevated TSH (may also be normal or low) and decreased T_3 (free and total). Abnormal results of thyroid function tests, without clinical signs of thyroid dysfunction, occur more often as the duration of treatment increases and drug accumulates.

Amiodarone may cause clinical hypothyroidism or thyrotoxicosis months to years after starting therapy. The effect of the drug depends on whether it has been given in the context of previous iodine deficiency or in the presence of overt or subclinical thyroid disease. In the first few weeks following initiation of amiodarone, the excess iodide load commonly inhibits thyroid hormone synthesis and release (Wolff–Chaikoff effect) (Newman et al., 1998). The normal thyroid is usually able to overcome this effect and thyroid hormone levels return to normal. However, if this does not happen hypothyroidism may result. Hypothyroidism secondary to amiodarone has been reported in 1–32% of patients on long-term therapy (Harjai and Licata, 1997). It is most prevalent in populations with high dietary iodine intake, such as the US, and is most common in females with pre-existing thyroid autoantibodies. Such women are about 14 times more likely than men without antibodies to present with hypothyroidism secondary to amiodarone (Harjai and Licata, 1997).

Symptoms of hypothyroidism include fatigue, intolerance of cold, mental and physical sluggishness and dry skin. Management involves either stopping the drug or, if this is not possible, T_4 replacement therapy. T_4 should be started at a dose of 25–50 µg and increased at 4–6-week intervals to maintain thyroid hormone levels at the upper end of the reference range.

In some circumstances, amiodarone may cause hyperthyroidism (thyrotoxicosis) which in some cases has been fatal. Possible mechanisms include the induction of autoantibodies by amiodarone in the presence of pre-existing antibodies or a direct toxic effect on the thyroid gland. The reported incidence of clinically significant hyperthyroidism ranges between 1 and 23% (Harjai and Licata, 1997). It is most common in populations with low iodine intake.

Patients with thyrotoxicosis secondary to amiodarone may present with unexplained weight loss, muscle weakness, goitre and tremor. They may also have an exacerbation of their pre-existing cardiac arrhythmia. Some classic symptoms (e.g. hyperactivity, heat intolerance and sweating) may be masked by the pharmacological properties of the drug. Symptoms are generally accompanied by a raised serum T_3 and T_4 and a suppressed TSH concentration or an absent TSH response to TRH. If thyrotoxicosis occurs, amiodarone should be stopped wherever possible. However, due to its long elimination half-life, it may take 8 months or more for the problem to resolve. In patients with serious cardiac arrhythmias, it may not be possible to stop amiodarone. In these cases, antithyroid therapy, such as carbimazole or propylthiouracil, and a beta-blocker may be given (Gittoes and Franklyn, 1995; Harjai and Licata, 1997). Corticosteroids (e.g. prednisolone 40–60 mg daily) may also be useful, particularly in patients with no previous history of thyroid disease (Bartalena *et al.*, 1996). Radioactive iodine is not usually a suitable treatment because high systemic iodine concentrations prevent uptake of radioactive iodine into the thyroid (Harjai and Licata, 1997).

Lithium

Lithium may also cause hypothyroidism or thyrotoxicosis. As with amiodarone, women with pre-existing thyroid autoantibodies are predominantly affected. Lithium-induced hypothyroidism is thought to involve inhibition of iodotyrosine and iodothyronine biosynthesis and inhibition of thyroid hormone release from the gland. As many as 30%

of patients treated are thought to develop subclinical hypothyroidism (Gittoes and Franklyn, 1995). However, long-term studies indicate that, although T_3 and T_4 tend to fall in the first few months of treatment, they return to pretreatment levels within 12 months and can exceed the pretreatment values afterwards (Yeung *et al.*, 1998). Conversely, TSH tends to rise in the first few months but gradually returns to pretreatment levels after more than 12 months. Only about 2% of patients develop clinical features of hypothyroidism requiring T_4 replacement.

Thyrotoxicosis due to lithium is rare. In most cases, symptoms develop several years after starting the drug and occasionally symptoms appear after it is stopped (Chow and Cockram, 1990). The mechanism is unclear, but in more than 50% of patients there is evidence of autoimmune thyroid disease. Several theories have been proposed, including over-compensation in response to abnormalities in iodine pharmacokinetics induced by lithium. When lithium treatment is stopped, rebound hyperthyroidism may occur, because thyroid hormone synthesis is no longer inhibited. Thyrotoxicosis may be treated by withdrawing the drug or by giving carbimazole (Becerra-Fernadez, 1995).

Interferon alfa

Hypothyroidism and thyrotoxicosis have been reported in patients receiving long-term treatment with recombinant interferon alfa (Roti *et al.*, 1996). The incidence is thought to be about 7% and 4%, respectively, and is highest in patients with chronic hepatitis C. Patients with thyroid autoantibodies are at greatest risk of thyroid disease but the exact mechanism is unclear. There is some evidence that interferon alfa may inhibit iodide organification in the thyroid, thus inhibiting thyroid hormone biosynthesis.

Drugs which may interfere with thyroid function tests

Many drugs affect thyroid function tests through alterations in the synthesis, transport and metabolism of thyroid hormones, as well as via influences on TSH synthesis and secretion (Davies and Franklyn, 1991). T_4 and T_3 are transported in the blood stream by three carrier proteins; only 0.03% of total T_4 and 0.3% of total T_3 circulate in the free or unbound form but it is this small fraction that is biologically active. The thyroid function tests used most widely are total plasma T_4 and T_3, plasma basal TSH and free T_4.

Often drugs have only a minor effect on thyroid function tests, so that results remain within the normal reference range. However, results outside the reference range can arise in the absence of any clinical evidence of thyroid dysfunction. It is important to be aware of the influence of drugs so that inappropriate investigations and therapy can be avoided. Some drugs that can interfere with thyroid function tests are shown in Table 6.2. Oestrogen, in combined oral contraceptives or hormone replacement therapy, results in a dose-dependent increase in TBG concentrations (Surks and Sievert, 1995). Serum T_4 concentrations are increased but the proportion of active free T_4 and TSH are unaltered and clinical hyperthyroidism is absent. TBG serum concentrations may also be increased in long-term heroin or methadone users or patients receiving fluorouracil. Conversely, androgens, including danazol and anabolic steroids, and glucocortiocoids decrease TBG concentrations (Surks and Sievert, 1995).

Table 6.2 Some drugs that can interfere with thyroid function tests

Amiodarone	Corticosteroids
Anabolic steroids	Heparin
Aspirin	Non-steroidal anti-inflammatory
Beta-blockers	drugs
Carbamazepine	Oestrogens
Contrast media	Phenytoin

Phenytoin, carbamazepine and rifampicin increase the metabolism and elimination of thyroid hormones, probably because of their ability to induce hepatic enzymes. This results in a fall in T_3 and T_4 serum concentrations but patients remain euthyroid and TSH is normal or only slightly raised (Davies and Franklyn, 1991).

Because of their high iodine content, radiographic contrast media may cause an increase in circulating T_4 which reaches a maximum 3–4 days after administration and returns to normal within 14 days. Care should be taken when interpreting thyroid function tests carried out within 2 weeks of exposure. However, clinical hyperthyroidism requiring treatment has been reported rarely (Martin *et al.*, 1993).

Heparin causes a rapid increase in the serum T_4 concentration, which peaks 15 minutes after injection but returns to normal by 60 minutes. For this reason, where possible, thyroid function tests should be postponed until after heparin therapy is stopped (Quin and Thomson, 1994). Corticosteroids are known to inhibit TSH release and small decreases in T_3 and T_4 may occur, although concentrations rarely fall outwith normal limits (Davies and Franklyn, 1991).

Drugs affecting adrenal function

Glucocorticoids

Cortisol production is stimulated by adrenocorticotrophic hormone (ACTH) produced by the pituitary gland. Cortisol in turn influences both corticotrophin-releasing factor production in the hypothalamus and ACTH release by the pituitary, by negative feedback. When steroids are given even for a few days, the feedback system is interrupted and suppression of the hypothalamic–pituitary–adrenal (HPA) system ocurs.

Cushing's syndrome occurs when there is adrenal hyperfunction due to chronic glucocorticoid excess. Administration of pharmacological doses of corticosteroids causes iatrogenic Cushing's syndrome. This usually occurs within 2 weeks of starting therapy at daily doses in excess of hydrocortisone 50 mg (or equivalent). However, there is great variability in patient response and some may exhibit symptoms at much lower doses. Symptoms are usually absent with doses of less than 20 mg hydrocortisone (Dukes, 1996). Typical signs include 'moon face' and 'buffalo hump', weight gain, psychiatric symptoms and skin thinning.

Prolonged administration of corticosteroids in excess of physiological doses (i.e. >7.5 mg prednisolone daily or equivalent) results in suppression of the HPA axis. In the absence of ACTH release, the adrenals become atrophied and can no longer synthesise and release glucocorticoids (Dukes, 1996). If corticosteroid therapy is stopped abruptly, a withdrawal syndrome may occur. Typically, patients experience headache, dizziness, joint pain, weakness and emotional changes but symptoms may be much more severe, particularly after long-term therapy, and fatalities have been reported.

It is therefore essential that patients treated with corticosteroids are counselled about the dangers of stopping treatment abruptly and that they carry a steroid warning card. Steroids should always be given for the shortest length of time at the lowest dose that is clinically necessary. Once-daily dosing in the morning and, if disease control will allow, alternate-day dosing may reduce suppression of the HPA axis (Page, 1997). Patients receiving long-term inhaled steroids in excess of 1.5 mg beclometasone dipropionate daily (or its equivalent) and those using high-potency topical preparations may also show signs of HPA suppression (Robinson and Geddes, 1996). Suppression of the HPA axis results in the adrenals responding inadequately to physiological stress. An increased dose of systemic corticosteroid must therefore be given during serious illness or surgery (Anon, 1999).

Patients stopping systemic corticosteroids after long-term treatment must have therapy withdrawn gradually. The British Thoracic Society asthma management guidelines advise that therapy may be stopped abruptly if the patient has been treated for less than 3 weeks with 40 mg prednisolone daily or less (British Thoracic Society, 1997). Patients at greatest risk of HPA suppression are those who have been treated for more than 3 weeks, had repeated courses of systemic corticosteroids, received more than 40 mg prednisolone daily or the equivalent, received a short course of steroids within 1 year of stopping long-term steroids, and those with underlying adrenocortical insufficiency. A reducing course of corticosteroids should be considered in all of these patients (Committee on Safety of Medicines, 1998). In patients treated with corticosteroids for 18 months or more, the HPA axis may take up to 1 year to recover (Page, 1997). When tailing off corticosteroids in patients on chronic high-dose therapy, a short Synacthen test may be useful in assessing the recovery of the HPA axis once a dose of 5 mg prednisolone is reached (Kountz and Clark, 1997).

Metyrapone/aminoglutethimide

Metyrapone and aminoglutethimide are both used in the treatment of Cushing's disease. They act by blocking corticosteroid biosynthesis and therefore when used in excess can result in hypoadrenalism (Yeung *et al.*, 1998).

Ketoconazole

Ketoconazole is a potent inhibitor of adrenal glucocorticoid synthesis. It acts at two enzyme steps in the adrenal steroid biosynthesis pathway: 11-beta-hydroxylase and conversion of cholesterol to pregnenolone. The effect seems to be dose-related, but adrenal insufficiency has been reported with oral doses of 200 mg twice daily after 2 days' treatment (Best *et al.*, 1987; Khosla *et al.*, 1989). Signs and symptoms include lethargy, anorexia, weight loss, hyponatraemia and hyperkalaemia. Patients may be treated by withdrawing the drug or by corticosteroid replacement therapy. Because of its effects on steroid biosynthesis, attempts have been made to use ketoconazole in the treatment of Cushing's syndrome in patients unresponsive to conventional therapy (Khanderia, 1991).

Rifampicin

Rifampicin has been reported to precipitate acute adrenal insufficiency in patients with pre-existing hypoadrenalism (Leuenberger and Sonntag, 1996). This is thought to be due to an increase in glucocorticoid metabolism secondary to hepatic microsomal enzyme induction. It is recommended that such patients should have their steroid replacement dose doubled or tripled on starting rifampicin.

Aldosterone synthesis

Aldosterone is the most potent mineralocorticoid secreted by the adrenal cortex; it increases sodium and water retention and potassium and hydrogen secretion by the kidney. Aldosterone production is regulated mainly by changes in blood volume, mediated through the renin–angiotensin system, which interacts with the sympathetic nervous system and prostaglandins. Other factors controlling its secretion include changes in potassium and ACTH. Some drugs that can cause hyperaldosteronism are shown in Table 6.3.

Table 6.3 Some drugs that may cause hyperaldosteronism

Carbenoxolone	Oral contraceptives
Lithium	Spironolactone
Loop diuretics	Thiazides

Angiotensin-converting enzyme (ACE) converts angiotensin I to angiotensin II, which, as well as being a potent vasoconstrictor, is the primary stimulator of aldosterone. ACE inhibitors can produce hyper-reninaemic hypoaldosteronism which manifests as hyperkalaemia with a hyperchloraemic metabolic acidosis. Angiotensin II receptor antagonists can also lead to a reduction in aldosterone. Non-steroidal anti-inflammatory drugs inhibit renin secretion, and thus aldosterone release, which can lead to a syndrome of hyporeninaemic hypoaldosteronism (Tan *et al.*, 1979; Clive and Stoff, 1984). Even at low doses, standard or low molecular weight heparins can produce hypoaldosteronism. Aldosterone suppression occurs within a few days of initiation of therapy, is reversible, and is independent of either anticoagulant effect or route of administration (Edes and Sunderrajan, 1985; Oster *et al.*, 1995). A clinically significant increase in the serum potassium level may occur in about 7% of patients. Certain types of patient seem to be more susceptible to the suppression of aldosterone secretion, such as those with diabetes mellitus, chronic renal impairment, pre-existing acidosis, raised plasma potassium or those taking potassium-sparing drugs (Committee on Safety of Medicines, 1999). Plasma potassium should be measured in at-risk patients before starting heparin and monitored regularly thereafter, particularly if heparin is to be continued for more than 7 days.

Drugs affecting gonadotrophin release and gonadal function

Glucocorticoids

Release of gonadotrophin-releasing hormones (GnRH or LH-RH) from the hypothalamus stimulates follicle-stimulating hormone (FSH) and luteinising hormone (LH) release from the pituitary. FSH and LH stimulate spermatogenesis and testosterone production in males and maturation of the follicle and production of oestrogen and progestogen in females. High doses of corticosteroids inhibit pituitary gonadotrophin release and result in ovarian and testicular dysfunction (Dukes, 1996).

Ketoconazole

Ketoconazole directly inhibits testicular steroidogenesis by inhibiting the 17-alpha-hydroxylase enzyme at doses of 400 mg daily (Tester-Dalderup, 1996). This is probably the mechanism by which ketoconazole causes gynaecomastia.

Danazol

Testosterone is transported in the body via sex hormone-binding globulin. Danazol decreases the ability of testosterone to bind to this protein, resulting in an increase in the free, active form of testosterone (Yeung *et al.*, 1998). This may explain the virilisation and hirsutism observed in patients treated with danazol, although the drug also has weak androgenic properties.

Gynaecomastia

Gynaecomastia is the abnormal accumulation of tissue in the male breast. It can occur physiologically in three phases of life: in the neonatal period, following exposure to maternal oestrogens; at puberty (in up to two-thirds of adolescent males); and in old age, due to a reduction in endogenous testosterone levels (Thomson and Reading Carter, 1993). About 50% of cases of gynaecomastia have a physiological cause and about 10–20% are secondary to drug therapy (Turner, 1997).

Drug-induced gynaecomastia may be very embarrassing and distressing for the patient but it is rarely a cause for alarm. A wide variety of drugs has been implicated, and for most the mechanism for the adverse effect is unknown. Two recognised mechanisms are firstly, increased serum oestrogen concentration or enhanced activity and secondly, blockade of testosterone's synthesis or effect (Thomson and Reading Carter, 1993). Table 6.4 lists drugs that have been reported to cause gynaecomastia and the proposed underlying mechanism. Drug-induced gynaecomastia usually develops soon after drug therapy is initiated and resolves when the drug is stopped (Lucas et al., 1987).

Table 6.4 Some drugs that can cause gynaecomastia

Drugs with oestrogenic activity
Clomifene
Digitalis glycosides
Oestrogens
Spironolactone

Drugs reducing testosterone synthesis or effects
Alcohol
Alkylating agents, e.g. vinblastine
Cimetidine
Cyproterone
Flutamide
Ketoconazole
Phenytoin
Spironolactone

Drugs where the mechanism is uncertain
Antipsychotics, e.g. chlorpromazine
Calcium channel blockers, e.g. verapamil, nifedipine
Isoniazid
Marijuana
Methadone
Methyldopa
Protease inhibitors (Melbourne et al., 1998)
Stavudine (Choi and Pai, 1998)
Tricyclic antidepressants

Hyperprolactinaemia

Prolactin is a hormone synthesised and released from the anterior pituitary. It has a major role in preparing the breast for lactation and maintenance of lactation. The release of prolactin from the pituitary is inhibited by dopamine from the hypothalamus and stimulated by the release of serotonin. Excess prolactin release (hyperprolactinaemia) may cause galactorrhoea, amenorrhoea, impotence or infertility. Galactorrhoea can be defined as the persistent discharge of milk or a milk-like substance from the breast in the absence of parturition or at least 6 months postpartum in mothers who are not breast-feeding (Yeung, 1993).

Drugs that have been implicated in the development of hyperprolactinaemia (Table 6.5) usually act in one of three ways. They may interfere with the production and release of dopamine from the hypothalamus. For example, reserpine and methyldopa deplete catecholamine stores in the hypothalamus, reducing the amount of dopamine available for release. Drugs may also cause hyperprolactinaemia by blocking dopamine receptors. The major tranquillisers, including the phenothiazines and the butyrophenones, are thought to cause hyperprolactinaemia and galactorrhoea in this way (Yeung, 1993; Dickson and Glazer, 1999). The atypical antipsychotics used in schizophrenia clozapine, olanzapine and quetiapine have a prolactin-sparing effect and are less likely to cause this problem. Hyperprolactinaemia may also be caused by drugs that interfere with serotonin reuptake or the sensitivity of postsynaptic serotonin receptors. Tricyclic antidepressants and selective serotonin reuptake inhibitors probably cause hyperprolactinaemia in this way.

Cimetidine and ranitidine may also cause hyperprolactinaemia and therefore it is likely that histamine also affects prolactin secretion. Other drugs reported to cause hyperprolactinaemia and galactorrhoea include oestrogens, morphine, methadone, benzodiazepines and verapamil.

Table 6.5 Some drugs that may cause hyperprolactinaemia

Analgesics, e.g. methadone, morphine
Antidepressants, e.g. amitriptyline, imipramine, fluoxetine
Antihypertensives, e.g. reserpine, methyldopa, verapamil
Antipsychotics, e.g. haloperidol, chlorpromazine
Antiulcer drugs, e.g. cimetidine, ranitidine
Benzodiazepines
Oestrogens

However, the exact mechanism for these adverse effects is unclear (Yeung *et al.*, 1998). Drug-induced hyperprolactinaemia and galactor-rhoea usually resolve within weeks of stopping the offending drug.

Syndrome of inappropriate secretion of antidiuretic hormone

Antidiuretic hormone (ADH, vasopressin) is released from the posterior pituitary, primarily in response to changes in osmotic pressure. When the plasma osmolality increases, e.g. during dehydration, ADH is released. ADH then acts on vasopressin-$_2$ receptors in the collecting duct of the renal tubule, resulting in an increase in the reabsorption of water and the formation of more concentrated urine. Syndrome of inappropriate secretion of antidiuretic hormone (SIADH) occurs when ADH is released from the pituitary under inappropriate circumstances, i.e. when the plasma osmolality is normal or low. This causes the extracellular fluid to become more dilute and to increase in volume.

Many of the symptoms of SIADH are secondary to hyponatraemia (serum sodium <125 mmol/l). Early symptoms include weakness, lethargy and weight gain. Headache, anorexia, nausea and vomiting may also be present. If the condition remains untreated, worsening hyponatraemia may result in confusion, convulsions, coma and death.

The three main causes of SIADH (Yamreudeewong *et al.*, 1991) are:

1   Release of ADH from sites other than the pituitary, e.g. malignancies such as oat cell lung carcinoma
2   Abnormal secretion of ADH due to central nervous system disorders such as a cerebrovascular accident
3   Drugs which may cause SIADH by enhancing the release of ADH or by increasing the responsiveness of the kidney to ADH release

Psychotropics

SIADH has been associated with various centrally acting, antipsychotic drugs, including phenothiazines, and with tricyclic antidepressants, selective serotonin reuptake inhibitors and venlafaxine (Spigset and Hedenmalm, 1995; Masood *et al.*, 1998). Diagnosis is complicated by the observation that patients with untreated psychiatric disease may drink large quantities of water but polydipsia alone does not usually result in clinical hyponatraemia (Spigset and Hedenmalm, 1995). The mechanism is thought to involve increased secretion or potentiation of the effects of ADH vasopressin. Hyponatraemia secondary to these drugs usually occurs soon after the drug is started, although in some cases symptoms may occur after several years.

Carbamazepine

SIADH secondary to carbamazepine is well known and the incidence may be as high as 22% in patients with epilepsy or trigeminal neuralgia (Spigset and Hedenmalm, 1995). Carbamazepine enhances release of ADH from the pituitary.

Cytotoxic agents

Cyclophosphamide, cisplatin, high-dose melphalan, vincristine, vinblastine and vinorelbine have all been reported to cause SIADH (Yamreudeewong *et al.*, 1991; Garrett and Simpson, 1998). The mechanism is unclear. With vincristine it has been suggested that the neurotoxic effect causes the osmoreceptors which control ADH to respond inappropriately (Yamreudeewong *et al.*, 1991).

Hypoglycaemic agents

Chlorpropamide and tolbutamide may cause hyponatraemia secondary to SIADH. The effect is more common with high doses but symptoms have been observed at doses as low as 125 mg chlorpropamide and 500 mg tolbutamide (Krans, 1980). The incidence of SIADH appears to be higher with chlorpropamide than with tolbutamide.

Chlorpropamide probably enhances the release of ADH from the pituitary and increases the sensitivity of the cyclic adenosine monophosphate–adenylate cyclase system in the ADH-sensitive cells of the kidney.

Treatment of SIADH

The mainstay of treatment of drug-induced SIADH is to remove the cause. It is also essential to restrict fluid intake to 500–1000 ml/day. This will result in a gradual increase in plasma sodium concentration and osmolality and an improvement in symptoms. In patients with severe, life-threatening symptoms, it may be necessary to administer hypertonic sodium chloride solution at a rate which increases the serum sodium by 1–2 mmol/l per hour, in addition to restricting fluid intake, until the serum sodium concentration exceeds 125 mmol/l. Some authors have recommended administration of a 3% sodium chloride solution for this purpose. Over-rapid correction of hyponatraemia, particularly in patients with hyponatraemia of more than 2 days' duration, can result in osmotic demyelinisation syndrome (bulbar palsy, paralysis of all limbs, coma and death) and therefore hypertonic sodium chloride solution should only be administered to patients with life-threatening symptoms. Osmotic demyelinisation syndrome does not usually occur in patients with acute-onset, severe hyponatraemia if the rate of correction of hyponatraemia does not exceed 24 mmol/l over 48 hours (Schulltz and Chitwood-Dagner, 1997).

In chronic SIADH, where other methods have proved ineffective, demeclocycline 900–1200 mg daily has been used successfully. Demeclocycline inhibits the renal effects of ADH. An initial response is usually observed within 1–2 weeks, after which the dose should be gradually reduced to the lowest possible at which the serum sodium concentration remains normal (Kinzie, 1987). It has been suggested that patients being initiated on drugs known to cause SIADH, particularly antipsychotics and carbamazepine, should have their serum sodium concentration measured before treatment is started and again after 1–4 weeks (Spigset and Hedenmalm, 1995).

 CASE STUDY

Mrs W is a middle-aged woman who seeks your advice about an embarrassing problem concerning her husband. He has recently been complaining of tenderness and swelling of the breasts but he refuses to seek medical advice. Since his recent retirement he has put on a lot of weight and is drinking more alcohol than usual. Mr W has been taking nifedipine for several years for hypertension and he has been taking cimetidine for the last couple of months for reflux oesphagitis.

What do Mr W's symptoms suggest and what are the possible causes?
This description is suggestive of gynaecomastia. Patients classically present with enlargement of the breast tissue and tenderness is often present. There are several possible causes:

1 Gynaecomastia may be a normal physical finding in older men due to decreased androgen activity.

→

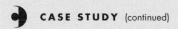 **CASE STUDY** (continued)

2 Liver disease due to alcohol excess may result in gynaecomastia. This is probably due to a reduction in hepatic clearance of androgens. Excess androgens are then converted to oestrogens which cause gynaecomastia. Prolonged alcohol abuse may also lead to testicular atrophy, resulting in low levels of endogenous testosterone.

3 Drugs: both nifedipine and cimetidine have been reported to cause gynaecomastia. The mechanism for calcium channel blocker-induced gynaecomastia is not clear. Cimetidine may cause gynaecomastia by blocking androgen receptors or by increasing the serum prolactin concentration.

Three per cent of cases of gynaecomastia are secondary to tumours, e.g. adrenal or testicular. Breast cancer may also occur rarely in men. Other possible causes such as hyperthyroidism, Cushing's syndrome and liver cirrhosis need to be ruled out.

What advice do you give Mrs W?
Mrs W should be reassured that most cases of breast enlargement in men are benign and do not suggest any serious underlying disease. However, she should encourage her husband to see his GP about the problem. Drug therapy is a possible contributory factor and, if so, it is likely that the problem will resolve when treatment is stopped. It is important to stress that medication should not be stopped without medical advice.

References

Anon. (1999). Drugs in the peri-operative period: 2. Corticosteroids and therapy for diabetes mellitus. *Drug Ther Bull* 37: 68-70.

Bartalena L, Brogioni S, Grasso L *et al.* (1996). Treatment of amiodarone-induced thyrotoxicosis, a difficult challenge: results of a prospective study. *J Clin Endocrinol Metab* 81: 2930–2933.

Becerra-Fernadez A (1995). Autoimmune thyrotoxicosis during lithium therapy in a patient with manic depressive illness. *Am J Med* 99: 575.

Best T R, Jenkins J K, Murphy F Y *et al.* (1987). Persistent adrenal insufficiency secondary to low dose ketoconazole therapy. *Am J Med* 82: 676–680.

British Thoracic Society, British Paediatric Association, Royal College of Physicians of London, The King's Fund Centre, National Asthma Campaign *et al.* (1997). Guidelines on the management of asthma. *Thorax* 52 (suppl 1): S1–S21.

Choi E, Pai H (1998). Gynecomastia associated with indinavir therapy. *Clin Infect Dis* 27: 1539.

Chow C C, Cockram C S (1990). Thyroid disorders induced by lithium and amiodarone: an overview. *Adverse Drug React Acute Poisoning Rev* 9: 207–222.

Clive D M, Stoff J S (1984). Renal syndromes associated with nonsteroidal anti-inflammatory drugs. *N Engl J Med* 310: 563–572.

Committee on Safety of Medicines (1998). Focus on corticosteroids. Withdrawal of systemic corticosteroids. *Curr Probl Pharmacovigilance* 24: 5–9.

Committee on Safety of Medicines (1999). Suppression of aldosterone secretion by heparin. *Curr Probl Pharmacovigilance* 25: 6.

Davies P H, Franklyn J A (1991). The effects of drugs on tests of thyroid function. *Eur J Clin Pharmacol* 40: 439–451.

Dickson R A, Glazer W M (1999). Neuroleptic-induced hyperprolactinaemia. *Schizophr Res* 35: S75–S86.

Drury P L (1994). Endocrinology. In: Kumar P, Clark M, eds. *Clinical Medicine*, 3rd edn. London: Baillière Tindall, chapter 16.

Dukes M N G (1996). Corticotrophins and corticosteroids. In: Dukes M N G, ed. *Meyler's Side Effects of Drugs*, 13th edn. Amsterdam: Elsevier, chapter 39.

Edes T E, Sunderrajan E V (1985). Heparin-induced hyperkalaemia. *Arch Intern Med* 145: 1070–1072.

Garrett C A, Simpson T A (1998). Syndrome of inappropriate antidiuretic hormone associated with vinorelbine therapy. *Ann Pharmacother* 32: 1306–1309.

Gittoes N J, Franklyn J A (1995). Drug-induced thyroid disorders. *Drug Safety* 13: 40–55.

Harjai K J, Licata A A (1997). Effects of amiodarone on thyroid function. *Ann Intern Med* 126: 63–73.

Khanderia U (1991). Use of ketoconazole in the treatment of Cushing's syndrome. *Clin Pharm* 10: 12–13.

Khosla S, Wolfson J S, Demerjian Z *et al.* (1989). Adrenal crisis in the setting of high-dose ketoconazole therapy. *Arch Intern Med* 149: 802–804.

Kinzie B J (1987). Management of the syndrome of inappropriate secretion of antidiuretic hormone. *Clin Pharm* 6: 625–633.

Kountz D S, Clark C L (1997). Safely withdrawing patients from chronic glucocorticoid therapy. *Am Fam Phys* 55: 521–525.

Krans H M J (1980). Insulin, glucagon and hypoglycaemic drugs. In: Dukes M N G, ed. *Side Effects of Drugs Annual 4*. Amsterdam: Excerpta Medica, 298–310.

Leuenberger P, Sonntag R (1996). Drugs used in tuberculosis and leprosy. In: Dukes M N G, ed. *Meyler's Side Effects of Drugs*, 13th edn. Amsterdam: Elsevier, chapter 30.

Lucas L M, Kumar K L, Smith D L (1987). Gynecomastia. A worrisome problem for the patient. *Postgrad Med* 82: 73–81.

Martin F I R, Tress B W, Colman P G (1993). Iodine-induced hyperthyroidism due to non-ionic contrast radiography in the elderly. *Am J Med* 95: 78.

Masood G R, Karki S D, Patterson W R (1998). Hyponatremia with venlafaxine. *Ann Pharmacother* 32: 49.

Melbourne K M, Brown S L, Silverblatt F J (1998). Gynaecomastia with stavudine treatment in an HIV-positive patient. *Ann Pharmacother* 32: 1108.

Newman C M, Price A, Davies D W *et al.* (1998). Amiodarone and the thyroid: a practical guide to the management of thyroid dysfunction induced by amiodarone. *Heart* 79: 121–127.

Oster J R, Singer I, Fishman L M (1995). Heparin-induced aldosterone suppression and hyperkalaemia. *Am J Med* 98: 575–586.

Page R C (1997). How to wean a patient off corticosteroids. *Prescribers' J* 37: 11–16.

Quin J D, Thomson J A (1994). Adverse effects of drugs on the thyroid gland. *Adverse Drug React Toxicol Rev* 13: 43–50.

Robinson D S, Geddes D M (1996). Inhaled corticosteroids: benefits and risks. *J Asthma* 33: 5–16.

Roti E, Minelli R, Giuberti T *et al.* (1996). Multiple changes in thyroid function in patients with chronic active HCV hepatitis treated with recombinant interferon-alpha. *Am J Med* 172: 482–487.

Schulltz N J, Chitwood-Dagner K K (1997). Body electrolyte homeostasis. In: Dipiro J T, Talbert R L, Yee G C *et al.*, eds. *Pharmacotherapy: A Pathophysiologic Approach*, 3rd edn. Stamford, Connecticut: Appleton and Lange, chapter 51.

Spigset O, Hedenmalm K (1995). Hyponatraemia and the syndrome of inappropriate antidiuretic hormone secretion (SIADH) induced by psychotropic drugs. *Drug Safety* 12: 209–225.

Surks M I, Sievert R (1995). Drugs and thyroid function. *N Engl J Med* 333: 1688–1694.

Tan S Y, Shapiro R, Franco R *et al.* (1979). Indomethacin-induced prostaglandin inhibition with hyperkalaemia. *Ann Intern Med* 90: 783–785.

Tester-Dalderup C B M (1996). Antifungal drugs. In: Dukes M N G, ed. *Meyler's Side-effects of Drugs*, 13th edn. Amsterdam: Elsevier, chapter 28.

Thomson D F, Reading Carter J (1993). Drug-induced gynecomastia. *Pharmacotherapy* 13: 37–45.

Turner H E (1997). Gynaecomastia. *Medicine* 25: 41–43.

Yamreudeewong W, Henann N E, Rangaraj U (1991). Drug-induced syndrome of inappropriate secretion of antidiuretic hormone. *J Pharm Technol* 7: 50–54.

Yeung V T F (1993). Drug-induced gynaecomastia and galactorrhoea. *Adverse Drug React Bull* 162: 611–614.

Yeung V T F, Chan W B, Cockram C S (1998). Endocrine disorders. In: Davies D M, Ferner R E, de Glanville H, eds. *Textbook of Adverse Drug Reactions*, 5th edn. London: Chapman and Hall Medical, 381–409.

7

Respiratory disorders

Karen Belton and Anne Lee

Adverse drug reactions affecting the respiratory system are uncommon but are often serious and sometimes fatal. This chapter reviews the types of respiratory reaction that can occur and the drugs most commonly implicated.

In a study of adverse drug reactions leading to hospitalisation, 3% of all reactions and 12% of those considered life-threatening involved the respiratory tract (Levy *et al.*, 1980). Because these reactions are potentially serious it is important that they are recognised early, although this is not easy as many mimic naturally occurring respiratory disease. Often the symptoms are non-specific, such as cough, wheeze or dyspnoea. Changes in pulmonary function, as measured by spirometry or lung function tests, and the radiological abnormalities seen on chest X-ray are usually non-specific. A high degree of vigilance is needed to detect adverse reactions involving the respiratory tract. A wide variety of drugs can be responsible and the underlying mechanisms are varied and often complex.

Nasal congestion

A number of drugs has been associated with nasal congestion (Table 7.1; Simon, 1995). These drugs can, by various mechanisms, cause dilation of the nasal vasculature which leads to tissue oedema and nasal congestion. Aspirin and non-steroidal anti-inflammatory drugs (NSAIDs) can also cause nasal congestion and rhinorrhoea in sensitive individuals. However, the commonest drug cause is the prolonged use of topical nasal decongestants containing vasoconstrictors such as ephedrine, xylometazoline and oxymetazoline (Diamond, 1998; Graf, 1999). These topical preparations cause vasoconstriction and decrease mucosal swelling by stimulating alpha-adrenergic receptors. With prolonged or repeated use of these decongestants, patients become tolerant; that is, more frequent applications and a greater dose are needed and this often results in rebound swelling and congestion. This rebound congestion (rhinitis medicamentosa) leads the patient to further use of the vasoconstrictor to gain relief and so a cycle of use and rebound congestion is set up. Several studies have shown that oxymetazoline and xylometazoline can cause rhinitis medicamentosa after just a few weeks of continued use.

Table 7.1 Some drugs associated with nasal congestion

Some antihypertensive agents
  e.g. methyldopa, prazosin, hydralazine, propranolol
Antidepressant/antipsychotic agents
  e.g. amitriptyline, thioridazine
Hormonal preparations
  e.g. oral contraceptives

The mechanisms responsible for rebound congestion are unclear. Theories proposed include desensitisation (down-regulation) of alpha-adrenoceptors and damage to the nasal mucosa. In addition, it has been shown that benzalkonium chloride, a preservative commonly added to decongestant solutions, can increase the severity of rhinitis medicamentosa (Graf, 1999). The use of topical vasoconstrictors to treat nasal congestion should be limited to a short course of no more than 7 days' duration to minimise the risk of this problem.

Neonates are particularly at risk from the excessive use of decongestant nose drops because they are obligate nasal breathers and do not develop oral breathing until aged between 2 and 6 months. Nasal obstruction can therefore cause severe respiratory distress. Topical nasal decongestants should preferably be avoided in babies less than 3 months old.

Airway obstruction

Bronchoconstriction, presenting as coughing, wheezing or worsening asthma, is the most common drug-induced respiratory problem. It can be caused by many drugs and may be part of a more generalised reaction, e.g. anaphylaxis. Patients affected nearly always have pre-existing bronchial hyperreactivity (i.e. asthma or chronic obstructive airways disease). These reactions can be caused by several mechanisms that ultimately result in the contraction of bronchial smooth muscle. Table 7.2 shows some of the proposed mechanisms and drugs commonly associated with each (Keaney, 1999).

Table 7.2 Proposed mechanisms of drug-induced airway obstruction and drugs commonly associated with them

Mechanism	Drugs
Drug acts as antigen	Pencillins, cephalosporins
Direct release of mediators	Iodine-containing contrast media, intravenous anaesthetics, muscle relaxants
Drug alters synthesis of mediators	Aspirin, non-steroidal anti-inflammatory drugs
Drug inhibits breakdown of mediators	Anticholinesterases, angiotensin-converting enzyme inhibitors
Antagonism of beta-adrenoceptor	Beta-blockers
Non-specific irritation	Some pharmaceutical excipients

Antibiotics

Penicillins are the most common cause of allergic drug reactions and anaphylaxis. The reaction is frequently accompanied by bronchospasm, pruritus, urticaria and angioedema (Anon, 1996; deShazo and Kemp, 1997). The true incidence of these reactions is difficult to determine, but it has been estimated that bronchospasm and acute severe dyspnoea will occur once in every 1000 to 10 000 treatment courses (Neftel *et al.*, 1996). There is almost always a history of a previous course of penicillin treatment with no sign of a reaction (Szczeklik and Nizankowska, 1989).

Patients sensitive to one penicillin should be considered sensitive to all penicillins. This reaction is most common in individuals with pre-existing asthma or other allergic conditions. A proportion of penicillin-sensitive patients will also be allergic to other beta-lactam antibiotics such as cephalosporins, carbapenems and monobactams. Estimates of cross-reactivity between penicillins and cephalosporins range from 10% for first-generation cephalosporins to 1–3% for third-generation cephalosporins (Kishiyama and Adelman, 1994; deShazo and Kemp, 1997).

Aspirin and NSAIDs

Aspirin and NSAIDs are another common cause of bronchoconstriction. Aspirin-induced asthma was first recognised in 1902, shortly after the drug's introduction (Kelly, 1997). Cross-sensitivity between aspirin and NSAIDs of diverse structure argues against an immunological basis for the reaction (deShazo and Kemp, 1997). Hypersensitivity is characterised by acute bronchospasm which is often accompanied by conjunctival irritation, rhinorrhoea, urticaria and flushing of the face and neck. A sensitive individual will exhibit any one, or a combination, of these symptoms typically within 30 minutes to 3 hours after ingestion of aspirin or NSAIDs. The reaction is severe and often life-threatening.

Aspirin sensitivity affects about 10% of all asthmatic patients (Settipane, 1983; Power, 1993; Szczeklik and Stevenson, 1999). The suggested mechanism relates to the inhibition of cyclooxygenase leading to an imbalance between prostaglandins and leukotrienes in the respiratory tract of sensitive individuals (Szczeklik, 1990; deShazo and Kemp, 1997). Patients with existing asthma, sinusitis, allergic rhinitis, nasal polyps or chronic urticaria have a greater frequency of hypersensitivity and women appear to be more susceptible than men (Oates *et al.*, 1988; Szczeklik and Stevenson, 1999). Desensitisation regimens are often unsuccessful and repeated treatments are needed to maintain any benefits. Pretreatment with leukotriene inhibitors such as zafirlukast and montelukast has been shown to attenuate aspirin-induced nasal and bronchial reactions (Szczeklik and Stevenson, 1999).

All potent inhibitors of cyclooxygenase will provoke respiratory symptoms in aspirin-sensitive asthmatic patients. It is important that patients with a previous history of bronchospasm, rhinorrhoea, rash or angioedema following aspirin or NSAID use be advised to avoid this group of drugs in the future (Ayres *et al.*, 1987; Chan, 1995). Paracetamol is usually a suitable analgesic in these patients, although cross-reactivity has been observed in some aspirin-sensitive patients (Settipane *et al.*, 1995). In this situation an opioid analgesic such as codeine may be recommended instead.

ACE inhibitors

Angiotensin-converting enzyme (ACE) inhibitors are associated with cough in 5–20% of all treated patients (Israili and Dallashall, 1992). The mechanism is not proven but is thought to involve the accumulation of prostaglandins, kinins (e.g. bradykinin) or substance P (the neurotransmitter present in respiratory C fibres) as a direct result of ACE inhibition (Overlack, 1996).

The cough is typically dry, persistent and non-productive. It can begin within a week of starting therapy, but in many patients the onset is delayed for up to a year. The cough usually disappears within several days of withdrawal of the ACE inhibitor, but can take as long as 4 weeks to subside. Pulmonary function does not seem to be affected. Cough usually recurs on rechallenge with the same or another ACE inhibitor. The cough can be debilitating, leading to sleep disturbances, vomiting, sore throat and voice changes. It does not respond to treatment with antitussives. Sodium cromoglicate, nifedipine and hydrochlorothiazide have been shown to ameliorate the cough in some studies (Overlack, 1996). Women may be affected more commonly than men. Asthma does not appear to be a predisposing factor. ACE inhibitors should generally be stopped in patients who experience a troublesome cough. The newer angiotensin II receptor antagonists, such as losartan and valsartan, do not seem to cause cough and may be suitable alternatives.

Beta-blockers

Beta-blockers can precipitate bronchoconstriction in patients with asthma or chronic obstructive airways disease and can interfere with the efficacy of adrenergic bronchodilators in such patients. This reaction is due to antagonism of the beta$_2$ adrenoceptors in the bronchi. Although beta$_1$ selective drugs, such as bisoprolol and atenolol, are theoretically safer, there are occasions when they have caused serious reductions in ventilatory function (Committee on Safety of Medicines, 1990). Bronchospasm has even been precipitated by the administration of timolol eye-drops for glaucoma in asthmatic patients. Beta-blockers should always be avoided in patients with a history of asthma or chronic obstructive airways disease, unless no alternative is available.

General anaesthesia

Allergic reactions occurring during anaesthesia are an important problem; the incidence is thought to be around 1 in 5000 anaesthetic episodes (Withington, 1994). In the UK it has been estimated that about 100 deaths during anaesthesia each year may be due to hypersensitivity reactions (McKinnon and Wildsmith, 1995). These reactions are more common in women and individuals with a history of atopy, asthma or previous complications during anaesthesia (Association of Anaesthetists of Great Britain and Ireland, 1995).

Bronchospasm occurs in up to 50% of affected patients. It may be either transient or severe, and in 3% may be the only presenting feature. Muscle relaxants are thought to account for about 70% of these reactions. Both depolarising agents, such as suxamethonium, and non-depolarising agents, such as atracurium, have been implicated, although suxamethonium is the most frequent cause (McKinnon and Wildsmith, 1995). The mechanism may involve release of mediators such as histamine or the development of specific antibodies.

Patients who may have experienced an allergic reaction during anaesthesia should be fully investigated to elucidate the cause. Skin prick testing may be useful. Where the reaction was caused by a muscle relaxant, cross-reactivity between drugs occurs in about 50% of patients. In the UK the Association of Anaesthetists of Great Britain and Ireland produces a useful booklet giving guidance on these reactions (Association of Anaesthetists of Great Britain and Ireland, 1995).

Other drugs

Radiocontrast media are a well-recognised cause of acute bronchospasm, usually as part of a generalised anaphylactic reaction. The reported adverse reaction rate to ionic contrast media is about 5% and to non-ionic contrast media about 1% (Board of the Faculty of Clinical Radiology, 1996). Most reactions are mild, although some are life-threatening; the incidence is thought to be greater in asthmatic patients (Hill, 1986). In the UK the Royal College of Radiologists has issued advice on the management of reactions to intravenous contrast media (Board of the Faculty of Clinical Radiology, 1996).

Some pharmaceutical excipients can cause hypersensitivity reactions featuring bronchospasm in susceptible individuals. Tartrazine was first identified as a cause of asthma in 1967. However, in double-blind placebo-controlled trials using pulmonary function testing, sensitivity to tartrazine was rare (Golightly *et al.*, 1988).

A small proportion of patients who develop hypersensitivity reactions with aspirin may show cross-sensitivity to tartrazine. Other excipients which have been implicated in these reactions include benzoates, phenylmercuric salts, parabens, benzalkonium chloride and metabisulphite. These reactions seem to occur almost exclusively in patients with pre-existing asthma (Golightly *et al.*, 1988; Uchegbu and Florence, 1996).

Parasympathomimetic drugs such as pilocarpine and carbachol, although now seldom used, have a direct effect on the vagal tone of the smooth muscles of the respiratory tract so can provoke bronchoconstriction. They should be used with caution in asthmatic patients (Keaney, 1998).

Respiratory disorders occur in 20% of patients who experience hypersensitivity reactions to the nucleoside reverse transcriptase inhibitor abacavir (Anon, 2000a). Hypersensitivity reactions affect about 3% of patients treated; they usually appear in the first 6 weeks of treatment but may occur at any time. Possible respiratory symptoms include dyspnoea, cough and pharyngitis. Signs of pneumonia or bronchitis have been observed in a high proportion of fatalities. Patients who experience a hypersensitivity reaction must never take the drug again due to the risk of a more severe, life-threatening reaction.

Exacerbation of asthma was recently reported in two patients taking interferon alfa for chronic hepatitis C infection (Bini and Weinshel, 1999). The severe asthmatic symptoms resolved promptly after the drug was discontinued and corticosteroid therapy initiated.

The findings of a recent UK case-control study suggested that frequent (daily or weekly) paracetamol use was associated with asthma (Shaheen, 2000), but whether or not there is a causal link remains uncertain.

Reflex bronchoconstriction

Paradoxical bronchoconstriction has been reported with a number of inhaled medicines, including beta-agonists, corticosteroids, ipratropium and cromoglicate. It is thought to result from non-specific irritation of the bronchial mucosa. The problem has occurred with both nebuliser solutions and metered-dose inhalers (Nicklas, 1990).

In the UK the Committee on Safety of Medicines warned about the risk of worsening airways disease in association with nebulised bronchodilator solutions in 1988 (Committee on Safety of Medicines, 1988). Formulation factors such as hypotonicity of the solution or the presence of preservatives, such as benzalkonium chloride, were implicated. Since most nebuliser solutions are now isotonic and preservative-free, this problem is much less common.

The hydrofluorocarbon propellants in metered-dose inhalers are frequently implicated in bronchoconstriction, although in some cases the drug itself may be responsible (Finnerty and Howarth, 1993). Bronchoconstriction has been described with delivery of the long-acting bronchodilator salmeterol by metered-dose inhaler but not after dry powder Diskhaler (Wilkinson *et al.*, 1992). It has been suggested that salmeterol's relatively slow onset of action may expose such bronchoconstriction, whereas agents with a faster onset of action may attenuate any bronchoconstriction that occurs. Bronchospasm has recently been reported after inhalation of zanamivir, the antiviral drug effective against influenza A or B infection (Anon, 2000b). The problem is more likely in patients with asthma or chronic bronchitis. If such patients are prescribed zanamivir they should be advised to keep a fast-acting bronchodilator to hand.

Lung parenchyma

Adverse drug reactions affecting the lung parenchyma can be classified into acute and chronic reactions, reflecting hypersensitivity and fibrosis respectively as the predominant mechanisms of toxic response. Hypersensitivity pneumonitis (sometimes termed alveolitis) and fibrotic pulmonary disease can be regarded as part of a spectrum of closely related disease states (Camus, 1989; Keaney, 1998). The aetiology and pathogenesis of these conditions, however, are poorly understood. Tables 7.3 and 7.4 show some of the drugs most frequently associated with hypersensitivity pneumonitis and pulmonary fibrosis (Hill, 1986; Banerjee and Honeybourne, 1996).

Table 7.3 Drugs typically associated with interstitial pneumonitis

Amiodarone	Paclitaxel
Gold	Penicillamine
Methotrexate	Sulfasalazine
Nitrofurantoin	

Table 7.4 Some drugs associated with pulmonary fibrosis

Amiodarone	Methysergide
Bleomycin	Mitomycin
Busulfan	Mycophenolate mofetil
Carmustine	Nitrofurantoin
Cyclophosphamide	Sulfasalazine
Gold	

Hypersensitivity pneumonitis

In general, these acute reactions are of an allergic nature, have a dramatic clinical presentation and require urgent diagnosis and withdrawal of the offending agent. With early treatment there is a high chance of a complete recovery. An adverse drug reaction may not be suspected with symptoms such as cough, breathlessness and wheeze, but the findings of other diagnostic techniques, such as bronchoscopic bronchoalveolar lavage, may help detect an iatrogenic cause. This technique involves the aspiration of buffered saline instilled into the bronchi via a broncho-scope. With this procedure it has proved possible to identify an increase in the cellular yield (pleocytosis) in hypersensitivity pneumonitis and eosinophilia and/or lymphocytosis in the fluid obtained. Pleural biopsy may be a useful investigation in some situations.

Hypersensitivity-type pneumonitis typically occurs acutely, between a few hours and a few weeks of starting therapy with the suspect drug (Wilkinson *et al.*, 1995). The main symptoms are cough, breathlessness and wheeze, sometimes accompanied by bronchospasm. A chest X-ray will normally reveal pulmonary infiltrates. If eosinophilia on a blood count is a feature of the clinical picture, allergy is certain and the patient's recent drug therapy should be reviewed (Keaney, 1999). Further diagnostic tests, in particular with bronchoscopic bronchoalve-olar lavage, may confirm the suspicion. Withdrawal of the suspect drug usually results in complete recovery. A course of corticosteroids can assist rapid symptom resolution (Keaney, 1999).

Nitrofurantoin

Nitrofurantoin is an important cause of respiratory reactions, causing both acute pneumonitis and, less commonly, chronic pulmonary fibrosis (D'Arcy, 1985). The frequency of acute severe pulmonary disease has been estimated at 1 in every 5000 first administrations (Malinverni *et al.*, 1996). These reactions seem to be more common in Scandinavia and South Africa than the UK, for unknown reasons. Women between 40 and 50 years of age are mainly affected. The mechanism of this reaction is thought to involve the production of free oxygen radicals that may damage the lung, although an immune mechanism may also be involved (Schattner *et al.*, 1999).

The acute reaction tends to occur within a month of starting treatment and is usually accompanied by eosinophilia (Holmbeag *et al.*, 1980). Symptoms include severe dyspnoea, tachypnoea, non-pro-ductive cough and fever. Recovery is usually rapid and complete after the drug is stopped. An allergic mechanism for the reaction has been postulated.

Chronic respiratory reactions with nitrofurantoin have a much slower onset and usually occur during long-term prophylactic therapy of 6 months or more. Recovery on drug withdrawal is usually good but not always complete; mortality is estimated at less than 1% (White and Ward, 1985).

Gold

Pulmonary reactions to gold therapy are thought to have an immunological basis rather than being a direct toxic effect (Tomioka and King, 1997; Brion *et al.*, 1989). The incidence is estimated at around 1% and the time to onset of the reaction is usually 5–16 weeks (White and Ward, 1985). The rate of complete recovery on withdrawal of treatment is about 50%, mortality is estimated at about 7% and the remaining patients will have some residual radiological and/or physiological effects (Tomioka and King, 1997).

Pulmonary fibrosis

Direct toxicity of the suspect drug causes cell damage which elicits an inflammatory fibrotic response, resulting in the distortion and subsequent destruction of the alveoli. This type of fibrotic reaction is frequently related to the length of time the patient has been taking the drug and/or the total cumulative dose received. The symptoms include malaise, a dry cough and increasing breathlessness, which progresses gradually over a period of weeks or months. Pulmonary function tests show reduced gas transfer and X-ray examination usually shows diffuse infiltrates. The withdrawal of the suspect drug, with or without corticosteroid treatment, does not always result in a complete resolution of the symptoms or cessation of the disease process. These reactions are associated with significant morbidity and mortality (White and Ward, 1985).

Bleomycin

Pulmonary fibrosis, with significant mortality, is a well-recognised complication of bleomycin therapy. The reported incidence of pulmonary toxicity with this drug ranges from 11 to 23% (Folb, 1996). Predisposing factors include impaired renal function, age over 70 years, concurrent radiotherapy and administration of high concentrations of oxygen (Cooper and Matthay, 1989). The high ambient oxygen tension in the lung facilitates the generation of superoxide radicals by bleomycin.

The risk of pulmonary toxicity rises with the total dose of bleomycin administered. At cumulative doses below 450 units (=450 000 units Ph Eur) about 3–5% of patients are affected. At doses above 450 units the rate of toxicity is about 13% and at doses above 550 units it is estimated at 17% (Cooper *et al.*, 1986). However, rapidly fatal pulmonary toxicity has occurred with doses as low as 100 units (Cooper *et al.*, 1986). Bleomycin is also associated with a hypersensitivity pneumonitis.

Busulfan

Busulfan is another cytotoxic drug commonly associated with pneumonitis and fibrosis; the incidence is estimated at about 1% (Cooper and Matthay, 1989). Features are similar to those seen with bleomycin, but a critical dose level or specific predisposing factors have not been demonstrated. In contrast to bleomycin, drug withdrawal rarely causes resolution; further progression of the fibrosis, resulting in death, is common (Rosenow *et al.*, 1992).

Amiodarone

Amiodarone is associated with both pneumonitis and pulmonary fibrosis. The incidence of pulmonary toxicity is reported to be about 5–10% (Dusman, 1990; Jessurun *et al.*, 1998). Affected patients usually present with insidious evolving, non-specific symptoms such as cough, dyspnoea, weight loss and chest pain. Non-specific complaints due to pulmonary toxicity may be masked by symptoms of cardiac failure, delaying recognition of the reaction. Several factors increase susceptibility to amiodarone lung damage, including dose, duration of therapy, advanced age and pre-existing pulmonary dysfunction (Banerjee and Honeybourne, 1996; Jessurun *et al.*, 1998). The cause of damage is probably multifactorial, involving direct damage, immune mechanisms and phospholipid accumulation in lung tissue. In most cases the reaction is reversible, if diagnosed at an early stage.

Clinical evidence suggests that the risk of a patient experiencing adverse effects with amiodarone increases as dose and duration of therapy increase. Most amiodarone-induced pulmonary manifestations are found to occur when the dose exceeds 400 mg daily administered for more than 2 months or when a lower dose is given for more than 2 years (Banerjee and Honeybourne, 1996; Jessurun *et al.*, 1998). However, several case studies and clinical trials of amiodarone have shown the possible occurrence of pulmonary toxicity during low-dose and short-duration therapy, suggesting that dose and duration of treatment are not the only determinants of risk (Jessurun *et al.*, 1998). For example, lung toxicity has been described after short-term amiodarone therapy in patients treated for acute respiratory distress syndrome on the intensive care unit (Donaldson *et al.*, 1998). Overall the mortality associated with pulmonary adverse reactions is estimated at about 10% (Wilson and Podrid, 1991), although may be lower now that clinicians are more aware of the problem (Kanji *et al.*, 1999). Management may consist of a dose reduction and pulmonary monitoring in mild cases of toxicity or complete withdrawal of amiodarone in more severe cases, although the potential for the recurrence of life-threatening arrhythmias on treatment discontinuation must be considered.

Up to 25% of patients with amiodarone-induced pulmonary damage may have bronchiolitis obliterans or bronchiolitis obliterans 'organising pneumonia'. Bronchiolitis obliterans organising pneumonia is characterised by destruction of the small airways by a non-specific inflammation. This type of reaction needs to be differentiated from other pulmonary conditions as it is associated with a more benign course and responds better to corticosteroids than the other infiltrative pulmonary diseases. Prednisolone treatment is recommended for all patients in case some areas of pneumonitis are of this nature and should probably be continued for at least 6 months after amiodarone is withdrawn because of its long half-life.

Healthcare professionals should be aware of the risk of pulmonary toxicity with amiodarone. Patients should be counselled to report the development of symptoms such as cough, dyspnoea and chest pain promptly. A chest X-ray may be advisable before amiodarone therapy is started. During treatment, if pulmonary toxicity is suspected, the chest X-ray should be repeated and lung function tests carried out.

Mycophenolate mofetil

The immunosuppresant drug mycophenolate mofetil has been shown to cause respiratory reactions ranging from cough and dyspnoea to acute respiratory failure and pulmonary fibrosis (Gross et al., 1997; Elli et al., 1998; Morrissey et al., 1998). These reactions have been reported with standard daily doses but are thought to be more likely with a 3 g daily dose and in patients with previous respiratory problems (Elli et al., 1998; Becker, 1999).

Pulmonary oedema

Non-cardiogenic pulmonary oedema or adult respiratory distress syndrome (ARDS) is thought to be due to increased pulmonary vascular permeability, resulting in extravasation of fluid and proteinaceous material into the alveoli (Hill, 1986; Reed and Glauser, 1991). The symptoms include acute breathlessness, cough and frothy sputum. Diffuse bilateral alveolar shadowing can be seen on chest X-ray (Banerjee and Honeybourne, 1996). The reaction seems to occur with therapeutic

Table 7.5 Some drugs associated with pulmonary oedema at therapeutic doses

Amphotericin	Naloxone
Diamorphine	Protamine
Epoprostenol	Ritodrine
Haloperidol	Salbutamol (IV)
Hydrochlorothiazide	Terbutaline (IV)
Indometacin	Vinorelbine
Methadone	

Table 7.6 Some drugs associated with pulmonary oedema in overdose

Aspirin	Dextropropoxyphene
Codeine	Dihydrocodeine
Colchicine	Tricyclic antidepressants

doses of some drugs and as a consequence of overdose with others (Humbert *et al.*, 1998; Keaney, 1998; Brooks, 1999; Cattan and Oberg, 1999; Farber *et al.*, 1999; see Tables 7.5 and 7.6).

Hydrochlorothiazide

Non-cardiogenic pulmonary oedema has been reported rarely with the thiazide diuretic hydrochlorothiazide (Almoosa, 1999; Bernal and Patarca, 1999). More than 30 cases have been described; most affected patients were women and most had been prescribed the drug for hypertension or fluid retention. In most cases, patients experienced an acute onset of dyspnoea, wheeze, cough, chest pain, sweating, nausea and vomiting within 30 minutes to 2 hours of ingestion of hydrochlorothiazide. In some cases the patient experienced recurrent episodes of pulmonary oedema before the link with drug therapy was made. The mechanism of the reaction is unknown, although an immunological basis has been suggested (Bernal and Patarca, 1999). Supportive therapy is the preferred management. In patients who have experienced this problem, furosemide (frusemide) may be given if subsequent diuretic therapy is needed.

Intravenous beta-agonists

The use of intravenous beta-agonists to suppress uterine contractions in premature labour is associated with pulmonary oedema. The incidence is thought to be as high as 4% (Reed and Glauser, 1991). A review of 58 cases associated with ritodrine, salbutamol and terbutaline suggested that most cases occurred during or within 24 hours of drug use (Pisani and Rosenow, 1989). Women improved rapidly when intravenous furosemide (frusemide) and oxygen were given. However, there were two maternal and three fetal deaths. Fluid overload is the single most important predisposing factor; others are multiple pregnancy, pre-existing cardiac disease and maternal infection. In the UK the Committee on Safety of Medicines has issued a reminder about the need for close monitoring of hydration in women receiving tocolytics (Committee on Safety of Medicines, 1995).

Pulmonary thromboembolism

Pulmonary thromboembolism occurs when a thrombus from the systemic veins embolises into the pulmonary arterial system. The clinical features of a large pulmonary embolism include sudden collapse, pleuritic pain, breathlessness, cyanosis and haemoptysis. Smaller emboli may present with increasing breathlessness and pleuritic pain (see Chapter 11).

Conditions leading to the formation of thrombi in the systemic veins can thus predispose to pulmonary embolism. It has been established that women taking the combined oral contraceptive pill have a higher risk of thromboembolic disease than those not taking it. Until recently this was thought to be related to the dose of oestrogen in the individual preparations but the progestogen component is now known to be a factor (see Chapter 11).

CASE STUDY

Mr C is a 70-year-old man with a history of prostate problems, a previous myocardial infarction and ventricular arrhythmias. His regular medication consists of terazosin 5 mg daily, aspirin 75 mg daily, amiodarone 400 mg daily and pravastatin 20 mg daily. Mr C has been troubled by a persistent cough over the past 6 weeks and has been feeling tired and breathless when out walking.

Could these symptoms be related to Mr C's medication?
Amiodarone can cause pulmonary toxicity which commonly presents with dyspnoea and non-productive cough. Aspirin can cause bronchospasm as part of a hypersensitivity syndrome in susceptible individuals, who usually have a history of asthma.

The incidence of lung toxicity with amiodarone is about 5–10% and the associated mortality is about 10%. Amiodarone probably causes lung damage by direct deposition of phospholipids in the lung tissue or by some immunologically mediated reaction.

What further information might help clarify the problem?
It would be helpful to know the dose and duration of amiodarone treatment. Pulmonary toxicity can occur at any time during treatment but the risk is greatest during the first year and in patients aged over 40 years. The problem is more likely with high doses of amiodarone or long-term use. Suspicion should be increased in patients who have taken low doses for several years or doses of 400 mg or more daily for more than 2 months. The risk of toxicity correlates better with the total cumulative dose than with the daily dose and plasma concentrations. The recommended maintenance dose of amiodarone should not exceed 200 mg daily (Jessurun and Crijns, 1997).

Other common presenting symptoms of amiodarone pulmonary toxicity are fever, nausea, fatigue, weight loss and pleuritic chest pain. Mr C should be asked whether he has experienced any of these symptoms in the past few weeks. He should be asked about the nature of the cough, which is typically non-productive, and whether he has any history of respiratory problems.

Mr C has had no fever, nausea or weight loss. The cough is non-productive and is getting worse, keeping him awake at night and causing chest soreness. He has been taking amiodarone 400 mg daily, initially prescribed by the consultant cardiologist, for the past 10 months. He is not due to see his consultant again for another 3 months. He has had no previous respiratory problems and does not smoke.

(continued overleaf)

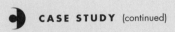

CASE STUDY (continued)

How would a diagnosis of pulmonary toxicity be confirmed in this patient?
Diagnosis of amiodarone pulmonary toxicity can be difficult. Other possible causes of the respiratory symptoms should be excluded, including congestive heart failure, pneumonia, pulmonary embolism or malignancy. Diagnostic tests that might be used to establish and confirm a diagnosis of pulmonary toxicity include chest X-ray, lung function tests and histological examination of lung tissue obtained by biopsy.

Chest X-ray may show interstitial alveolar infiltrates. Pulmonary function tests are characterised by a restrictive ventilatory defect with impaired gas diffusion. Bronchial lavage fluids may show the presence of lymphocytes and 'foamy' macrophages which are believed to contain amiodarone. However, these lipid-laden alveolar macrophages may be found in patients taking amiodarone with no evidence of pulmonary toxicity. The absence of these macrophages counts against the diagnosis. Lung biopsy may reveal phospholipidosis. In addition, the erythrocyte sedimentation rate may be high in more than 50% of cases (Fraire et al., 1993).

How should the problem be managed?
The preferred management of suspected amiodarone pulmonary toxicity is discontinuation of the drug. If this is done, symptoms usually resolve slowly over several months, due to the long half-life of the drug (up to 45 days). However, stopping the drug may put the patient at risk of sudden death from recurrence of arrhythmia. Some patients improve after the dose of amiodarone is reduced. Corticosteroid therapy is usually given.

References

Almoosa K F (1999). Hydrochlorothiazide-induced pulmonary edema. *South Med J* 92: 1100–1102.

Anon. (1996). Penicillin allergy. *Drug Ther Bull* 34: 87–88.

Anon. (2000a). Abacavir: risks limit the value. *Prescrire Int* 9: 67–69.

Anon. (2000b). Bronchospasm with zanamivir. *Prescrire Int* 9: 80.

Association of Anaesthetists of Great Britain and Ireland and British Society of Allergy and Clinical Immunology (1995). *Suspected Anaphylactic Reactions Associated with Anaesthesia*, 2nd edn. London: Association of Anaesthetists of Great Britain and Ireland and British Society of Allergy and Clinical Immunology.

Ayres J G, Fleming D M, Whittington R M (1987). Asthma death due to ibuprofen. *Lancet* i: 1082.

Banerjee D J, Honeybourne D (1996). Drug induced pulmonary alveolar disease. *Adverse Drug React Bull* 181: 687–690.

Becker B N (1999). Mycophenolate mofetil. *Transplant Proc* 31: 2777–2778.

Bernal C, Patarca R (1999). Hydrochlorothiazide-induced pulmonary edema and associated immunologic changes. *Ann Pharmacother* 33: 172–174.

Bini E J, Weinshel E (1999). Severe exacerbation of asthma: a new side effect of interferon-α in patients with asthma and chronic hepatitis C. *Mayo Clin Proc* 74: 367–370.

Board of the Faculty of Clinical Radiology/the Royal College of Radiologists (1996). *Advice on the Management of Reactions to Intravenous Contrast Media.* London: Royal College of Radiologists.

Brion N, Legros V, Adnenifer C *et al.* (1989). Pneumonitis induced by rheumatological drugs. In: Akoun G M, White J P, eds. *Treatment Induced Respiratory Disorders.* Amsterdam: Elsevier, 132–149.

Brooks J C (1999). Noncardiogenic pulmonary oedema immediately following rapid protamine administration. *Ann Pharmacother* 33: 927–930.

Camus P (1989). Pathophysiology of drug induced lung disease. In: Akoun G M, White J P, eds. *Treatment Induced Respiratory Disorders.* Amsterdam: Elsevier, 24–46.

Cattan C E, Oberg K C (1999). Vinorelbine tartrate-induced pulmonary edema confirmed on rechallenge. *Pharmacotherapy* 19: 992–994.

Chan T Y K (1995). Severe asthma attacks precipitated by NSAIDs. *Ann Pharm* 29: 199.

Committee on Safety of Medicines (1988). Nebuliser solutions and paradoxical bronchoconstriction. *Curr Probl* 22: 2.

Committee on Safety of Medicines (1990). Bronchospasm associated with cardio-selective and topical beta-blockers. *Curr Probl* 28: 2–3.

Committee on Safety of Medicines (1995). Reminder: ritodrine and pulmonary oedema. *Curr Probl* 21: 7.

Cooper J A D, Matthay R A (1989). Pneumonitis induced by cytotoxic drugs. In: Akoun G M, White J P, eds. *Treatment Induced Respiratory Disorders.* Amsterdam: Elsevier, 51–73.

Cooper J A D, White D A, Matthay R A (1986). Drug induced pulmonary disease. Part 1: cytotoxic drugs. *Am Rev Respir Dis* 133: 321–340.

D'Arcy P F (1985). Nitrofurantoin. *Drug Intell Clin Pharm* 19: 540–547.

deShazo R D, Kemp S F (1997). Allergic reactions to drugs and biologic agents. *JAMA* 278: 1895–1906.

Diamond C (1998). Ear, nose and throat disorders. In: Davies D M, Ferner R E, de Glanville H, eds. *Textbook of Adverse Drug Reactions*, 5th edn. London: Chapman and Hall Medical, 643–668.

Donaldson L, Grant I S, Naysmith M R *et al.* (1998). Acute amiodarone-induced lung toxicity. *Intens Care Med* 24: 626–630.

Dusman R E (1990). Clinical features of amiodarone-induced pulmonary toxicity. *Circulation* 82: 51–59.

Elli A, Aroldi A, Montagnino G *et al.* (1998). Mycophenolate mofetil and cough. *Transplantation* 66: 409.

Farber H W, Graven K K, Kokolski G *et al.* (1999). Pulmonary edema during acute infusion of epoprostenol in a patient with pulmonary hypertension and limited scleroderma. *J Rheumatol* 26: 1195–1196.

Finnerty J P, Howarth P H (1993). Paradoxical bronchoconstriction with nebulised salbuterol but not with terbutaline. *Am Rev Respir Dis* 148: 512–513.

Folb P I (1996). Cytostatics and immunosuppressive drugs. In: Dukes M N G, ed. *Meyler's Side Effects of Drugs*, 13th edn. Amsterdam: Elsevier, chapter 45.

Fraire A E, Guntupalli K K, Greenberg S D *et al.* (1993). Amiodarone pulmonary toxicity: a multidisciplinary review of current status. *South Med J* 86: 67–77.

Golightly L K, Smolinske S S, Bennett M L *et al.* (1988). Pharmaceutical excipients: adverse effects associated with inactive ingredients in drug products (part I). *Med Toxicol* 3: 128–165.

Graf P (1999). Adverse effects of benzalkonium chloride on the nasal mucosa: allergic rhinitis and rhinitis medicamentosa. *Clin Ther* 21: 1749–1755.

Gross D C, Sasaki T M, Buick M K *et al.* (1997). Acute respiratory failure and pulmonary fibrosis secondary to administration of mycophenolate mofetil. *Transplantation* 64: 1607–1609.

Hill L E (1986). Iatrogenic lung disease. In: D'Arcy P F, Griffin J P, eds. *Iatrogenic Diseases*, 3rd edn. Oxford: University Press.

Holmbeag L, Boman G, Bottiger L E *et al.* (1980). Adverse reactions to nitrofurantoin: analysis of 921 reports. *Am J Med* 69: 733.

Humbert M, Maitre S, Capron F *et al.* (1998). Pulmonary edema complicating continuous intravenous prostacyclin in pulmonary capillary hemangiomatosis. *Am J Respir Crit Care Med* 157: 1681–1685.

Israili Z H, Dallashall W (1992). Cough and angioneurotic edema associated with angiotensin-converting enzyme inhibitor therapy. *Ann Intern Med* 117: 234–242.

Jessurun G A J, Crijns H J G M (1997). Amiodarone pulmonary toxicity. *Br Med J* 314: 619–620.

Jessurun G A J, Boersma W G, Crijns H J G M (1998). Amiodarone-induced pulmonary toxicity. *Drug Safety* 18: 339–344.

Kanji Z, Sunderji R, Gin K (1999). Amiodarone-induced pulmonary toxicity. *Pharmacotherapy* 19: 1463–1466.

Keaney N P (1998). Respiratory disorders. In: Davies D M, Ferner R E, de Glanville H, eds. *Textbook of Adverse Drug Reactions,* 5th edn. London: Chapman and Hall Medical, 202–233.

Keaney N P (1999). Drug induced lung disease. In: Walker R, Edwards C, eds. *Clinical Pharmacy and Therapeutics*, 2nd edn. London: Churchill Livingstone, 202–233.

Kelly H W (1997). Drug-induced pulmonary diseases. In: Dipiro J T, Talbert R L, Yee G C *et al.,* eds. *Pharmacotherapy: A Pathophysiologic Approach*, 3rd edn. Connecticut: Appleton & Lange, chapter 28.

Kishiyama J L, Adelman D C (1994). The cross-reactivity and immunology of β-lactam antibiotics. *Drug Safety* 10: 318–327.

Levy M, Kewitz H, Altwein W *et al.* (1980). Hospital admissions due to adverse drug reactions: a comparative study from Jerusalem and Berlin. *Eur J Clin Pharmacol* 17: 25–31.

Malinverni R, Hoigne R, Sonntag R (1996). Sulfonamides, other folic acid antagonists and miscellaneous antibacterial drugs. In: Dukes M N G, ed. *Meyler's Side Effects of Drugs*, 13th edn. Amsterdam: Elsevier, chapter 29.

McKinnon R P, Wildsmith J A W (1995). Histaminoid reactions in anaesthesia. *Br J Anaesth* 74: 217–228.

Morrissey P, Gohh R, Madras P *et al.* (1998). Pulmonary fibrosis secondary to administration of mycophenolate mofetil. *Transplantation* 65: 1414.

Neftel K A, Zoppi M, Cerny A *et al.* (1996). Reactions typically shared by more than one class of beta-lactam antibiotic. In: Dukes M N G, ed. *Meyler's Side Effects of Drugs*, 13th edn. Amsterdam: Elsevier, 678–692.

Nicklas R A (1990). Paradoxical bronchospasm associated with the use of inhaled beta-agonists. *J Allergy Clin Immunol* 85: 959–964.

Oates J A, Fitzgerald G A, Branch R A *et al.* (1988). Clinical implications of prostaglandin and thromboxane formation. *N Engl J Med* 319: 689.

Overlack A (1996). ACE inhibitor-induced cough and bronchospasm: incidence, mechanisms, and management. *Drug Safety* 15: 72–78.

Pisani R J, Rosenow E C (1989). Pulmonary edema associated with tocolytic therapy. *Ann Intern Med* 110: 714–718.

Power I (1993). Aspirin-induced asthma (editorial). *Br J Anaesth* 71: 619–621.

Reed C R, Glauser F L (1991). Drug-induced non-cardiogenic pulmonary oedema. *Chest* 100: 120–124.

Rosenow E C, Myers J L, Swenson S J *et al.* (1992). Drug-induced pulmonary disease: an update. *Chest* 102: 239–250.

Schattner A, Von Der Walde J, Kozak N *et al.* (1999). Nitrofurantoin-induced immune-mediated lung and liver disease. *Am J Med Sci* 317: 336–340.

Settipane G A (1983). Aspirin and allergic diseases: a review. *Am J Med* 74 (suppl 6a): 102–109.

Settipane R A, Schrank P J, Simon R A *et al.* (1995). Prevalence of cross-sensitivity with acetaminophen in aspirin-sensitive asthmatic subjects. *J Allergy Clin Immunol* 96: 480–485.

Shaheen S O, Sterne J A C, Songhurst C E *et al.* (2000). Frequent paracetamol use and asthma in adults. *Thorax* 55: 266–270.

Simon P A (1995). Acute and chronic rhinitis. In: Young L Y, Koda Kimble M A, eds. *Applied Therapeutics: The Clinical Use of Drugs*, 6th edn. Vancouver: Applied Therapeutics, 21.1–21.22.

Szczeklik A (1990). The cyclo-oxygenase theory of aspirin-induced asthma. *Eur Respir J* 3: 588.

Szczeklik A, Nizankowska E (1989). Drug induced asthma and bronchospasm. In: Akoun G M, White J P, eds. *Treatment Induced Respiratory Disorders*. Amsterdam: Elsevier, 189–209.

Szczeklik A, Stevenson D D (1999). Aspirin-induced asthma: advances in pathogenesis and management. *J Allergy Clin Immunol* 104: 5–13.

Tomioka H, King T E (1997). Gold-induced pulmonary disease: clinical features, outcome, and differentiation from rheumatoid lung disease. *Am J Respir Crit Care Med* 155: 1011–1020.

Uchegbu I F, Florence A T (1996). Adverse drug events related to dosage forms and delivery systems. *Drug Safety* 14: 39–67.

White J P, Ward M J (1985). Drug induced adverse pulmonary reactions. *Adverse Drug React Acute Poisoning Rev* 4: 183–211.

Wilkinson J R W, Roberts J A, Bradding P *et al.* (1992). Paradoxical bronchoconstriction in asthmatic patients after salmeterol by metered dose inhaler. *Br Med J* 305: 931–932.

Wilkinson W, Dang B and Kelly H W. (1995). Drug induced pulmonary disorders. In: Young L Y, Koda Kimble M A, eds. *Applied Therapeutics: The Clinical Use of Drugs*, 6th edn. Vancouver: Applied Therapeutics, 22.1–22.10.

Wilson J S, Podrid P J (1991). Side effects from amiodarone. *Am Heart J* 121: 158–171.

Withington D E (1994). Allergy, anaphylaxis and anaesthesia. *Can J Anaesth* 41: 1133–1139.

8

Musculoskeletal disorders

Philip Young

Some drugs have adverse effects on muscle, bone or connective tissue. The resulting problems include symptoms such as cramps, aches and pains in the limbs, or, less often, osteoporosis, fractures and tendinitis (Shetty *et al.*, 1998). These problems can be disabling but they can also be an early indication of potentially serious drug-induced disorders. For example, myalgia is often a precursor of rhabdomyolysis. Symptoms and signs relating to the musculoskeletal system are very common complaints in general practice, so it is important to remember drug therapy as a possible cause of such problems (Anon, 1971). This chapter reviews the most common drug-induced musculoskeletal disorders.

Muscle disorders

Myalgia (muscle pain) and cramps, usually in the legs and mainly at night, are a very common complaint. They may be an early symptom of drug-induced polyneuropathy, myopathy or extrapyramidal disorders (see Chapter 7; Shetty *et al.*, 1998). Drug-induced retroperitoneal fibrosis may similarly present with aching in the legs and back in the early stages, because of vascular compression. Mild muscle aches and pain can occasionally be caused by fluid retention; this has been described with oral contraceptives. Diuretics, calcium channel blockers and beta-2-agonists can cause muscle cramps. With diuretics, the problem may be related to electrolyte disturbances.

Myalgia is clinically characterised mainly by muscle pain, tenderness and/or muscle weakness. It may be accompanied by an increase in the enzyme creatine phosphokinase (CPK) in serum, which may be an indicator of muscle damage. The main source of CPK is skeletal muscle and the myocardium. Myositis, with or without CPK elevations in the serum, is usually self-limiting and is characterised by muscle weakness. Biopsy usually indicates cell damage with muscle fibre necrosis and inflammatory cell infiltration.

Suxamethonium causes myalgia in up to 50% of patients following surgery. The pain occurs mainly in the neck, shoulders, back and chest, and seems to be more common in women. The frequency and severity of muscle pain may be reduced by giving a small dose of a non-depolarising muscle relaxant just before suxamethonium.

Severe and widespread myalgia and joint pain may occur after corticosteroid withdrawal. Symptoms have been reported after stopping more than 10 mg prednisone (or equivalent) taken daily for at least 30 days. In some cases a syndrome resembling lupus erythematosus has developed, but it has been suggested that stopping the steroid therapy may have unmasked a pre-existing condition (Shetty *et al.*, 1998).

Drug-induced acute or subacute myopathy is characterised by a syndrome of muscle pain, tenderness and weakness, mainly of the proximal limb, but at times it may be more generalised (Ucar *et al.*, 2000). Muscle biopsy may reveal muscle fibre necrosis. Factors that may contribute to myopathy include electrolyte disturbance (e.g. hypercalcaemia, hypokalaemia) or endocrine abnormalities. Usually, affected patients recover fully after the causative agent is withdrawn. Serious muscle toxicity (myopathy) can be clinically defined as muscle pain, tenderness and/or muscle weakness, accompanied by abnormal elevations in CPK. Myopathy should be considered when serum CPK levels are more than 10 times the upper limit of normal or in patients with diffuse myalgia, muscle tenderness and a marked increase in CPK.

A focal myopathy consisting of local muscle inflammation may follow the intramuscular injection of any drug as a result of traumatic necrosis, haematoma formation or low-grade infection (needle myopathy). This has been described after chronic intramuscular injection of opioids such as pentazocine and pethidine (Oh *et al.*, 1975; Louis *et al.*, 1994; Kim and Song, 1996).

Rhabdomyolysis is an acute, fulminating, potentially fatal condition of skeletal muscle featuring destruction of skeletal muscle leading to myoglobinaemia (the presence of myoglobin, an oxygen transport protein, in the blood) and myoglobinuria (Ucar *et al.*, 2000). The serum CPK level usually rises to at least 10 times the upper limit of normal. Rhabdomyolysis generally has an acute onset featuring severe muscle weakness, tenderness and swelling. It may lead to seizures, coma, hyperkalaemia and acute renal failure due to tubular necrosis (see Chapter 5).

Lipid-lowering drugs such as the fibrates and statins can have adverse effects on muscle. Myalgia, muscle weakness and increased levels of CPK have been reported with these drugs. If myopathy is not recognised and treatment discontinued, it can proceed to rhabdomyolysis and acute renal failure. Renal impairment, acute serious illness, infections, major trauma, hypoxia and, possibly, hypothyroidism are risk factors for serious toxicity (Pedersen and Tobert, 1996; Ucar *et al.*, 2000). However, the incidence of rhabdomyolysis with statin or fibrate therapy is low (about one case in every 100 000 treatment years) (Committee on Safety of Medicines, 1995). Concomitant treatment with ciclosporin, erythromycin, danazol, itraconazole, keto-conazole, nefazodone or nicotinic acid increases the risk and severity of rhabodomyolysis. Concomitant treatment with a fibrate and a statin is also thought to increase the risk of serious muscle toxicity. It is important that combinations of these drugs are avoided wherever possible.

Patients who are treated with both fibrates and statins should be advised to report any muscle aches, pains or weakness immediately to their doctor. Levels of CPK should also be monitored in these patients. There appears to be no relationship between the magnitude of the CPK elevation and the intensity of symptoms. If a patient taking a statin or fibrate develops symptoms of muscle toxicity the drug should be withdrawn and the patient monitored carefully. With increased prescribing of statins for primary and secondary prevention of coronary heart disease, it is important that healthcare professionals are aware of this rare adverse effect.

Table 8.1 lists drugs that have been associated with myalgia or myopathy.

Table 8.1 Some drugs that may cause myalgia or myopathy

Amiodarone	Opioids
Carbimazole	Penicillamine
Ciclosporin	Quinine, chloroquine
Cimetidine	Quinolones
Colchicine	Statins
Corticosteroids (on withdrawal)	Suxamethonium
Danazol	Taxanes (docetaxel, paclitaxel)
Diuretics	Vincristine
Fibrates	Zidovudine
Nicotinic acid	

Eosinophilia–myalgia syndrome

Eosinophilia–myalgia syndrome (EMS) is characterised by severe, incapacitating myalgia and a raised blood eosinophil count (more than 1.0×10^9 cells per litre) (Swygert et al., 1990). Other features include arthralgia, rash, cough, dyspnoea, oedema, abnormal liver function tests and fever. Following the first documented case in 1989, over 1500 cases, some fatal, were reported in one year in the US. Almost all the affected patients had taken dietary supplements containing tryptophan. The median dose ingested was 1.5 g daily for periods ranging between a few weeks and several years. Women were more frequently affected than men; more than 80% of initial reports involved women. The course of the disease was variable. In some patients it resolved quickly after discontinuation of tryptophan preparations, but in most it was chronic, severe and disabling. In some cases, symptoms progressed after drug withdrawal. A contaminant in the tryptophan manufacturing process is believed to have been responsible but this has not been confirmed (Belongia et al., 1990). In 1990, the Committee on Safety of Medicines recommended the withdrawal of products containing tryptophan in the UK, despite only a few reports of EMS in Europe (Committee on Safety of Medicines, 1990). Tryptophan was later reintroduced for the adjunctive treatment of severe and disabling resistant depression. It should only be prescribed by hospital specialists and treatment must be closely monitored.

Bone

Bone is a metabolically active tissue, with 10–15% of bone surfaces remodelling at any one time in adults (Robinson and Geddes, 1996). Drugs can interfere with the metabolism of calcium, phosphate, vitamin D or bone to cause metabolic bone disease such as osteoporosis or osteomalacia (Jones and Sambrook, 1994).

Osteoporosis

Osteoporosis is characterised by microarchitectural deterioration of bone tissue and low bone mass, resulting in increased bone fragility and susceptibility to fracture. Bone is considered to be osteoporotic when bone mineral denisty is 2.5 standard deviations or more below the young adult mean value. Those at increased risk of osteoporosis include postmenopausal women, small thin women, women with a premature menopause, smokers, those with a family history of the disease and long-term steroid users (i.e.

those taking 7.5 mg prednisolone or equivalent or more daily for 6 months or longer) (Picado and Luengo, 1996). Pain caused by drug-induced osteoporosis is usually acute in onset and commonly affects the back because of vertebral compression and collapse. It may also occur elsewhere due to spontaneous fractures of the ribs, pelvis or other bones. Sudden or gradual spine deformity is another possible feature of osteoporosis.

Corticosteroids have been known to affect bone for over 50 years but how they induce bone loss is not fully understood (Spector and Sambrook, 1993; Stevenson, 1998). The main contributory factor is probably suppressed osteoblastic activity and reduced osteoblast lifespan (Bialas and Routledge, 1998). Reduced testosterone and adrenal androgen levels and increased renal calcium excretion and reduced calcium absorption from the gut with resultant secondary hyperparathyroidism may also contribute. Exposure to high doses of systemic corticosteroids will lead to rapid loss of bone mass, with rates approaching 4–10% per year (Jones and Sambrook, 1994). Bone loss is greatest in the first year, but probably continues for as long as treatment is given (Spector and Sambrook, 1993). The extent of bone loss depends on the cumulative dose of corticosteroid given and is influenced by factors such as age, sex and menopausal status.

Oral corticosteroids are associated with an increased fracture rate (Adinoff and Hollister, 1983). The trabecular bone of the vertebrae and ribs is most commonly affected, but other sites, including the neck of the femur, may be involved. Patients taking long-term oral therapy are most at risk; the effects of intermittent short courses and topical or inhaled therapy are less clear. With the increasing use of inhaled corticosteroids in asthma treatment, the long-term effects on bone have been questioned (Robinson and Geddes, 1996). Studies in this area are difficult to interpret due to confounding factors such as previous oral steroid treatment. Nevertheless, there is some evidence linking inhaled therapy with osteoporosis. It has been suggested that long-term use of inhaled doses greater than beclometasone dipropionate 800 µg daily (or equivalent) may contribute to the development of osteoporosis.

Preventive measures should be considered in patients at risk of corticosteroid-induced osteoporosis (Stevenson, 1998). The lowest effective dose should always be used for the minimum duration and topical or inhaled therapy used when possible. Patients should be advised to stop smoking and to limit their alcohol consumption, to take regular exercise and to ensure an adequate calcium intake. Those deficient in vitamin D, the frail elderly and the housebound should be considered for vitamin D supplements (Bialas and Routledge, 1998). In the UK the Committee on Safety of Medicines has advised that patients with osteoporosis and other diseases such as diabetes and congestive heart failure should be closely monitored if systemic corticosteroid treatment is given (Committee on Safety of Medicines, 1997).

Several studies have shown the benefits of oestrogen replacement therapy, bisphosphonates and calcitriol in the prevention of osteoporosis due to long-term corticosteroid therapy (Bialas and Routledge, 1998). However, studies indicate that only a small proportion of patients treated with oral corticosteroids are co-prescribed therapy to prevent bone loss (Peat *et al.*, 1995; Walsh *et al.*, 1996). Guidelines on the prevention and management of corticosteroid-induced osteoporosis were recently published in the UK (National Osteoporosis Society, 1998). For patients in whom treatment is indicated, bisphosphonates are the recommended option. There is now evidence that etidronate, alendronate and risedronate are effective for this indication.

Osteoporosis and fractures have been reported, rarely, in patients treated long-term with heparin (Griffith *et al.*, 1965; Swaminathan, 1998). Osteoporotic vertebral fractures have also been described in pregnant women treated with heparin (Dahlman, 1993). Osteopenia is thought to be related to the dose and duration of therapy, particularly where heparin is given in a daily dose of at least 10 000 units for 3 months or longer. This problem is mainly associated with unfractionated heparin, although a case of vertebral fracture in a young woman treated with low molecular weight heparin has been reported (Sivakumaran *et al.*, 1996). The bone loss appears to be reversible in about 70% of patients with improvement within 6–12 months of stopping heparin. It has been suggested that, where possible, bone density should be monitored in patients being treated for longer than 3 months; however, this may be impractical (Jones and Sambrook, 1994). The mechanism of heparin-induced osteoporosis is not clear; increased bone resorption and decreased bone formation have been implicated but the results of published studies are conflicting.

Loss of oestrogens is associated with accelerated bone loss and low oestrogen concentrations may result from treatment with long-acting gonadotrophin-releasing hormone (GnRH) agonists or neuroleptics (Swaminathan, 1998). Drugs associated with osteoporosis are shown in Table 8.2.

Table 8.2 Some drugs that may cause osteoporosis

Corticosteroids
Heparin
Thyroid hormones

Osteomalacia

Osteomalacia is the condition that results from a lack of vitamin D or a disturbance of its metabolism; it is often referred to as rickets. Severe calcium deficiency or hypophosphataemia can also lead to osteomalacia. The main histological feature is defective mineralisation of bone matrix and the main symptoms are bone pain and tenderness and muscle weakness. Patients with osteomalacia may also experience fractures either spontaneously or as a consequence of trauma.

Long-term administration of antiepileptics can cause bone disease with features of osteomalacia (Hoikka *et al.*, 1981). This has been attributed to the induction of hepatic enzymes which metabolise vitamin D to biologically inactive derivatives, although a direct effect on bone resorption and formation may be involved (Swaminathan, 1998).

It is most common in patients undergoing long-term therapy with at least two of the drugs phenobarbital, primidone and phenytoin; carbamazepine is thought not to cause the problem, although available data are conflicting (Tjellesen *et al.*, 1983). This complication is most likely to affect patients with other factors contributing to vitamin D deficiency, such as poor diet or lack of exposure to sunlight (Morijiri and Sato, 1981).

Aluminium can produce adverse effects on bone through impairment of bone mineralisation and effects on osteoblast function. The problem was first documented in patients with chronic renal failure on haemodialysis (Goodman and Duarte, 1991). The high aluminium content of water used in the dialysis fluid was subsequently found to be responsible. Patients developed symptoms of osteomalacia not responsive to vitamin D. The use of aluminium salts as phosphate binders in patients with chronic renal failure can lead to osteomalacia (Kaye, 1983). The prevalence of aluminium-induced bone disease in renal patients has reduced markedly since the problem was recognised.

Prolonged ingestion of large quantities of aluminium-containing antacids has resulted in osteomalacia and pseudofractures (areas of bone resembling fractures on X-ray) in patients with normal renal function (Spencer and Kramer, 1983; Woodson, 1998).

Histological osteomalacia may occur with chronic fluoride ingestion, chronic etidronate overdosage and aluminium and gallium nitrate toxicity (Boyce *et al.*, 1984; Stamp, 1997). Osteomalacia is also a potential complication of long-term parenteral nutrition. Metabolic bone disease has been reported to affect 42–100% of patients treated at home (Hurley and McMahon, 1990). There are many possible contributory factors, including inadequate calcium and phosphate supplementation, aluminium over-

Table 8.3 Some drugs that may cause osteomalacia

Aluminium salts	Phenytoin
Barbiturates	Total parenteral nutrition
Bisphosphonates	

load and hypercalciuria (Klein and Coburn, 1994). Patients on long-term parenteral nutrition should be carefully monitored. Table 8.3 lists some drugs that may cause osteomalacia.

Avascular bone necrosis (osteonecrosis)

Avascular necrosis of bone, or osteonecrosis, is an uncommon clinical problem. It occurs when there is impairment of blood supply to a specific region of bone leading to the death of osteocytes (Capell, 1992). The condition can occur at all ages, but often affects people in their 30s and 40s. There are several predisposing factors, including exposure to high barometric pressures (e.g. in divers), sickle cell disease, alcohol abuse and drug therapy. The most common iatrogenic cause is systemic corticosteroids, although adrenocorticotrophic hormone (ACTH) and heparin have also been implicated (Shetty et al., 1998). Osteonecrosis has been observed in patients on steroid therapy for a variety of clinical problems. Patients with systemic lupus erythematosus (SLE) and rheumatoid arthritis appear to be most at risk, but the problem has occurred in inflammatory bowel disease, organ transplant recipients and patients receiving chemotherapy for Hodgkin's disease. In corticosteroid-induced cases, dose appears to be the major risk factor. In some case series, a high steroid dose taken over a short period of time has proved more likely to produce osteonecrosis than chronic low-dose treatment. Recent studies in renal transplant patients suggest a relationship between osteonecrosis of the femoral head and the total dose of methylprednisolone given as pulse therapy to treat episodes of acute rejection (Saisu et al., 1996; Kubo et al., 1998). The pathogenesis of steroid-induced osteonecrosis is unclear. It has been suggested that steroids induce a vasculitis of the small vessels supplying the affected part of the bone.

Severe joint pain and stiffness are the usual presenting symptoms. The head of the femur is the commonest site of involvement, but the head of the humerus, the tibia, the condyle of the mandible and the carpal bones may also be affected (Erill, 1991). The characteristic lesion may be seen on X-ray after a few weeks, when a well-demarcated area of increased bone density is visible. In the femur this lies at the upper pole of the femoral head; joint collapse is likely. Management of confirmed osteonecrosis is difficult. In general, attempts to promote healing in adults by resting the joint are relatively unsuccessful. Surgical core decompression techniques have been used successfully but many patients with femoral head collapse will require hip joint replacement (Capell, 1992; Spencer *et al.*, 1999).

Joints

Mild arthralgia (joint pain) may accompany almost any drug-induced skin eruption and more severe joint pain with swelling are an essential component of 'serum sickness' which may be induced by certain drugs (e.g. penicillin or barbiturates). Arthralgia and arthropathy of small peripheral joints have been reported after rubella vaccination. Rubella vaccination, like natural rubella infection, can cause acute joint symptoms; adult women are more likely to be affected than children (Weibel and Benor, 1996; Slater, 1997). Whether rubella vaccination can cause chronic arthropathy and musculoskeletal symptoms has been the subject of much controversy. The most recent epidemiological studies suggest that any increased risk is small (Weibel and Benor, 1996; Ray *et al.*, 1997; Slater, 1997). The use of intradermal and intravesical BCG for immunotherapy in cancer patients has been linked with arthritis (Hughes *et al.*, 1989; Price, 1994; Missioux *et al.*, 1995). Arthritis, mainly affecting the knees, occurs in about 0.5% of patients receiving intravesical BCG (Lamm *et al.*, 1992). Following intradermal BCG, arthritis occurs after an average duration of 32 weeks and predominantly affects the hands (Missioux *et al.*, 1995). A single case report describes arthritis after intradermal BCG vaccination in a healthy adult (Kodali and Clague, 1998). Other vaccines reported to cause joint complications include influenza and hepatitis B (Cathebras *et al.*, 1996; Thurairajan *et al.*,1997; Pope *et al.*, 1998). Table 8.4 lists some drugs associated with arthralgia or arthritis. There is no evidence that rheumatoid arthritis is ever drug-induced, but a number of drugs have been reported to exacerbate the condition, including sodium aurothiomalate, levamisole and interferon (Shetty *et al.*, 1998).

Table 8.4 Some drugs associated with arthralgia

Calcium channel blockers	Quinidine
Carbimazole	Quinolone antibiotics
Isoniazid	Rubella vaccine
Procainamide	

Severe joint pain may also be caused by the arthritis of acute gout, which can be precipitated by certain drugs. Gout, resulting from hyperuricaemia, may be induced by low-dose salicylate therapy, diuretics, pyrazinamide and ciclosporin. Published case reports have suggested an association between omeprazole and gout (Kraus and Flores-Suarez, 1995), but a recent cohort study could not confirm such a relationship (Meier and Jick, 1997).

Vasculitis may present with polyarthralgia and polyarthritis. This uncommon disease may arise spontaneously or be induced by drugs (see Chapter 2; Jennette and Falk, 1997; Merkel, 1998).

Quinolone antibiotics

In studies in young dogs, prolonged administration of high doses of quinolone antibiotics has caused erosions of articular cartilage and permanent damage to the weight-bearing joints (Stahlmann *et al.*, 1993). Quinolones have also been linked with joint disease in humans and this has led to restrictions in their use. They are contraindicated in children, growing adolescents and during pregnancy. The mechanism of quinolone arthrotoxicity has not been confirmed.

Quinolone-related arthropathy usually affects adults of less than 30 years of age. The overall incidence has been estimated at around 1% (Hayem and Carbon, 1995). Stiffness, pain and synovial swelling are the main symptoms, which occur within the first few days after starting treatment. Symptoms usually resolve on stopping treatment. Where quinolones have been used for specific restricted indications in children, arthrotoxicity seems to be relatively rare. Limited outcome data after exposure during human pregnancy have so far been reassuring. It is important that quinolones are not used inappropriately in children.

Connective tissue

The potential for quinolone antibiotics to damage articular cartilage was recognised before these agents were marketed. Since then it has become apparent that these drugs can also have toxic effects on tendons (Hayem and Carbon, 1995; Poon and Sundaram, 1997; West and Gow, 1998; Lewis *et al.*, 1999). Quinolone tendinopathy differs greatly from arthropathy. The mean age of the population affected is over 50 years of age; renal impairment and corticosteroid therapy are risk factors (Harrell, 1999; Lewis *et al.*, 1999). Ofloxacin may be associated with a higher risk of this complication than other quinolones (van der Linden *et al.*, 1999). The main site affected is the Achilles tendon, although the shoulder, knee and hand have also been affected. Tendon lesions can lead to rupture, or at least to prolonged disability. A magnetic resonance imaging (MRI) scan is useful in diagnosing tendinopathy and tendon rupture. At the first sign of painful or inflamed tendons, patients taking quinolone antibiotics should discontinue therapy. Treatment involves rest, physiotherapy and tendon repair, if appropriate. Tendinitis usually resolves in several weeks but can persist for 3 months. Tendon rupture may take up to 6 months to heal.

Tendinopathy may complicate corticosteroid treatment, if infiltration of the periarticular tissues or intra-articular injections are used. The Achilles tendon is most often involved, but the patellar tendon can also rupture.

Retroperitoneal fibrosis is a disorder characterised by fibrous tissue proliferation behind the peritoneum. Fibrosis may also occur around the lungs and pericardium. The disorder has been observed in patients being treated for migraine with vasoconstrictor agents. Methysergide is the most likely cause, but ergotamine or dihydroergotamine may also have been involved. Patients commonly describe persistent pain in the loins and groins, oliguria, pain on micturition, myalgia and oedema. Withdrawal of treatment results in symptom improvement. Several beta-blockers have also been associated with retroperitoneal fibrosis, including atenolol, propranolol, oxprenolol and sotalol (MacDonald and McDevitt, 1991). Several other drugs have been linked with retroperitoneal fibrosis (see Table 8.5), but a causal relationship has not been established.

Table 8.5 Some drugs that may cause retroperitoneal fibrosis

Aspirin	Ergotamine
Beta-blockers	Haloperidol
Bromocriptine	Methysergide
Codeine	

Drug-induced lupus

SLE is an autoimmune disease of the connective tissue, the cause of which remains unknown. Since a syndrome resembling SLE was first reported with sulfadiazine in 1945, many medications have been implicated as a cause of lupus (Price and Venables, 1995; Pramatarov, 1998; Rubin, 1999). The various terms used for this condition include lupus-like syndrome, drug-induced lupus erythematosus, drug-related lupus and lupus erythematosus medicamentosa. There are no specific diagnostic criteria for drug-induced lupus, but the diagnostic criteria listed in Table 8.6 generally apply.

Table 8.6 Guidelines for identifying drug-induced lupus

- Continuous treatment with suspect drug for at least 1 month and usually much longer
- Common presenting symptoms are arthralgias, myalgias, malaise, fever, serositis (pleurisy and pericarditis)
- Abnormal laboratory profile: presence of antihistone antibodies, especially immunoglobulin G antibodies directed against the histone H2A–H2B complex (although not always present)
- Symptom improvement within days or a few weeks of discontinuation of the suspect drug

Drug-induced lupus usually occurs after several months or years of continued therapy. Although symptom onset can be rapid, patients frequently present with mild lupus-like symptoms, which typically worsen the longer the patient is on the implicated drug. Features resemble those of naturally occurring SLE and include arthralgia and/or arthritis (80–90%), myalgia (up to 50%), fever, pleurisy and pericarditis. Some patients also have mild leukopenia, thrombocytopenia, anaemia and elevated erythrocyte sedimentation rate. Some of the features characterising SLE are seldom seen in drug-induced lupus, such as malar or discoid rash, oral ulcers, alopecia and renal or neurological disorders. Cutaneous manifestations feature in about 25% of cases of drug-induced lupus (Breathnach and Hintner, 1992; Gough *et al.*, 1996). The typical manifestations of SLE (i.e. erythematous 'butterfly' eruption, discoid lesions and mucosal ulcers) are usually absent. These skin manifestations may occur in drug-induced lupus, but erythema multiforme-like lesions, papular skin lesions and purpura also occur. Involvement of the kidney and central nervous system is much rarer than in idiopathic SLE.

Gender does not appear to be an important factor in drug-induced lupus, whereas more females than males are affected by idiopathic SLE. Again, in contrast to idiopathic SLE, drug-induced lupus often occurs in older age groups. Drug-induced lupus must be distinguished from drug-induced autoimmunity, in which drug therapy results in asymptomatic development of autoantibodies, elevated immunoglobulin levels and other laboratory abnormalities. Although a large number of patients develop laboratory features of autoimmunity, such as the production of antinuclear antibodies, a very small proportion of them develop drug-induced lupus.

Drug-induced lupus develops between 1 month and 5 years after starting the causative drug. Drug withdrawal is usually followed by resolution of symptoms and laboratory abnormalities within days or weeks, although they may persist for months or years in some patients. There have been occasional reports of fatalities. The prompt resolution of symptoms is of particular value in the diagnosis of drug-induced lupus. Non-steroidal anti-inflammatory agents should not be used in patients who may have drug-induced lupus as this may confound the diagnosis. However, some patients may require short-term treatment with low-dose corticosteroids (Pramatarov, 1998; Rubin, 1999).

Many drugs have been implicated as a cause of drug-induced lupus, although for some of these the risk may be very low or the causality uncertain (Table 8.7). By far the highest-risk drugs are procainamide and hydralazine. About 20% of patients treated with procainamide develop symptoms, as do about 5–8% of those treated with hydralazine during 1 year of therapy at currently used doses (Rubin, 1999). Both these drugs are inactivated by acetylation; there is a genetic polymorphism of N-acetyltransferase. The risk of drug-induced lupus is greater in women and in those who are slow acetylators or possess the HLA-DR4 genotype. Pleuritis and pericarditis are frequent characteristics of procainamide-induced lupus and glomerulonephritis and rash may be seen in hydralazine-induced lupus. Patients taking long-term hydralazine or procainamide should be carefully monitored; every 3 months a full blood count should be carried out and erythrocyte sedimentation rate and antinuclear antigen measured.

Table 8.7 Some drugs associated with systemic lupus erythematosus

High-risk	Methyldopa
Hydralazine	Nitrofurantoin
Procainamide	Penicillamine
	Phenytoin
Low-risk	Quinidine
Beta-blockers	Sulfasalazine
Carbamazepine	Sulphonamides
Chlorpromazine	Tetracyclines (including minocycline)
Disopyramide	Thiazide diuretics
Isoniazid	Thiouracils

For other drugs associated with lupus-like disease, the risk is probably considerably less than 1% of patients treated. Quinidine can be considered moderate-risk, whereas chlorpromazine, penicillamine, methyldopa, carbamazepine, isoniazid, captopril, propylthiouracil and minocycline incur a relatively low risk. Other drugs have been noted to exacerbate pre-existing SLE; the onset of problems usually occurs within hours of drug exposure (Rubin, 1999).

The mechanism behind drug-induced lupus is not yet fully understood; it has been suggested that certain drugs act as immunogens in genetically predisposed individuals. There is a strong suggestion that the problem is mediated by drug metabolites. Several lupus-inducing drugs are known to undergo oxidative metabolism by activated neutrophils, including procainamide, hydralazine, phenytoin, quinidine, dapsone, propylthiouracil and carbamazepine. This hypothesis is in keeping with the finding that individuals with rapid acetylator status are less likely to develop drug-induced lupus with procainamide or hydralazine. N-acetylation of these drugs in the liver is known to compete with neutrophil-mediated N-oxidation, blocking the generation of oxidised drug metabolites (Rubin, 1999). Further research into the mechanisms underlying drug-induced lupus is in progress.

Minocycline, the most widely prescribed systemic antibiotic for acne, has recently been linked with drug-induced lupus (Gough *et al.*, 1996; Knights *et al.*, 1998; Angulo *et al.*, 1999; Elkayam *et al.*, 1999). In total over 30 well-documented cases of minocycline-induced lupus have been reported (Elkayam *et al.*, 1999). Most of the affected patients were young women, with a mean age of 17 years. The dosage of minocycline was 50–200 mg daily for a mean duration of 30 months. The indication for which the drug was prescribed was acne in all cases. Arthralgia was a feature in all cases. Fever, rash, pleuritic pain and hepatitis were seen in some cases. Although laboratory tests showed an increased erythrocyte sedimentation rate in most patients, antihistone antibodies were present in only four patients. In most patients the syndrome resolved rapidly after minocycline was discontinued. In some cases there was a long time period before the link with minocycline therapy was made. Interestingly, minocycline is increasingly being used as a second-line drug in rheumatoid arthritis but no reports of autoimmune syndromes among these patients have been published (Langevitz *et al.*, 2000). Healthcare professionals should have a high index of suspicion in young patients taking minocycline who develop features of autoimmune syndromes.

> **CASE STUDY**

Mrs H is a 58-year-old woman who has had asthma for many years. She is on the following medication:

> Salbutamol inhaler prn
> Beclometasone inhaler 500 μg bd
> Salmeterol inhaler 50 μg bd
> Prednisolone 30 mg od (reducing course over a week)

Mrs H has just spent 4 days in hospital following an asthma attack and the dose of her steroid inhaler was increased. She is still smoking about five cigarettes a day. Mrs H tells you she is worried about taking the steroid tablets because she knows they can 'soften your bones' and her mother, who died recently, suffered from osteoporosis.

What risk factors for osteoporosis does Mrs H have?
There are several risk factors. Mrs H is postmenopausal, has a family history of osteoporosis and is a smoker. She should be asked about her history of fractures, whether she takes regular exercise and about her calcium and alcohol intake, as these factors are all important.

What advice do you give about the concern that corticosteroids 'soften' bones?
Mrs H should be informed that taking oral steroids for prolonged periods increases the risk of osteoporosis. It is possible that the occasional short courses of oral steroids together with regular inhaled therapy needed for her asthma may have some adverse effect on her bones, but the risk is probably fairly small. Mrs H should be encouraged to stop smoking and could be advised to increase her dietary intake of calcium and vitamin D. If possible, she should try to take some regular exercise if her asthma allows. After a few months, Mrs H may be able to step down her inhaled steroid dosage, in line with the British Thoracic Society guidelines on asthma (British Thoracic Society, 1997), which will minimise the risk of adverse effects.

References

Adinoff A D, Hollister J R (1983). Steroid-induced fractures and bone loss in patients with asthma. *N Engl J Med* 309: 265–268.

Angulo J M, Sigal L H, Espinoza L R (1999). Minocycline induced lupus and autoimmune hepatitis. *J Rheumatol* 26: 1420–1421.

Anon. (1971). Drug induced aches and pains. *Adverse Drug React Bull* 30.

Belongia E A, Hedberg C W, Gleich G J *et al.* (1990). An investigation of the eosinophilia–myalgia syndrome associated with tryptophan use. *N Engl J Med* 323: 357–365.

Bialas M C, Routledge P A (1998). Adverse effects of corticosteroids. *Adverse Drug React Toxicol* 17: 227–235.

Boyce B F, Smith L, Fogelman I *et al.* (1984). Focal osteomalacia due to low-dose diphosphonate therapy in Paget's disease. *Lancet* i: 821–824.

Breathnach S M, Hintner H (1992). *Adverse Drug Reactions and the Skin*. Oxford: Blackwell Scientific Publications.

British Thoracic Society, British Paediatric Association, Royal College of Physicians of London, The Kings Fund Centre, National Asthma Campaign *et al.* (1997). The British guidelines on asthma management. *Thorax* 52 (suppl 1): S1–S20.

Capell H (1992). Selected side-effects: 5. Steroid therapy and osteonecrosis. *Prescribers' J* 32: 32–35.

Cathebras P, Cartry O, Lafage-Proust M H *et al.* (1996). Arthritis, hypercalcemia and lytic bone lesions after hepatitis B vaccination. *J Rheumatol* 23: 558–560.

Committee on Safety of Medicines (1990). Update on L-tryptophan and eosinophilia–myalgia syndrome. *Curr Probl* 29: 2.

Committee on Safety of Medicines (1995). Rhabdomyolysis associated with lipid lowering drugs. *Curr Probl Pharmacovigilance* 21: 3.

Committee on Safety of Medicines (1997). Using long-term systemic corticosteroids safely. *Curr Probl Pharmacovigilance* 23: 4.

Dahlman T C (1993). Osteoporotic fractures and the recurrence of thromboembolism during pregnancy and the puerperium in 184 women undergoing thromboprophylaxis with heparin. *Am J Obstet Gynecol* 168: 1265–1270.

Elkayam O, Yaron M, Caspi D (1999). Minocycline-induced autoimmune syndromes: an overview. *Semin Arth Rheum* 29: 392–397.

Erill S (1991). Corticotrophins and corticosteroids. In: Dukes M N G, Aronson J K, eds. *Meyler's Side Effects of Drugs Annual 15*. Amsterdam: Elsevier, chapter 41.

Goodman W G, Duarte M E L (1991). Aluminium: effects on bone and role in the pathogenesis of renal osteodystrophy. *Miner Electrolyte Metab* 17: 221–232.

Gough A, Chapman S, Wagstaff K *et al.* (1996). Minocycline induced autoimmune hepatitis and systemic lupus erythematosus-like syndrome. *Br Med J* 312: 169–172.

Griffith G C, Nichols G, Asher J D *et al.* (1965). Heparin osteoporosis. *JAMA* 193: 91–94.

Harrell R (1999). Fluoroquinolone-induced tendiopathy: what do we know? *South Med J* 92: 622–625.

Hayem G, Carbon C (1995). A reappraisal of quinolone tolerability. The experience of their musculoskeletal adverse effects. *Drug Safety* 13: 338–342.

Hoikka V, Savolainen K, Alhava M *et al.* (1981). Osteomalacia in institutionalised epileptic patients on long-term anticonvulsant therapy. *Acta Neurol Scand* 64: 122.

Hughes R A, Allard S A, Maini R N (1989). Arthritis associated with adjuvant mycobacterial treatment for carcinoma of the bladder. *Ann Rheum Dis* 48: 432–434.

Hurley D L, McMahon H M (1990). Long-term parenteral nutrition and metabolic bone disease. *Endocrinol Metab Clin North Am* 19: 113.

Jennette J C, Falk R J (1994). Small vessel vasculitis. *N Engl J Med* 337: 1512.

Jones G, Sambrook P N (1994). Drug-induced disorders of bone metabolism. Incidence, management and avoidance. *Drug Safety* 10: 480–489.

Kaye M (1983). Oral aluminium toxicity in a non-dialyzed patient with renal failure. *Clin Nephrol* 20: 208.

Kim H A, Song Y W (1996). Polymyositis developing after prolonged injections of pentazocine. *J Rheumatol* 23: 1644–1646.

Klein G L, Coburn J W (1994). Total parenteral nutrition and its effects on bone metabolism. *Crit Rev Clin Lab Sci* 31: 135.

Knights S E, Leandro M J, Khamashta M A, Hughes G R (1998). Minocycline-induced arthritis. *Clin Exp Rheumatol* 16: 587–590.

Kodali V R R, Clague R B (1998). Arthritis after BCG vaccine in a healthy woman. *J Int Med* 244: 183–187.

Kraus A, Flores-Suarez L F (1995). Acute gout associated with omeprazole. *Lancet* 345: 461–462.

Kubo T, Fujioka M, Yamazoe S *et al.* (1998). Relationship between steroid dosage and osteonecrosis of the femoral head after renal transplantation as measured by magnetic resonance imaging. *Transplant Proc* 30: 3039–3040.

Lamm D L, Van Der Merijden A D P M, Morales A *et al.* (1992). Incidence and complications of bacillus Calmette-Guerin intravesical therapy in superficial bladder cancer. *J Urol* 147: 596–600.

Langevitz P, Livneh A, Bank I *et al.* (2000). Benefits and risks of minocycline in rheumatoid arthritis. *Drug Safety* 5: 405–414.

Lewis J R, Gums J G, Dickensheets D L (1999). Levofloxacin-induced bilateral achilles tendonitis. *Ann Pharmacother* 33: 792–795.

Louis E D, Bodner R A, Challenor Y B, Brust J C (1994). Focal myopathy induced by chronic intramuscular heroin injection. *Muscle Nerve* 17: 550–552.

MacDonald T M, McDevitt D G (1991). Anti-anginal and beta-adrenoceptor blocking drugs. In: Dukes M N G, ed. *Meyler's Side Effects of Drugs*. Amsterdam: Elsevier, chapter 19.

Meier C R, Jick H (1997). Omeprazole, other antiulcer drugs and newly diagnosed gout. *Br J Clin Pharmacol* 44: 175–178.

Merkel P A (1998). Drugs associated with vasculitis. *Curr Opin Rheumatol* 10: 45–50.

Missioux D, Hermabessiere J, Sauvezie B (1995). Arthritis and iritis after bacillus Calmette-Guerin therapy. *J Rheumatol* 22: 2010.

Morijiri Y, Sato T (1981). Factors causing rickets in institutionalised handicapped children on anticonvulsant therapy. *Arch Dis Child* 56: 446.

National Osteoporosis Society (1998). *Guidance on the Prevention and Management of Corticosteroid-induced Osteoporosis*. Bath: National Osteoporosis Society.

Oh S J, Rollins J L, Lewis I (1975). Pentazocine-induced fibrous myopathy. *JAMA* 231: 271–273.

Peat I D, Healy S, Reid D M *et al.* (1995). Prevention of steroid induced osteoporosis. A missed opportunity? *Ann Rheum Dis* 54: 66–68.

Pedersen T R, Tobert J A (1996). Benefits and risks of HMG–CoA reductase inhibitors in the prevention of coronary heart disease. *Drug Safety* 14: 11–24.

Picado C, Luengo M (1996). Corticosteroid-induced bone loss: prevention and management. *Drug Safety* 15: 347–359.

Poon C C H, Sundaram N A (1997). Spontaneous bilateral achilles tendon rupture associated with ciprofloxacin. *Med J Aust* 166: 665.

Pope J E, Stevens A, Howson W *et al.* (1998). The development of rheumatoid arthritis after recombinant hepatitis B vaccination. *J Rheumatol* 25: 1687–1693.

Pramatarov K D (1998). Drug-induced lupus erythematosus. *Clin Dermatol* 16: 368–377.

Price G E (1994). Arthritis and iritis after BCG therapy for bladder cancer. *J Rheumatol* 21: 564–565.

Price E J, Venables P J W (1995). Drug-induced lupus. *Drug Safety* 12: 283–290.

Ray P, Black S, Shinefield H (1997). Risk of chronic arthropathy among women after rubella vaccination. *JAMA* 278: 551–556.

Robinson D S, Geddes D M (1996). Inhaled corticosteroids: benefits and risks. *J Asthma* 33: 5–16.

Rubin R L (1999). Etiology and mechanisms of drug-induced lupus. *Curr Opin Rheumatol* 11: 357–363.

Saisu T, Sakamoto K, Yamada K *et al.* (1996). High incidence of osteonecrosis of femoral head in patients receiving more than 2g of intravenous methylprednisolone after renal transplantation. *Transplant Proc* 28: 1559–1560.

Shetty H G M, Routledge P A, Davies D M (1998). Disorders of muscle, bone, and connective tissue. In: Davies D M, Ferner R E, de Glanville H, eds. *Davies's Textbook of Adverse Drug Reactions*, 5th edn. London: Chapman and Hall Medical, chapter 18.

Sivakumaran M, Ghosh K, Zaidi Y *et al.* (1996). Osteoporosis and vertebral collapse following low-dose, low molecular weight heparin therapy in a young patient. *Clin Lab Haematol* 18: 55.

Slater P E (1997). Chronic arthropathy after rubella vaccination in women. *JAMA* 278: 594–595.

Spector T D, Sambrook P N (1993). Steroid osteoporosis. A pragmatic approach is needed while prospective trials are awaited. *Br Med J* 307: 519–520.

Spencer H, Kramer L (1983). Antacid-induced calcium loss. *Arch Intern Med* 143: 657.

Spencer C, Smith P, Rafla N *et al.* (1999). Corticosteroids in pregnancy and osteonecrosis of the femoral head. *Obstet Gynecol* 94: 848.

Stahlmann R. Forster C, Sickle D V (1993). Quinolones in children. Are concerns over arthropathy justified? *Drug Safety* 9: 397–403.

Stamp T (1997). Rickets and osteomalacia. *Medicine* 25: 71–73.

Stevenson J C (1998). Management of corticosteroid-induced osteoporosis. *Lancet* 352: 1327–1328.

Swaminathan R (1998). Disorders of metabolism 2. In: Davies D M, Ferner R E, de Glanville H, eds. *Davies's Textbook of Adverse Drug Reactions*, 5th edn. London: Chapman and Hall Medical, chapter 17.

Swygert L A, Maes E F, Sewell L E *et al.* (1990). Eosinophilia–myalgia syndrome. Results of national surveillance. *JAMA* 264: 1698–1703.

Thurairajan G, Hope-Ross M W, Situnayake R D *et al.* (1997). Polyarthropathy, orbital myositis and posterior scleritis: an unusual adverse reaction to influenza vaccine. *Br J Rheumatol* 36: 120–123.

Tjellesen L, Nilas L, Christiansen C (1983). Does carbamazepine cause disturbances in calcium metabolism in epileptic patients? *Acta Neurol Scand* 68: 13–19.

Ucar M, Mjorndal T, Dahlquist R (2000). HMG–CoA reductase inhibitors and myotoxicity. *Drug Safety* 6: 441–457.

van der Linden P D, van de Lei J, Nab H W *et al.* (1999). Achilles tendinitis associated with fluoroquinolones. *Br J Clin Pharmacol* 48: 433–437.

Walsh L J, Wong C A, Pringle M *et al.* (1996). Use of oral corticosteroids in the community: a cross sectional study. *Br Med J* 313: 344–346.

Weibel R E, Benor D E (1996). Chronic arthropathy and musculoskeletal symptoms associated with rubella vaccines. *Arth Rheum* 39: 1529–1534.

West M B, Gow P (1998). Ciprofloxacin, bilateral achilles tendonitis and unilateral tendon rupture – a case report. *NZ Med J* 111: 18–19.

Woodson G C (1998). An interesting case of osteomalacia due to antacid use associated with stainable bone aluminum in a patient with normal renal function. *Bone* 22: 695–698.

9

Blood disorders

Moira McMurray

Although drug-induced blood disorders (dyscrasias) are comparatively rare, they are always serious and have a high incidence of morbidity and mortality. As with other adverse drug reactions (ADRs), their exact incidence is not easy to determine, mainly because of difficulties in assessing the risk with particular drugs and in proving a causal relationship. The high incidence of blood dyscrasias with some drugs, for example remoxipride, has led to their withdrawal from the market. Any suspected adverse reaction involving the blood should be reported to the appropriate regulatory authority.

Like other ADRs, those affecting the blood can be divided into type A and type B reactions. Type A reactions are predictable from the known pharmacology of the drug. Bone marrow suppression by cytotoxics and other immunosuppressants is a common type A effect. Although serious and potentially fatal, appropriate monitoring and management limit the impact of this kind of reaction. This chapter discusses the main adverse effects of drugs on blood, focusing on type B (unpredictable) reactions. Healthcare professionals should be aware of the most important symptoms associated with haematological ADRs, the drugs most commonly implicated and the drugs that require routine blood count monitoring. Patients receiving high-risk drugs should be advised of the symptoms of blood dyscrasias and be told to seek advice immediately should any of these symptoms develop. In practice, patients will often present with a sore throat, mouth ulcers, bruising or bleeding, fever, malaise, rash or non-specific illness. Early recognition of these signs of a potentially fatal reaction is crucial.

For some drugs the risk of a haematological reaction is high enough to warrant regular routine monitoring of the blood count (Table 9.1). This list is not exhaustive and it does not include cytotoxic and other myelosuppressant drugs. There are other drugs with a known risk of blood dyscrasias for which regular monitoring is not considered worthwhile, such as carbimazole (Anon, 1997). This is because the

Table 9.1 Some drugs requiring regular blood count monitoring

Amphotericin	Mefenamic acid (prolonged)
Apomorphine (when given with levodopa)	Mianserin
	Nalidixic acid (for > 2 weeks)
Chloramphenicol	Penicillamine
Clozapine	Phenylbutazone (for > 7 days)
Co-trimoxazole (prolonged)	Phenytoin
Cyproterone acetate	Pyrimethamine (prolonged)
Felbamate (US market)	Rifampicin (prolonged or if patient has hepatic disorder)
Gold	
Heparin (for > 5 days)	Sulfasalazine
Indometacin (prolonged)	Tacrolimus
Interferon alfa	Ticlopidine
Interferon beta	Tryptophan
Leflunomide	Zidovudine

adverse effect develops too quickly for regular monitoring to be of value.

In humans, normal haemopoiesis takes place only in the bone marrow. One type of undifferentiated stem cell (pluripotential) develops into a number of progenitor cells which are responsible for the three main marrow cell lines: erythroid (red cells); granulocytic and monocytic (white cells); and megakaryocytic (platelets) (Hoffbrand and Pettit, 1993).

The normal ranges of blood components are shown in Table 9.2. A reduction below the normal range in the peripheral blood cell count of any particular cell type is known as a cytopenia. Reductions may be caused either by a decrease in the production rate of that cell type or by a reduced lifespan of the cells in the circulation (Carey, 1995). Drugs can cause blood dyscrasias by acting at different stages of haemopoiesis, from the stem cell through to the mature cell. The number of cell types affected depends on where in the process the effect takes place. Damage to a stem cell will affect most cell lines, while damage to the mature cell may be specific to that cell line. Damage to the earliest progenitor cells usually takes more than 2 weeks for recovery, while damage to one of the later precursors is associated with recovery within a few days (Patton and Duffull, 1994).

Depending on the type of cell line affected and the severity of the reaction, haematological ADRs usually manifest as one or more of the following: signs of anaemia, bleeding and/or bruising and infection (often fever, sore throat, mouth ulcers). For many of the type B reactions the underlying mechanisms are either toxic or immune in nature (Patton and Duffull, 1994).

Table 9.2 Normal ranges of blood components

Component	Males and females	
Haemoglobin	13.5−17.5 g/dl (males)	11.5−15.5 g/dl (females)
Red cells	$4.5−6.5 \times 10^{12}/l$ (males)	$3.9−5.6 \times 10^{12}/l$ (females)
White cells total	$4.0−11.0 \times 10^9/l$	
Neutrophils	$2.5−7.5 \times 10^9/l$	
Lymphocytes	$1.5−3.5 \times 10^9/l$	
Monocytes	$0.2−0.8 \times 10^9/l$	
Eosinophils	$0.04−0.44 \times 10^9/l$	
Basophils	$0.01−0.1 \times 10^9/l$	
Platelets	$150–400 \times 10^9/l$	

Aplastic anaemia

Aplastic anaemia describes a peripheral blood picture with suppression of red cells (anaemia), white cells (leukopenia) and platelets (thrombocytopenia) due to hypoplasia of the bone marrow. The incidence in Europe and America has been estimated at between two and five per million of the population per year (Gordon-Smith, 1996). Aplastic anaemia can be congenital but most cases are acquired from drugs, chemicals, radiation or viral infection (Young, 1995). This reaction is rarer than agranulocytosis or thrombocytopenia but, in contrast to these, it often persists and worsens despite drug withdrawal. It is characterised by symptoms and signs of anaemia, infection and bleeding. The onset of drug-induced aplastic anaemia can be acute or, more commonly, chronic. Acute cases usually present with severe bleeding and sometimes with infection. When the onset is insidious, weakness, fatigue and pallor are the predominant symptoms.

A number of drugs are associated with an unpredictable (type B) aplastic anaemia (Table 9.3).

Table 9.3 Some drugs strongly associated with aplastic anaemia

Group	Examples
Antidiabetics	Chlorpropamide, tolbutamide
Antiepileptics	Carbamazepine, phenytoin, felbamate, lamotrigine
Anti-inflammatory drugs	Diclofenac, gold, indometacin, penicillamine, phenylbutazone, piroxicam, sulindac, sulfasalazine
Antimalarials	Pyrimethamine
Antimicrobials	Chloramphenicol, co-trimoxazole, sulphonamides
Antiplatelet agents	Ticlopidine
Antipsychotics	Chlorpromazine
Antithyroid drugs	Carbimazole, propylthiouracil

However, it is often difficult to prove a causal association, particularly because there may be a significant delay between exposure to the drug and development of the reaction. The reaction can occur months after the causative drug has been stopped (Gordon-Smith, 1996). It is also more likely to occur after two or more exposures to the drug than after the initial exposure. Chloramphenicol was one of the first agents to be associated with aplastic anaemia (Rich *et al.*, 1950). Large doses produce mild, reversible bone marrow depression in all patients; this mainly affects red cells and is thought to be due to mitochondrial injury (Yunis, 1973). This is a predictable, type A reaction.

The type B aplastic anaemia is rare, unpredictable and frequently irreversible and fatal. It has been reported to occur days, months or even years after an initial exposure to chloramphenicol and in some cases has terminated in leukaemia (Holt *et al.*, 1993). The incidence is thought to be between $1:25\,000$ and $1:60\,000$. The mortality rate is about 70%, with only 10% of affected patients making a full recovery. There is some evidence that genetic predisposition is involved. It is thought that the nitrobenzene ring on the chloramphenicol molecule undergoes nitroreduction in susceptible individuals to a toxic intermediate which causes stem cell damage (Yunis, 1989). In the UK, systemic chloramphenicol is reserved for life-threatening infections. Regular blood count monitoring before and during systemic chloramphenicol treatment is essential.

The link between ocular chloramphenicol and aplastic anaemia is controversial (Rayner and Buckley, 1996). Several published studies do not support the view that the use of chloramphenicol eye drops is inadvisable due to the risk of aplastic anaemia (Lancaster *et al.*, 1998; Wiholm *et al.*, 1998). A recent epidemiological estimate of the risk found that, although an association between ocular chloramphenicol and aplastic anaemia could not be excluded, the absolute risk was very low, in the order of less than one per million treatment courses (Laporte *et al.*, 1998). The *British National Formulary* states that chloramphenicol is the drug of choice for superficial eye infections.

Since the use of systemic chloramphenicol has declined, non-steroidal anti-inflammatory drugs (NSAIDs), as a therapeutic group, are thought to be the most frequent cause of drug-induced aplastic anaemia (Gordon-Smith, 1996). Due to its association with aplastic anaemia and agranulocytosis, the use of phenylbutazone is restricted to hospital treatment of ankylosing spondylitis unresponsive to other therapy (Inman, 1977).

Many of the second-line or disease-modifying antirheumatic drugs (DMARDs) have the potential to cause haematological toxicity, including aplastic anaemia. Patients receiving gold, penicillamine, sulfasalazine or immunosuppressants must undergo regular blood monitoring. Platelet and neutrophil counts usually fall first in these patients, so regular monitoring may help avoid development of aplastic anaemia (Jackson and Proctor, 1991).

The antiepileptic agent, felbamate, is only available for restricted use on the US market because of associated cases of aplastic anaemia and acute liver failure. By 1997, 34 cases of felbamate-associated aplastic anaemia had been reported, 13 of which had been fatal. It should only be used for patients with epilepsy refractory to other antiepileptics, especially patients with the Lennox–Gastaut syndrome, and full blood counts should be carried out before the patient starts treatment and regularly during treatment (Pellock and Brodie, 1997). Aplastic anaemia can occur after felbamate has been discontinued, so patients should continue to be monitored. Felbamate is not licensed in the UK.

The antiplatelet agent ticlopidine has also been associated with aplastic anaemia with 19 cases reported by early 1998 (Yeh *et al.*, 1998). The effect occurred 3.5 weeks to 5 months after starting therapy and in some cases was fatal. The mechanism may be idiosyncratic or may be a direct toxic effect on marrow cells. In some cases the development of aplastic anaemia was preceded by agranulocytosis or thrombocytopenia (Love *et al.*, 1998).

The diagnosis of aplastic anaemia is assisted by examination of peripheral blood and bone marrow. Patient management involves two main principles: supporting and protecting the patient to improve the chance of a spontaneous recovery, and accelerating the recovery process. Any drug therapy that may be implicated in the reaction must be stopped. Supportive care involves transfusion of blood and platelet concentrates and antibiotic treatment or prophylaxis. The anabolic steroid nandrolone is licensed for the treatment of aplastic anaemia but its use is controversial due to uncertain efficacy. Another anabolic steroid oxymetholone (unlicensed in the UK) has also been used with mixed results. When some marrow function remains, anabolic steroids may increase cell lines but there is no evidence of improved patient survival (Gordon-Smith, 1996). Immunosuppression with antilymphocyte globulins achieves a response in about half of acquired cases but recovery is slow and may be incomplete. Ciclosporin has produced an improvement in some patients with aplastic anaemia and a 50% response rate in patients refractory to antilymphocyte globulins has been reported. A recent study has reported improved response in terms of haematological parameters, quality of response and early mortality when antithymocyte globulin was used in combination with ciclosporin compared with ciclosporin alone. Patients had previously untreated non-severe aplastic anaemia (Marsh *et al.*, 1999). High-dose corticosteroids can induce a response but other treatments are preferred (Young and Barrett, 1995).

Administration of recombinant human growth factors (granulocyte colony-stimulating factor (GCSF) or granulocyte–macrophage colony-stimulating factor (GM-CSF)) tends to increase the neutrophil count only. When used alone, they have generally not produced a sustained response. Their use after bone marrow transplantation can reduce the neutropenic period (Young and Barrett, 1995). Preliminary results of treatment of aplastic anaemia with G-CSF and erythropoietin indicate an increase in neutrophil and red cell counts in some patients (Yonekura *et al.*, 1997). Allogenic bone marrow transplantation may be an option for some – particularly young – patients (Reiter *et al.*, 1997) and peripheral stem cell transplantation has also been reported to be successful (Manley *et al.*, 1997).

Agranulocytosis

Drugs can cause a reduction in total white cell count (leukopenia) but selective reduction in granulocytes, which include neutrophils, eosinophils and basophils, is more common. Agranulocytosis is defined as a profound decrease in the number of circulating granulocytes, resulting in a neutrophil count of less than 0.5×10^9/l. Patients with neutropenia of this severity are susceptible to serious and sometimes fatal infection. More modest reductions in the neutrophil count are referred to as neutropenia or granulocytopenia.

Agranulocytosis is usually drug-induced but a few clinical conditions may occasionally be responsible, including viral infection, lymphomas or leukaemia. The aetiology is believed to be either autoimmune or direct toxicity to the bone marrow cells (Heimpel, 1988). Immune-mediated destruction of neutrophils or suppression of granulopoiesis is probably the most common mechanism and this may result in severe neutropenia of rapid onset, often within a few months of starting therapy. This mechanism is believed to be involved in agranulocytosis caused by sulphonamides, antithyroid agents, quinidine and phenytoin (Heimpel, 1988). Complete recovery may occur 2–3 weeks after the drug is withdrawn but the patient is then sensitised so that further drug exposure initiates a prompt recurrence.

Toxic-mediated agranulocytosis has also been reported. Chlorpromazine has been shown to produce a dose-dependent inhibition of granulopoiesis in this way. Severe, symptomatic and potentially fatal agranulocytosis is believed to occur in about 0.1% of patients taking chlorpromazine in standard doses. This effect is usually delayed in onset (Vincent, 1986).

Antithyroid drugs (i.e. carbimazole and propylthiouracil) appear to incur a relatively high risk of agranulocytosis; some studies have estimated this risk to be in the order of 1.9–3 per 10 000 users per year (International Agranulocytosis and Aplastic Anaemia Study, 1988; van der Klauw *et al.*, 1999).

Ticlopidine is thought to inhibit reversibly myeloid colony growth leading to neutropenia. In the UK, the initial clinical trials with ticlopidine were suspended because of neutropenia. The incidence of neutropenia was 2.4%, with 0.85% of patients described as severely neutropenic (neutrophil count less than $0.45 \times 10^9/l$). Most cases tended to develop within the first 3 months of treatment. Full blood counts are therefore recommended at the start of ticlopidine therapy and then every 2 weeks for 3 months (Yeh *et al.*, 1998).

Drugs most strongly associated with agranulocytosis are listed in Table 9.4; there is considerable overlap with those implicated in aplastic anaemia.

Patients with drug-induced agranulocytosis usually become suddenly unwell with fever and sometimes rigors, sore throat, mouth ulcers, headache and malaise. Most patients develop septicaemia and some have evidence of pneumonia, oropharyngeal candidiasis or skin infection.

The potential severity of agranulocytosis is indicated by an analysis of reports to the UK regulatory authority (Committee on

Table 9.4 Some drugs strongly associated with agranulocytosis

Group	Examples
Antibacterials	Penicillins, cephalosporins, co-trimoxazole, chloramphenicol, sulphonamides
Antidepressants	Imipramine, clomipramine, desipramine, mianserin
Antiepileptics	Carbamazepine, phenytoin
Anti-inflammatory drugs	Gold, leflunomide, penicillamine, sulfasalazine, non-steroidal anti-inflammatory drugs
Antimalarials	Pyrimethamine
Antipsychotics	Chlorpromazine, thioridazine, clozapine
Antithyroid drugs	Carbimazole, propylthiouracil
Cardiovascular drugs	Captopril, procainamide, ticlopidine

Safety of Medicines) during the period 1963–1993 (Committee on Safety of Medicines, 1993a). There were 912 cases of agranulocytosis, 30% of which had a fatal outcome. Of 1499 cases of neutropenia, 3.5% were fatal. Six drug classes accounted for half the reports of agranulocytosis and a third of the reports of neutropenia. These were antithyroid drugs, beta-lactam antibiotics, NSAIDs, phenothiazines, sulphonamides and tricyclic antidepressants. The individual drugs most commonly implicated were carbimazole, co-trimoxazole, chlorpromazine, clozapine, mianserin, phenylbutazone, sulfasalazine and thioridazine.

Clozapine is associated with a 2–3% incidence of neutropenia. Consequently, in the UK its use is restricted to patients registered with a mandatory blood monitoring programme (the Clozaril Patient Monitoring Service). This ensures that the drug is not given if the total white cell count falls below $3 \times 10^9/l$ or if the neutrophil count is less than $1.5 \times 10^9/l$.

Any patient with suspected drug-induced agranulocytosis should be admitted to hospital immediately for full blood count monitoring. A full drug history, including exposure to over-the-counter medicines, should be taken. If agranulocytosis is confirmed, any drug that may be implicated should be stopped immediately. In most cases there is spontaneous recovery within 2 weeks of drug withdrawal. Patients who are febrile or have other evidence of infection should be treated promptly with broad-spectrum antibiotics, including one with good activity against *Pseudomonas aeruginosa*. Antifungal therapy should be added if fever continues after 3–4 days of antibiotic therapy and there is some evidence that prophylactic use may be of benefit (Anon, 1997).

Death is more likely when agranulocytosis is severe or prolonged and in such cases recombinant human growth factors have been used to accelerate neutrophil recovery. The efficacy of these agents (GCSF or GM-CSF) in this situation has not been assessed in clinical trials but there are numerous case reports (Sprinkkelman *et al.*, 1994) in which therapy appears to have improved the recovery time. Recombinant human growth factors are not licensed for this indication.

Patients prescribed drugs with a significant risk of causing agranulocytosis should be advised to see the doctor immediately if fever, sore throat, mouth ulcers or excessive tiredness develop. They should be aware that a blood test will be necessary and that the medicine will be stopped if the white blood cell count is low. If patients are unable to see their general practitioner immediately, they should go to the local hospital accident and emergency department.

Thrombocytopenia

Thrombocytopenia is defined as a reduction in the platelet count to less than $150 \times 10^9/l$. The main presenting feature is haemorrhage, which is most commonly seen in the skin, giving rise to purpura and petechiae, and in the gastrointestinal and genitourinary tracts. Cerebral haemorrhage is the most common cause of death. Haemorrhage is unlikely to develop unless the platelet count is below $20 \times 10^9/l$ (Machin, 1996). In thrombocytopenia the bleeding time is prolonged, although coagulation tests (e.g. international normalised ratio, prothrombin time) remain normal.

Thrombocytopenia can result from a reduction in platelet production due to suppression or failure of the bone marrow. The platelet count usually falls 7–10 days after initiation of the offending drug. An autoimmune mechanism may also be responsible; autoimmune antibodies reduce the lifespan of platelets in the circulation from 7–10 days to several hours (Liesner, 1997). Table 9.5 lists the drugs most commonly associated with thrombocytopenia.

A study in Denmark from 1969 to 1991 found the most commonly implicated drugs were sodium aurothiomalate, co-trimoxazole, quinidine, valproate and penicillamine. NSAIDs were the class of drug most commonly involved (Pedersen-Bjergaard *et al.*, 1996). Different drugs appear to produce different clinical pictures of thrombocytopenia. Severe thrombocytopenia was associated with gold salts, NSAIDs, sulphonamides, antibiotics, quinine and quinidine. Valproic acid-induced thrombocytopenia tended to be mild, dose-dependent, and of gradual onset (Pedersen-Bjergaard *et al.*, 1998).

Removal of the responsible drug is often sufficient to restore the platelet count within several days. Platelet transfusions may be needed if the count is very low. Corticosteroids may also be beneficial in

Table 9.5 Some drugs associated with thrombocytopenia

Effect	*Examples*
Decreased platelet production	Chloramphenicol, co-trimoxazole, idoxuridine, phenylbutazone, penicillamine
Increased platelet consumption	Acetazolamide, chlorpropamide, diazepam, digoxin, furosemide (frusemide), gold, heparin, methyldopa, oxprenolol, penicillins, quinine, quinidine, rifampicin, sodium valproate, sulphonamides, thiazide diuretics, tolbutamide, trimethoprim

immune-mediated cases. Future exposure to the likely causative agent should be avoided. Aspirin and NSAIDs should be avoided as they decrease the effectiveness of the remaining platelets (Magee and Beeley, 1994).

Heparin causes thrombocytopenia in about 5% of patients (Caron *et al.*, 1996). Two clinical types have been defined. Type I is characterised by a mild, frequent thrombocytopenia occurring on the first few days of heparin administration. The platelet count does not usually fall below $100 \times 10^9/l$ and it is not associated with an increased risk of thrombosis. Monitoring is needed but therapy can usually be continued and thrombocytopenia regresses.

Type II heparin-induced thrombocytopenia is less frequent. This type is of more clinical importance because thromboembolic events are the main complication. This reaction has an immunological basis, involving the formation of a complex between heparin and a specific antibody. This can trigger platelet activation, coagulation activation and thrombin generation (Warkentin and Barkin, 1999).

The onset of the reaction is usually within 5–8 days of starting heparin therapy. Patients usually have mild to moderate thrombocytopenia (platelet counts $20–150 \times 10^9/l$), although sometimes the platelet count does not fall below the standard threshold for thrombocytopenia ($150 \times 10^9/l$). None the less, these patients are at risk of thrombotic events. Deep vein thrombosis and pulmonary embolism are the most common complications. Heparin-induced thrombocytopenia is less likely to occur with low molecular weight heparins than with unfractionated heparin (Warkentin *et al.*, 1995). Heparin should be stopped immediately if this reaction is suspected. The recommended treatment is an agent that reduces thrombin generation; this may be achieved with the new agents lepirudin or danaparoid (Warkentin and Barkin, 1999). New evidence suggests that warfarin should not be used because of the risk of warfarin-induced venous limb gangrene. Platelet transfusions should be avoided in these patients since they may precipitate thrombotic events (Warkentin and Barkin, 1999). Thrombocytopenia usually remits within a few days of stopping heparin treatment.

Pure red cell aplasia

Pure red cell aplasia is characterised by anaemia with a marked reduction in reticulocytes (immature red cells). In most cases the mechanism remains unclear, with possible immune- or toxic-mediated cell destruction. Patients experience weakness, lethargy and pallor. About 5% of reported cases are thought to be drug-induced. Over 30 drugs have been implicated by one or two case reports to cause pure red cell aplasia but those associated with several reports include phenytoin, azathioprine and isoniazid. Other associated drugs include penicillamine, chlorpropamide and chloramphenicol. Some patients will respond to corticosteroid therapy and others to immunosuppressants such as cyclophosphamide (Thompson and Gales, 1996).

Haemolytic anaemia

Haemolytic anaemia is anaemia resulting from an increased rate of red cell destruction. Anaemia may not develop until the rate of red cell destruction has increased several-fold as initially erythropoiesis will increase to compensate. The red cell normally survives for about 120 days but in haemolytic anaemia the lifespan may be reduced to only a few days (Hoffbrand and Pettit, 1993).

Immune or metabolic mechanisms may be responsible for drug-induced haemolytic anaemia. The immune type may be further divided into hapten–membrane association, immune complex formation and autoimmune haemolysis. Penicillins, cephalosporins, tetracyclines and insulin have been reported to act as haptens which stimulate antibody production after binding to components of the red blood cell membrane. Antibodies are formed during initial exposure to the drug. During subsequent administration, the formed drug–antibody complexes activate the complement mechanism on the red cell membrane, resulting in cell lysis. In immune complex formation, the drug forms a complex with an immunoglobulin and a drug membrane-binding site. Activation of the complement cascade usually results in intravascular haemolysis with haemoglobinaemia and haemoglobinuria. Isoniazid, methotrexate, quinidine, quinine, rifampicin and sulphonylureas have been implicated. Haemolysis develops after the second or subsequent exposure to the drug (Gordon-Smith and Contreras, 1996).

In autoimmune haemolysis, the drug alters immune regulation so that autoantibodies are expressed against normal red blood cell antigens. This is more common than immune complex formation and has been associated with methyldopa, levodopa, mefenamic acid and azapropazone (Carey, 1995).

The Coombs test, which detects the presence of antibodies on red cells, can distinguish these immune mechanisms from other disorders which reduce the lifespan of red blood cells.

Red blood cells can also be damaged by drugs which have an oxidant effect on the cell membrane. These metabolic effects can occur in normal individuals but are more common in those deficient in glucose-6-phosphate dehydrogenase (G6PD), an enzyme required for the stability of red blood cells. Many drugs have been associated with haemolysis in G6PD deficiency, but only a few of these have proven haemolytic potential. Drugs which should be avoided in susceptible patients include nitrofurantoin, nalidixic acid, sulfamethoxazole and sulfasalazine (Lee and Rawlins, 1994). The *British National Formulary* gives further details.

Patients with haemolytic anaemia usually present acutely with symptoms of anaemia. They often have jaundice, haemoglobinuria (which may be marked enough to make the urine black in colour) and some will have renal impairment. Any implicated drug therapy should be withdrawn. Red cells usually return to normal within 2–3 weeks. Corticosteroid therapy is sometimes beneficial and some patients will require dialysis (Machin, 1996).

Megaloblastic anaemia

Megaloblastic anaemia results from impaired DNA synthesis while protein and RNA synthesis remain normal. It is usually due to folate or vitamin B_{12} deficiency. The mechanisms through which drugs cause megaloblastic anaemia are either by inhibiting DNA synthesis, for example, cytotoxic agents and zidovudine, or by reducing vitamin B_{12} or folate levels, for example, trimethoprim and antiepileptics (Love *et al.*, 1998). Table 9.6 lists implicated drugs.

The condition is characterised by a high mean cell volume (macrocytosis) and disordered maturation of haemopoietic cells. As a result,

Table 9.6 Drugs associated with megaloblastic anaemia

Aciclovir	Pentamidine
Alcohol	Proguanil
Antiepileptics	Pyrimethamine
Cycloserine	Sulfasalazine
Methotrexate	Triamterene
Nitrofurantoin	Trimethoprim
Oral contraceptives	

patients generally develop progressive symptoms of anaemia but, in severe cases, may also have leukopenia and thrombocytopenia. Neurological symptoms, such as neuropathy, may also be present with the legs more likley to be affected than the arms (Hoffbrand and Provan, 1997).

When given at therapeutic doses, folate reductase inhibitors, such as trimethoprim and pyrimethamine, do not normally induce megaloblastic anaemia but may worsen folate deficiency. Methotrexate-induced cases are dose-related and high doses require rescue therapy with calcium leucovorin. If megaloblastic anaemia develops in patients on antiepileptics, folic acid supplements are recommended (Machin, 1996).

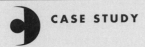

CASE STUDY

Mr P is a 38-year-old man who asks his community pharmacist to recommend something for influenza. On questioning, he has a sore throat, possibly a temperature and feels tired and miserable. The patient has a recent history of ulcerative colitis for which he takes sulfasalazine 500 mg four times a day and occasional loperamide.

What drug-induced disorder could the symptoms suggest?
Sore throat, malaise and fever are possible features of a blood dyscrasia. Haematological reactions are well recognised during sulfasalazine therapy and include agranulocytosis, aplastic anaemia, leukopenia, neutropenia and thrombocytopenia. The Committee on Safety of Medicines has warned that fatalities still occur despite the reaction being well established (Committee on Safety of Medicines, 1993b). The *British National Formulary* recommends that differential white cell, red cell and platelet counts are carried out initially and at monthly intervals for the first 3 months of sulfasalazine therapy. Some sources also recommend monitoring at 3-monthly intervals thereafter (Anon, 1997).

What information would help clarify the problem?
It is important to know how long Mr P has been taking sulfasalazine, whether he has seen a doctor about his current symptoms, and when he last had his blood count checked.

The pharmacist's patient medication records show that Mr P has been taking sulfasalazine for about 8 months. Mr P knows that his blood count has been checked regularly since he started taking the drug and that the results have always been normal. His blood count was normal at his last hospital appointment, which was only 3 weeks ago. His symptoms have been much better controlled recently and his consultant is pleased with his response to sulfasalazine.

Mr P feels sure that he has flu and that nothing more sinister is responsible for his symptoms. His wife has been in bed for the past 2 days with exactly the same symptoms. He has not been to see his GP.

What advice is appropriate?
Most cases of blood dyscrasia due to sulfasalazine will occur during the first 3 months after starting therapy but reactions can occur after months of treatment. The onset of these reactions can be very rapid and a normal blood count 3 weeks previously cannot be taken as reassurance that an adverse reaction has not occurred.

Mr P should be advised to see his GP as soon as possible to have his blood count checked. It is quite possible that he may have a viral infection but it is vital that any adverse effect of his medication is ruled out.

References

Anon. (1997). Drug-induced agranulocytosis. *Drug Ther Bull* 35: 49–52.

Carey P J (1995). Drug-induced haemocytopenias. *Adverse Drug React Bull* 175: 663–666.

Caron J, Libersa C, Thomas C (1996). Drugs affecting blood clotting, fibrinolysis and haemostasis. In: Dukes M N G, ed. *Meyler's Side Effects of Drugs*, 13th edn. Amsterdam: Elsevier Science, chapter 35.

Committee on Safety of Medicines (1993a). Drug-induced neutropenia and agranulocytosis. *Curr Probl Pharmacovigilance* 19: 10–11.

Committee on Safety of Medicines (1993b). Sulphasalazine and fatal blood dyscrasias. *Curr Probl Pharmacovigilance* 19: 6.

Gordon-Smith E C (1996). Aplastic anaemia and other causes of bone marrow failure. In: Weatherall D J, Ledingham J G G, Warrell D A, eds. *Oxford Textbook of Medicine*, 3rd edn. Oxford: Oxford Medical Publications, 3441–3449.

Gordon-Smith E C, Contreras M (1996). Acquired haemolytic anaemia. In: Weatherall D J, Ledingham J G G, Warrell D A, eds. *Oxford Textbook of Medicine*, 3rd edn. Oxford: Oxford Medical Publications, 3541–3551.

Heimpel H (1988). Drug-induced agranulocytosis. *Med Toxicol* 3: 449–462.

Hoffbrand V, Pettit J E (1993). *Essential Haematology*, 3rd edn. Oxford: Blackwell Scientific Publications.

Hoffbrand V, Provan D (1997). ABC of clinical haematology. Macrocytic anaemias. *Br Med J* 314: 430–433.

Holt D, Harvey D, Hurley R (1993). Chloramphenicol toxicity. *Adverse Drug React Toxicol Rev* 12: 83–95.

Inman W H W (1977). Study of fatal bone marrow depression with special reference to phenylbutazone and oxyphenbutazone. *Br Med J* i: 1500.

International Agranulocytosis and Aplastic Anaemia Study (1988). Risk of agranulocytosis and aplastic anaemia in relation to use of antithyroid drugs. *Br Med J* 297: 262–265.

Jackson G H, Proctor S J (1991). Disorders of blood cells. In: Davies D M, ed. *Textbook of Adverse Drug Reactions*, 4th edn. Oxford: Oxford University Press, chapter 22.

Lancaster T, Swart A M, Jick H (1998). Risk of serious haematological toxicity with use of chloramphenicol eye drops in a British general practice database. *Br Med J* 316: 667.

Laporte J-R, Vidal X, Ballarin E *et al.* (1998). Possible association between ocular chloramphenicol and aplastic anaemia – the absolute risk is very low. *Br J Clin Pharmacol* 46: 181–184.

Lee A, Rawlins M D (1994). Adverse drug reactions. In: Walker R, Edwards C, eds. *Clinical Pharmacy and Therapeutics*. London: Churchill Livingstone, chapter 3.

Liesner R J, Machin S J (1997). Platelet disorders. *Br Med J* 314: 809–812.

Love B B, Biller J, Gent M (1998). Adverse haematological effects of ticlopidine. *Drug Safety* 19: 89–98.

Machin S J (1996). Disorders of the blood. In: Weatherall D J, Ledingham J G G, Warrell D A, eds. *Oxford Textbook of Medicine,* 3rd edn. Oxford: Oxford University Press, 3373–3702.

Magee P, Beeley L (1994). Drug-induced blood disorders. In: Walker R, Edwards C, eds. *Clinical Pharmacy and Therapeutics*. London: Churchill Livingstone, chapter 46.

Manley R, Fearnley D, Patton W N *et al.* (1997). Syngeneic peripheral blood stem cell transplantation for severe aplastic anaemia. *Bone Marrow Transplant* 20: 1009–1010.

Marsh J, Schrezenmeier H, Marin P *et al.* (1999). Prospective randomised multicenter study comparing cyclosporin alone versus the combination of antithymocyte globulin and cyclosporin for treatment of patients with nonsevere aplastic anemia: a report from the European Blood and Marrow Transplant (EBMT) Severe Aplastic Anaemia Working Party. *Blood* 93: 2191–2195.

Patton W N, Duffull S B (1994). Idiosyncratic drug-induced haematological abnormalities. Incidence, pathogenesis, management and avoidance. *Drug Safety* 11: 445–462.

Pedersen-Bjergaard U, Andersen M, Hansen P B (1996). Thrombocytopenia induced by noncytotoxic drugs in Denmark 1968–91. *J Intern Med* 239: 509–515.

Pedersen-Bjergaard U, Andersen M, Hansen P B (1998). Drug-specific characteristics of thrombocytopenia caused by non-cytotoxic drugs. *Eur J Clin Pharmacol* 54: 701–706.

Pellock J M, Brodie M J (1997). Felbamate: 1997 update. *Epilepsia* 38: 1261–1264.

Rayner S A, Buckley R J (1996). Ocular chloramphenicol and aplastic anaemia. Is there a link? *Drug Safety* 14: 273–276.

Reiter E, Keil F, Brugger S *et al.* (1997). Excellent long-term survival after allogenic marrow transplantation in patients with severe aplastic anaemia. *Bone Marrow Transplant* 19: 1191–1196.

Rich M L, Ritterhoff R J, Hoffman R J (1950). A fatal case of aplastic anaemia following chloramphenicol therapy. *Ann Intern Med* 33: 1459–1467.

Sprinkkelman A, de Wolf J T M, Vellenga E (1994). The application of haemapoietic growth factors in drug-induced agranulocytosis: a review of 70 cases. *Leukemia* 8: 2031–2036.

Thompson D F, Gales M A (1996). Drug-induced pure red cell aplasia. *Pharmacotherapy* 16: 1002–1008.

van der Klauw M M, Goudsmit R, Halie R *et al.* (1999). A population-based case-cohort study of drug-associated agranulocytosis. *Arch Intern Med* 159: 369–374.

Vincent P C (1986). Drug-induced aplastic anaemia and agranulocytosis. Incidence and mechanisms. *Drugs* 31: 52–63.

Warkentin T E, Barkin R L (1999). Newer strategies for the treatment of heparin-induced thrombocytopenia. *Pharmacotherapy* 19: 181–195.

Warkentin T E, Levine M N, Hirsh J *et al.* (1995). Heparin-induced thrombocytopenia in patients treated with low-molecular-weight heparin or unfractionated heparin. *N Engl J Med* 332: 1330–1335.

Wiholm B E, Kelly J P, Kaufman D *et al.* (1998). Relation of aplastic anaemia to use of chloramphenicol eye drops in two international case-control studies. *Br Med J* 316: 666.

Yeh S P, Hsueh E J, Wu H *et al.* (1998). Ticlopidine-associated aplastic anemia. A case report and review of literature. *Ann Hematol* 76: 87–90.

Yonekura S, Kawada H, Watanabe S *et al.* (1997). Hematologic response in patients with aplastic anaemia after long-term administration of recombinant human granulocyte colony-stimulating factor and erythropoietin. *Clin Ther* 19: 1394–1407.

Young N S (1995). Aplastic anaemia. *Lancet* 346: 228–232.

Young N S, Barrett A J (1995). The treatment of severe acquired aplastic anaemia. *Blood* 12: 3367–3377.

Yunis M (1973). Chloramphenicol-induced bone marrow suppression. *Semin Hematol* 10: 225–234.

Yunis M (1989). Chloramphenicol toxicity: 25 years of research. *Am J Med* 87: 44–48.

10

Mental health disorders

Susan Bishop

Drug-induced mental health disorders, which are relatively common, include depression, mania, psychosis and confusion. This chapter discusses the types of mental health problem that may occur and the drugs most commonly implicated. Neuroleptic malignant syndrome and the serotonin syndrome are briefly reviewed, as is the problem of psychiatric morbidity due to drug misuse.

Most adverse psychiatric effects of drugs are classified as type A reactions, as they are dose-related or predictable, based on the drug's pharmacological profile, although a few are idiosyncratic type B reactions. The relationship between the time the causative drug was started and the appearance of psychiatric symptoms can be unpredictable, occurring either insidiously or abruptly during drug use. Psychiatric symptoms are also a common feature of withdrawal reactions, which can occur after certain drug therapy is stopped, particularly when the drug is stopped abruptly.

The risk of an individual experiencing a psychiatric reaction to a drug is greater if mental illness is already present or has occurred in the past. Other predisposing factors include impaired cerebral function, as in the elderly or patients with brain damage, alcohol or drug abuse, concurrent physical disease and stressful environments, such as intensive treatment units (Davison and Hassanyeh, 1991). There may also be more than one predisposing factor; for example, people with mental health disorders are more likely to misuse alcohol and other substances (Hall and Farrell, 1997).

There are many difficulties associated with the recognition and diagnosis of drug-induced mental health disorders. In patients with a history of mental health problems, symptoms may be attributed to underlying illness rather than drug therapy. In addition, affected patients may be unable to give a reliable history of their symptoms and the stigma attached to mental illness may hinder an accurate diagnosis. The inconsistent use of terms to describe, or classify, psychiatric and personality disorders is another issue. Greater awareness and use of the existing classification systems might improve identification, recording and recognition of these reactions. Underlying physical problems, such as dehydration or thyroid dysfunction, should be excluded before confirming a drug-related event (Table 10.1).

Table 10.1 Some conditions that may cause or mimic mental illness

Cushing's syndrome	Pernicious anaemia
Electrolyte imbalance	Renal dysfunction
Neurological disorders	Thyroid disease

Many drugs implicated in psychiatric reactions can cause more than one type of effect. For example, levodopa can cause delirium, depression, paranoid delusional psychosis and mania (Saint-Cyr *et al.*, 1993), and phenytoin can cause delirium, hallucinations and psychoses (Reynolds and Trimble, 1985). With some medications, mood disorder is the predominant change, and some may lead to psychosis. Drug-induced mental health disorders are usually considered serious reactions; in the UK the Committee on Safety of Medicines classifies confusion, depression, drug dependence, hallucinations, psychosis and withdrawal syndromes as serious reactions.

Depression

Depressive reactions to drugs vary from, at one end of the scale, mild mood changes to more severe mood change featuring sleep disturbance, loss of appetite and weight, and suicidal ideas at the other extreme. Depression is common and an association with prescribed drugs may be coincidental. However, a number of drugs have been consistently implicated in a large number of cases (Table 10.2). If the symptoms resolve following withdrawal of the suspect drug, this suggests that the drug may have been responsible.

Abnormalities in the neurotransmitter systems involving noradrenaline (norepinephrine), serotonin and dopamine are thought to underlie depression. Some older antihypertensives, probably because of their effects on these neurotransmitters, can induce or worsen depression. For example, methyldopa, which causes central depletion of serotonin and dopamine, may cause depressive symptoms in up to 10% of patients (Beers and Passman, 1990). It should not be used in patients with a history of depression.

Table 10.2 Some drugs that may cause depression

Antimicrobials Ciprofloxacin Sulphonamides	Carbamazepine Levodopa Phenothiazines
Cardiovascular drugs Beta-blockers Calcium channel blockers Digoxin Methyldopa Statins	**Hormones** Corticosteroids Oestrogens Progestogens
Drugs acting on the central nervous system Alcohol Amantadine Amfetamines (withdrawal) Benzodiazepines	**Miscellaneous** Disulfiram Interferon alfa Isotretinoin Mefloquine Metoclopramide Non-steroidal anti-inflammatory drugs

Mood changes, as well as sleep disturbances, delirium and hallucinations, have also been linked with beta-blockers (Lim and MacDonald, 1996). These effects may occur irrespective of whether or not the drug crosses the blood–brain barrier. Ophthalmic administration of beta-blockers in glaucoma leads to systemic absorption and is not devoid of these effects. Beta-blockers can also cause physical complaints such as lethargy and fatigue which may be mistaken for symptoms of depression.

Calcium channel blockers have been reported to cause depression and have been linked to an increased risk of suicide (Hullett *et al.*, 1988; Eccleston and Cole, 1990; Lyndon *et al.*, 1991; Lindberg *et al.*, 1998). Whether the relationship is causal or not requires confirmation. Calcium is believed to have a role in the pathophysiology of both depression and mania. Calcium channel blockers are sometimes used for their mood-stabilising properties in patients with bipolar or rapid cycling disorder who have not responded to conventional treatments such as lithium or carbamazepine. The use of calcium channel blockers in this indication is not licensed in the UK and should only be undertaken with caution and careful monitoring of efficacy and adverse effects.

The potential for cholesterol-lowering drugs such as simvastatin, pravastatin and lovastatin to affect mood has received a lot of attention. In 1996 psychiatric disorders represented 15% of all reactions to statins recorded in Norway's database of spontaneous reports. Adverse effects included aggression, nervousness, depression, anxiety and sleep distur-bances. The effect of statins on mental health has been investigated (Harrison and Ashton, 1994; Muldoon *et al.*, 2000). Researchers have also considered the risk of depression and suicide associated with lower-ing serum cholesterol by other means such as diet and in populations with a baseline of low serum cholesterol (Wardle *et al.*, 2000). A large prospective epidemiological study in Finland examined the association between serum total cholesterol, self-reported depression and hospital admission. The results suggested that depression is the primary event and that the decline in serum total cholesterol is a secondary occurrence. It was postulated that low serum cholesterol may be used to predict the subsequent risk of admission to hospital because of depression or suicide (Partonen *et al.*, 1999). Other experimental work has deter-mined an association between serotonin, which has a role in the causa-tion of depression, and impulsive behaviour and low cholesterol (Kaplan *et al.*, 1997; Buydens-Branchey *et al.*, 2000).

In the UK the Committee on Safety of Medicines highlighted the observation that 5% of all reported reactions to the retinoid isotretinoin are psychiatric reactions, including depression and suicide (Committee on Safety of Medicines, 1998). Although such problems could be more common among patient populations suffering from severe acne, a posi-tive rechallenge was reported in some patients (Anon, 1998b).

Depression may develop in the context of substance abuse. For example, people who use amphetamines may have flashbacks, which are acute hallucinations or recurrence of the initial drug experience. This may cause acute distress, evolving into panic disorder, depression and suicide. Withdrawal from amfetamines can precipitate depression, irri-tability, fatigue, insomnia or hypersomnia or anxiety.

Psychosis

Characteristic features of psychosis include distorted personality, delu-sions and hallucinations. Delusions are firmly sustained, false personal beliefs. Paranoid delusions feature persecution. Delusions may occur with or without hallucinations. Hallucinations are uncontrolled false sensory perceptions which have no real external stimuli. Visual halluci-nations are more commonly induced by drugs than auditory hallucina-tions. Table 10.3 lists some drugs that may cause psychosis.

There is a high incidence (10–30%) of psychiatric effects with drugs used in the management of Parkinson's disease. Antimuscarinic agents such as trihexyphenidyl (benzhexol) and procyclidine can cause

Table 10.3 Some drugs that may cause psychosis

Amantadine	Ganciclovir
Amfetamines	Histamine H_2-receptor antagonists
Anticholinergics	Isoniazid
Antiepileptics	Levodopa
Bromocriptine	Mefloquine
Chloroquine	Non-steroidal anti-inflammatory drugs
Clonidine	Quinidine
Digoxin	Quinolone antibiotics
Disulfiram	Zolpidem

disorientation, agitation and visual hallucinations. Levodopa has been associated with a much wider range of effects, including acute confusion, depression, delirium, delusions, euphoria, hallucinations, inappropriate sexual behaviour and mania (Saint-Cyr et al., 1993). Confusion, agitation, delusions and hallucinations are encountered more often in older patients. The overall incidence of hallucinations is believed to be about 20%. Psychoses, visual hallucinations and confusional states are serious enough to warrant drug discontinuation in about 10% of patients. The effects are usually dose-related and resolve on discontinuation. These complications are more common in patients with a previous psychiatric history and sometimes arise after many months of successful levodopa therapy. A withdrawal syndrome can develop on treatment discontinuation, featuring lethargy, anxiety, nightmares, depression and suicidal ideas. The possibility of levodopa-induced adverse effects illustrates how challenging the diagnosis of drug-induced mental health disorders can be.

Other dopaminergic drugs used in treating Parkinson's disease, such as bromocriptine, lisuride and pergolide, can cause hallucinations and other psychiatric effects.

Disulfiram is used as an aid to the management of alcohol misuse. It has been reported to cause psychosis and delirium (Daniel et al., 1987; Murthy, 1997). These effects are postulated to be due to inhibition of the dopamine beta-hydroxylase enzyme, leading to excess concentrations of dopamine. The rare delusion, Capgras syndrome, in which a relative or friend has been replaced by an identical double, has been reported (Daniel et al., 1987). Disulfiram should be discontinued if psychosis occurs; short-term use of benzodiazepines may be effective in its management.

Substance misuse is always considered in the differential diagnosis of a person who presents with psychotic symptoms. In the UK the misuse of drugs with the potential to cause psychosis is common, especially in people between the ages of 16 and 29 years.

Amfetamines produce a hallucinogenic experience, often referred to as psychedelic. LSD, methylenedioxymethamfetamine (MDMA or Ecstasy) and other amfetamine-related substances stimulate dopamine-sensitive adenylcyclase, leading to increased dopamine activity, and are also serotonin antagonists. Acute intoxication can result in short-lived psychotic symptoms which resolve within a day. Usually delusions, hallucinations and panic last for two days or more. Making the decision that these symptoms are associated with amfetamine intoxication is often difficult because there can be a delay between taking the drug and onset of psychosis. Long-term use of amfetamines may lead to development of a chronic psychosis: paranoid ideas, bizarre thinking (often with religious content and grandiosity), disturbed memory, hallucinations and illusions.

Khat (also called qat or miraa) is a plant substance which is widely used, normally chewed, in some cultures. It contains cathinone, which has stimulant effects. Cathinone is controlled under the Misuse of Drugs Act (1971) but khat is not. A reaction similar to amfetamine psychosis has been reported. Other psychological reactions include sleep disturbance, anxiety and depression (Griffiths *et al.*, 1997).

Cannabis-induced psychosis is characterised differently with symptoms of acute paranoid psychosis and feelings of panic. Many people with schizophrenia may abuse substances as a form of self-medication of distressing symptoms. Substance abuse is a common co-morbidity in as many as 50% of people with schizophrenia. Although substance abuse can precipitate relapse in a person predisposed to mental illness, it has not been conclusively shown to cause schizophrenia (Poole and Brabbins, 1996). Table 10.4 summarises the psychiatric symptoms that may be induced by drugs of abuse.

An association between the acetylcholinesterase inhibitor, donepezil, used to delay cognitive deterioration in Alzheimer's disease, and psychiatric disturbances, including hallucinations, agitation and aggressive behaviour, has recently been suggested (Anon, 1998a). Since psychiatric disturbances may coexist with Alzheimer's disease, these adverse effects may remain undetected.

For many years, chloroquine has been known to cause psychosis and behavioural toxicity, especially in the higher doses used to treat malaria (Philips-Howard and ter Kuile, 1995). The link between mefloquine and neuropsychiatric reactions has attracted much debate particularly about whether or not the risk of neuropsychiatric disorders is unacceptably high. Large observational studies suggest that

Table 10.4 Psychiatric symptoms induced by drugs of abuse

Cannabis
Dysphoria, anxiety, agitation and suspicion, distortions of time and space, reduced
  vigilance and unco-ordination, psychosis with confusion, hallucinations, delusions and emotional lability

CNS stimulants
High doses – agitation, panic attacks, impaired concentration. Transient or
  prolonged psychosis persisting for a few days after the drug is stopped

CNS depressants
Very high doses of benzodiazepines – amnesia, psychomotor impairment, aggressive and disinhibited behaviour

Hallucinogenic drugs
Alter perception, thoughts and feelings, causing pseudohallucinations (illusions)
  and hallucinations
May uncover mental illness
Prolonged use of LSD may lead to prolonged psychosis, resembling schizophrenia

---

severe neuropsychiatric reactions to prophylactic mefloquine occur at a frequency of around 1 in 10 000 to 1 in 20 000 patients (Committee on Safety of Medicines, 1996). Various reactions have been reported, including depression, anxiety, panic, confusion, hallucinations, paranoid delusions and convulsions. These reactions can be severe and protracted. Patients should be counselled about the risk of psychiatric symptoms with mefloquine and advised to seek medical advice promptly if these should develop. Prophylactic mefloquine is contraindicated in patients with a history of neuropsychiatric disturbance, including depression or convulsions.

Mania

The main clinical characteristic of mania is an elevated mood. Other features include overactivity, insomnia, rapid speech, grandiose ideas and disinhibition. Less severe forms of mania are termed hypomania (Peet and Peters, 1995). Drug-induced mania is rare, but symptoms of agitation or delirium may be misclassified as mania.

Usually the patients affected have a history of mood disorder. This was illustrated in a small study examining the effect of donepezil in reversing memory loss induced by antidepressants and mood stabilisers. Mania was triggered in two patients with pre-existing, but stabilised, bipolar disorder (Jacobsen and Comas-Diaz, 1999). Insomnia was also reported as an adverse effect of donepezil in this study. Studies with older cholinergic agonist drugs suggest that acetylcholine has a multi-faceted neurophysiological role in mood disorders, behaviour and sleep (Sunderland *et al.*, 1988).

Drugs with a clear tendency to cause manic symptoms include levodopa, corticosteroids and anabolic androgens (see Table 10.5). The onset of manic symptoms usually occurs early in the course of treatment or soon after a dose increase. Management involves stopping the offending drug and treating the remaining manic symptoms with an antipsychotic.

Mania may be precipitated by introducing or, more commonly, by increasing the dose of an antidepressant. All antidepressants probably have the potential to cause mania and it is a well-known adverse effect of tricyclic antidepressants. A switch from depression into mania has been reported in up to 10% of patients with bipolar disorder (Knight Laird and Benefield, 1995). Rapid cycling disorder, where there is a short period between manic and depressive episodes, may also be triggered. If the symptoms are recognised early enough, reducing the antidepressant dose may be sufficient to stabilise mood.

On rare occasions, withdrawal of an antidepressant can cause mania (Goldstein and Frye, 1999).

Manic episodes are among the most important manifestations of corticosteroid-induced psychiatric toxicity and there are many published case reports (Patten and Neutel, 2000). In one study, corticosteroid therapy was judged responsible for 54% of cases of mania seen by a psychiatric consultation service (Rundell and Wise, 1989). A prospective study investigated the neuropsychological effects of 8 days' treatment with oral methylprednisolone or fluorocortolone (dose ranging between 50 and 150 mg daily) in 50 ophthalmological patients (Naber *et al.*, 1996). The authors reported that 13 of 50 participants developed manic-like episodes and five developed a depressive syndrome. None of the episodes were severe and none were associated with psychotic symptoms.

Although this study was uncontrolled, the reported incidence of problems is much greater than expected. There are no clear predisposing factors for corticosteroid-induced psychiatric disturbances. However,

Table 10.5 Some drugs that may cause mania

Baclofen	Isoniazid
Bromocriptine	Levodopa
Chloroquine	Monoamine oxidase inhibitors
Corticosteroids	Tricyclic antidepressants
Dopaminergic agents	

there is good evidence of a dose–response relationship; doses above prednisone 40 mg daily (or equivalent) may be associated with an increased risk of problems (Patten and Neutel, 2000). Information relating to the management of such problems derives mainly from case reports; antidepressants, antipsychotics, lithium and electroconvulsive therapy have all been used. Eight patients from a chest clinic who were interviewed about their experience of long-term corticosteroid therapy indicated that they would have preferred to have been warned about the possibility of psychiatric adverse effects (Reckart and Eisendrath, 1990). Healthcare professionals should be more proactive in discussing the possibility of corticosteroid psychiatric adverse effects.

Behavioural toxicity

Drug-related disturbances in behaviour are common. Features include aggression, drowsiness, insomnia, vivid dreams, nightmares, restlessness, irritability and excitement. These symptoms may be the precursors of a more florid psychiatric disorder, such as delirium.

There is now greater awareness of the behavioural effects of antiepileptic drugs. These adverse effects may be the result of the action of these drugs on central gamma-aminobutyric acid neurotransmission producing inhibition, or on the excitatory glutamate system. Barbiturates can produce drowsiness, depression and delirium. Recognition of the behavioural toxicity of the barbiturates, particularly in children, means they are seldom used in children with epilepsy (Ferrari *et al.*, 1983). Lamotrigine has been associated with sleep disturbance, agitation and confusion, irritability and aggression. Aggressive behaviour was reported in a series of patients with learning disability who required dose reduction or discontinuation of treatment.

Vigabatrin is associated with drowsiness and fatigue, but in children excitation and agitation are more often seen. In addition, some patients have experienced confusion and memory disturbance. Post-marketing surveillance has identified more severe effects on mental health, including aggression, depression, psychosis and mania. Consequently vigabatrin should be used with caution in people with a history of psychosis or behavioural problems. However, pre-existing mental illness is not a prerequisite for these effects to ocur.

Agitation and insomnia are now being recognised as adverse effects of acetylcholinesterase inhibitors used in the management of Alzheimer's disease (Dooley and Lamb, 2000; Greenberg *et al.*, 2000; Spencer and Noble, 1998).

The new-generation antihistamines and antipsychotics that have been developed have resulted in drugs with fewer effects on behaviour. For example, traditional antihistamines such as diphenhydramine cross the blood–brain barrier and cause drowsiness and impaired attention, memory and psychomotor functioning (Kay *et al.*, 1997). In contrast, the non-sedating antihistamine loratadine has been shown to have effects on fatigue, cognitive functioning and driving performance similar to placebo.

Newer atypical antipsychotics such as olanzapine and risperidone seem to have fewer adverse effects on behaviour (insomnia, restlessness, bizarre dreams, social withdrawal and cognitive impairment) than conventional antipsychotics (Hollister, 1961).

Confusion

Patients suffering from an acute confusional state have a short attention span. They often appear perplexed or bewildered and have difficulty following questions or commands. There may also be disorientation and poor memory. The main risk factors for confusional states (including delirium and dementia) are old age, pre-existing cognitive impairment, severe chronic illness and unfamiliar surroundings. Acute confusion may be induced by psychotropic drugs but many other drug classes, including histamine H_2-receptor antagonists, beta-blockers, corticosteroids and non-steroidal anti-inflammatory drugs may be responsible. Most drug-induced confusional states resolve on withdrawal of the implicated drug, although resolution may be complicated by drugs given for symptom control.

Delirium

Delirium may be defined as a disturbance of consciousness (reduced clarity of awareness of the environment) and change in cognition that develop over a short period of time (Mayou, 1996). As in confusion, there is disorientation and reduced attention but the picture is more florid and the disorientation more profound. The patient may become frightened, bewildered, restless and often hostile. Delirium is frequently under-recognised and may be misdiagnosed as dementia or other psychiatric illness or attributed to the ageing process. The hallmark of delirium is an acute onset and a fluctuating course (Gray *et al.*, 1999). In contrast, the cognitive deficits associated with dementia tend to develop insidiously and do not fluctuate throughout the day. The incidence of delirium is difficult to determine because of major differences in available studies in design, methodology and study population (Carter *et al.*, 1996; Gray *et al.*, 1999). It is estimated that 10–16% of elderly patients have delirium at the time of hospital admission and 18–38% experience delirium during the hospital stay (Gray *et al.*, 1999).

Drugs may be the most frequent single cause of delirium and very often they are important where there are multiple contributing factors. In practice, patients with delirium are often taking multiple medications, several of which may be a possible cause.

Epidemiological studies that have evaluated several drug classes as risk factors for delirium have shown inconsistent results. However, benzodiazepines, opioids, anticholinergics and tricyclic antidepressants are probably the worst offenders.

Dementia

Dementia presents as a deterioration of intellect, memory and personality. Consciousness is not impaired. Anxiety, lability of mood and depression may develop. The prevalence of dementia increases significantly with age, affecting 25–48% of those older than 85 years of age (Gray *et al.*, 1999). Compared with delirium, even less is known about the prevalence of drug-induced dementia. Drug toxicity may contribute to symptoms in more than 10% of patients presenting with dementia (Moore and O'Keeffe, 1999). Among 308 outpatients with dementia, 35 were found to have an adverse drug reaction that contributed to the cognitive impairment (Larson *et al.*, 1987). In about two-thirds of these patients additional causes of impairment were identified (e.g. Alzheimer's disease). Discontinuation or modification of the suspect drug(s) resulted in improvement in cognition for all patients.

Symptoms of depression in the elderly are occasionally mistaken for dementia. This is known as pseudodementia and this diagnosis should be excluded before considering a drug-related cause for dementia. There is considerable overlap between the features of dementia and delirium. Many drug classes can cause delirium or dementia in susceptible individuals, but some drug classes are associated with a greater risk. Drugs implicated as a cause of delirium or dementia are shown in Table 10.6.

Atropine and other anticholinergic drugs are well known to cause delirium, as well as disorientation, confusion and visual hallucinations or pseudohallucinations. These effects can occur together with physical symptoms, such as urinary retention and narrow pupils, known as the central anticholinergic syndrome (Longo, 1966). Features resolve quickly when the causative drug is withdrawn. Procyclidine and orphenadrine are known to have abuse potential, probably due to their euphoric effect. Misuse may cause hallucinations, intensified perceptions, impaired judgement, delusional disorder, anxiety and depression. The use of anticholinergics to relieve the extrapyramidal side-effects of antipsychotics should be minimised and their use should be subject to ongoing review. Sedative antihistamine preparations, such as diphenhydramine which is marketed as a hypnotic in some countries, produce signs of central anticholinergic toxicity when taken in excess. Many other drug classes have anticholinergic properties, including tricyclic antidepressants, antipsychotics and antiarrhythmics.

Delirium is a possible consequence of toxicity due to lithium and digoxin. Postoperative analgesic-induced confusion and delirium is also a significant problem.

Steps that may be taken to minimise the incidence of delirium, particularly in elderly patients, include avoiding medication known to cause delirium wherever possible, using the lowest effective dose and monitoring carefully those patients receiving more than one drug with central nervous system effects. Effective management of delirium involves early recognition of the condition, identification and withdrawal of the causative drug, management of agitation and disruptive behaviour and supportive care. Drugs that may produce confusion should be stopped or the dosage reduced where possible. Supportive care, such as ensuring adequate sleep, nutrition, hydration, and providing emotional reassurance is important for managing the patient with delirium (Gray *et al.*, 1999). If symptoms cannot be managed with supportive care, pharmacological treatment may be required (Carter *et al.*, 1996). Treatment may be required for aggression, risk of harm to self or others, hallucinations, distress or insomnia. Benzodiazepines (diazepam or lorazepam) and/or a short-acting antipsychotic may be used. The use of psychotropic medication can further complicate the assessment of mental state and diagnosis in delirious patients (Meagher *et al.*, 1996).

Table 10.6 Some drugs that may cause delirium or dementia

Antiarrhythmics	Benzodiazepines
Antibacterials	Corticosteroids
Anticholinergic agents	Disulfiram
Antidepressants	Dopaminergic agonists
Antiepileptics	Histamine H_2-antagonists
Antipsychotics	Lithium
Antituberculous drugs	Opioid analgesics

Psychiatric manifestations of drug withdrawal reactions

Adverse effects can be caused by withdrawal of treatment with several classes of drug (Table 10.7). The key to identifying a true withdrawal effect is to determine whether symptoms are alleviated by readministration of the drug, but this is not always clinically indicated or necessary. The mechanisms behind drug withdrawal reactions are unclear but are thought to involve loss of normal homoeostatic control in the nervous, endocrine, haematological and cardiovascular systems (Routledge and Bialas, 1997). Stopping a drug with complex effects on body systems may induce an imbalance in these body systems, resulting in both psychological and physical symptoms.

Delirium tremens, experienced within 48–72 hours of stopping chronic excessive alcohol intake, is characterised by disorientation, hallucinations, convulsions and increased psychomotor and autonomic activity (Johns, 1996).

Rapid withdrawal after short-term use of benzodiazepines may cause rebound insomnia and anxiety. Withdrawal after chronic use (4–6 weeks or longer) gives rise to significant and often intolerable symptoms, including severe anxiety, perceptual changes, convulsions or delirium (Menkes and Laverty, 1991). Up to 90% of long-term (more than 3 months) benzodiazepine users experience symptoms on discontinuation, especially if stopped abruptly. Gradual withdrawal over a period of weeks or months will reduce the risk of withdrawal reactions.

A withdrawal syndrome can occur when tricyclic antidepressants are stopped suddenly. Symptoms include anxiety, nightmares, nausea and vomiting, dizziness, headache, muscular aches and akathisia (Garner *et al.*, 1993). In addition to these symptoms, abrupt withdrawal of monoamine oxidase inhibitors (MAOIs) can lead to delirium, auditory and visual hallucinations, and schizophreniform psychosis. The incidence of this syndrome has been reported to be as high as 32% (Tyrer, 1984). Chronic administration of MAOIs leads to down-regulation and subsensitisation of $alpha_2$ and dopamine autoreceptors which control the release of noradrenaline and dopamine. Sudden withdrawal

Table 10.7 Some drugs implicated in withdrawal reactions

Alcohol	Barbiturates
Anticholinergic agents	Benzodiazepines
Antidepressants	Sympathomimetics
Baclofen	

of the MAOI leads to release of noradrenaline (norepinephrine) and dopamine. This mechanism is thought to be similar to that underlying amphetamine withdrawal syndromes (Joyce and Walsh, 1983; Liskin *et al.*, 1985; Naylor *et al.*, 1987; Dilsaver, 1988).

Symptoms due to withdrawal of tricyclic and MAOI antidepressants usually arise within a few days to two weeks after stopping treatment. This helps to differentiate withdrawal symptoms from relapse of depression, which tends to take longer to appear. Abrupt withdrawal of selective serotonin reuptake inhibitors (SSRIs) can lead to sleep disturbance, dizziness, behavioural disturbance, tremor and dyskinesias (Pacheco *et al.*, 1996; Young *et al.*, 1997). All SSRIs have been associated with a withdrawal syndrome, although the problem appears to be more common with paroxetine (Price *et al.*, 1996). In a recent randomised controlled trial in 242 patients receiving maintenance treatment with fluoxetine, sertraline or paroxetine, therapy was interrupted with placebo for 5–8 days (Rosenbaum *et al.*, 1998). Significantly fewer patients on fluoxetine experienced new somatic and psychological symptoms. It has been postulated that paroxetine is more likely to cause withdrawal symptoms than other SSRIs due to its shorter half-life and its more potent anticholinergic effects.

Because of the potential for withdrawal phenomena, antidepressants should not be stopped abruptly (unless a serious adverse effect has occurred). Instead, treatment should be tapered gradually. There is no fixed timescale for this but, if symptoms occur, restarting the antidepressant and subsequently withdrawing it more slowly should resolve the problem. It is also important to reassure patients who experience these effects that antidepressants are not addictive.

Serotonin syndrome

Serotonin syndrome is a rare condition which is becoming increasingly well recognised in patients receiving combinations of serotonergic drugs. It arises as a result of the pharmacodynamic interaction that can occur when two or more drugs that increase serotonin are given at the same time or after one such drug is stopped and another started. It is characterised by a variety of symptoms, including confusion, disorientation, abnormal movements, exaggerated reflexes, fever, sweating, diarrhoea and hypotension or hypertension (Sporer, 1995). Diagnosis is made when three or more of these symptoms are present and no other cause can be found. Symptoms usually develop within hours of starting the second drug but occasionally they can occur later.

Drug-induced serotonin syndrome is generally mild and resolves when the offending drugs are stopped. However, it can be severe and deaths have occurred (Gravlin, 1997). A large number of drugs has been implicated, including tricyclic antidepressants, MAOIs, SSRIs, pethidine, dextromethorphan and lithium. The most severe type of reaction has occurred with the combination of SSRIs and MAOIs. Both non-selective MAOIs, such as phenelzine, and selective MAOIs, such as moclobemide and selegiline, have been implicated (Lane and Baldwin, 1997).

Serotonin syndrome is best prevented by not using serotonergic drugs in combination, although occasionally combination therapy is used intentionally. Special care is needed when changing from an SSRI to an MAOI and vice versa. The SSRIs, particularly fluoxetine, have long half-lives and serotonin syndrome may occur if a sufficient wash-out period is not allowed. When changing from an SSRI to an MAOI, the guidance in manufacturers' summaries of product characteristics should be followed. When changing from an MAOI to an SSRI, a 2-week gap should be allowed before starting the SSRI.

It may be difficult to distinguish serotonin syndrome from the clinical features of depression, adverse effects and withdrawal effects. However, healthcare professionals should be aware of this rare but potentially serious problem and the combinations of drugs that can cause it. Special care should be taken with over-the-counter cough and cold remedies containing dextromethorphan, as serotonin syndrome has been reported when this was given in combination with MAOIs or the SSRIs paroxetine and fluoxetine (Stockley, 1999).

Neuroleptic malignant syndrome

Neuroleptic malignant syndrome is a rare but life-threatening adverse reaction to antipsychotic drugs. It is characterised by fever, rigidity, altered mental status and autonomic dysfunction (Najib, 1997). Laboratory investigations usually reveal a leukocytosis together with markedly raised levels of creatine phosphokinase. The syndrome is believed to be due to depletion of dopamine both centrally and peripherally. Virtually all dopamine receptor antagonists have been associated with the syndrome, although phenothiazines and butyrophenones are most frequently implicated. Potential risk factors include dehydration, mood disorder, Parkinson's disease, male gender, high dosage and intramuscular drug administration.

Neuroleptic malignant syndrome appears to affect 0.4–1.4% of patients on antipsychotic drugs (Cranston, 1996). It frequently occurs within a week of the initiation of an oral antipsychotic or within 4 weeks of the first dose of a depot preparation. It can lead to various complications, including rhabdomyolysis, aspiration pneumonia, renal failure and disseminated intravascular coagulation. Neuroleptic malignant syndrome is a medical emergency; the associated mortality is 15–25%.

Antipsychotic drug treatment should be withdrawn immediately if the syndrome is suspected. Management in an intensive care facility may be needed to deal with cardiovascular, respiratory and renal complications. Supportive care is the mainstay of treatment, including temperature reduction and fluid and electrolyte replacement. There is no known specific treatment but bromocriptine has been used, with variable efficacy, in an attempt to restore brain dopaminergic function. Dantrolene is often given to reduce muscle rigidity and its use appears to be beneficial. The syndrome can last for up to 10 days after drug discontinuation, or longer if depot preparations have been given. Patients who have recovered from the syndrome can be cautiously restarted on another antipsychotic, if treatment is essential.

Management of drug-induced psychiatric disturbances

Healthcare professionals have an important role in preventing psychiatric morbidity due to prescribed or over-the-counter medicines. The general principles of ensuring that drug therapy is needed, avoiding polypharmacy and using the minimum effective dose are important. In addition, drugs to be prescribed should be screened for their potential central nervous system effects. Drugs known or suspected to have psychiatric adverse effects should be introduced and withdrawn gradually whenever possible.

When a psychiatric reaction to a drug is suspected, the drug should be withdrawn wherever possible. There may be reluctance to do this when a patient is being treated with the drug for an existing mental health problem. Correspondingly, rechallenge may be more often attempted in such patients. Specialists (e.g. psychiatrists or clinical pharmacists) will be able to review previous drug treatment and advise on future treatment options and the risks of rechallenge. In addition, pharmacists will be able to give guidance on how to taper medication to minimise the risk of withdrawal reactions and how best to go about switching from one drug to another.

Most psychiatric adverse drug events resolve quickly. Short-term use of minor tranquillisers, or non-drug treatments, may be sufficient management options. If the symptoms persist and present a danger to the health of the patient or others, treatments such as electroconvulsive therapy for depressive symptoms and antipsychotics may be necessary.

 CASE STUDY

Mrs K, an elderly woman, asks for advice about her husband as over the past few weeks she has become increasingly concerned about his state of mind. Mr K is 72 years old and was diagnosed with Parkinson's disease 2 years ago. He has seemed a bit confused recently, is not sleeping well and, most worrying of all, he has started to complain of seeing people in the house who are not really there. Mrs K is worried that her husband may be suffering from dementia, although his memory seems fine. He has never had any mental illness in the past. Mr K began treatment for Parkinson's disease about 18 months ago and he is currently taking co-beneldopa.

Could Mr K's problem be drug-induced?
Levodopa can cause many psychiatric manifestations, including confusion (about 13% of patients), sleep disturbances (20%) and hallucinations (30%). Hallucinations often occur at night, are usually visual and are not threatening initially but may in time become frightening. Auditory hallucinations are rare. Psychotic features and dementia can also complicate Parkinson's disease, irrespective of the prescribed medication.

Mr K will probably need to see the specialist who is treating his Parkinson's disease to discuss his drug therapy. It is important that Mr K does not change his medication in the meantime.

What changes to Mr K's drug therapy might be appropriate?
In patients with moderate or advanced Parkinson's disease, stopping levodopa therapy may be impossible because this may cause inability to walk, speak or swallow. A reduction in levodopa dose may help the hallucinations and it may be possible to titrate the dose downward until a compromise between neuropsychiatric and motor symptoms is obtained.

If necessary, which antipsychotic can be recommended for a patient with Parkinson's disease?
The management of psychosis in a patient with Parkinson's disease is a challenging clinical problem, as most antipsychotics are potent dopamine antagonists and can worsen Parkinson's disease. If an antipsychotic is indicated, an agent which is less selective for dopamine, such as risperidone or olanzapine, may be tried.

References

Anon. (1998a). Donepezil update. *Drug Ther Bull* 36: 60–61.

Anon. (1998b). Isotretinoin-associated depression. *WHO Drug Inf* 12: 84.

Beers M H, Passman L J (1990). Antihypertensive medications and depression. *Drugs* 40: 792–799.

Buydens-Branchey L, Branchey M, Hudson J, Fergeson P (2000). Low HDL cholesterol, aggression and altered central serotonergic activity. *Psychiatry Res* 93: 93–102.

Carter G L, Dawson A H, Lopert R. (1996). Drug-induced delirium: incidence, management and prevention. *Drug Safety* 15: 291–301.

Committee on Safety of Medicines (1996). Mefloquine (Lariam) and neuropsychiatric reactions. *Curr Probl Pharmacovigilance* 22: 6.

Committee on Safety of Medicines (1998). In focus. Isotretinoin (Roaccutane). *Curr Probl Pharmacovigilance* 24: 12.

Cranston W L (1996). Drug-induced diseases of body temperature. In: Weatherall D J, Ledingham J G G, Warrell D A, eds. *Oxford Textbook of Medicine*, 3rd edn. Oxford: Oxford University Press, 1181–1182.

Daniel D G, Swallows A, Wolff F (1987). Capgras delusion and seizures in association with therapeutic dosages of disulfiram. *South Med J* 80: 1577–1579.

Davison K, Hassanyeh F (1991). Psychiatric disorders. In: Davies D M, ed. *Textbook of Adverse Drug Reactions*, 4th edn. Oxford: Oxford University Press, chapter 21.

Dilsaver S C (1988). Monoamine oxidase inhibitor withdrawal phenomena: symptoms and pathophysiology. *Acta Psychiatr Scand* 78: 1–7.

Dooley M, Lamb H M (2000). Donepezil: a review of its use in Alzheimer's disease. *Drugs Aging* 16: 199–226.

Eccleston D, Cole A J (1990). Calcium channel blockade and depressive illness. *Br J Psychiatry* 156: 889–891.

Ferrari M, Barabas G, Schempp Matthews W (1983). Psychologic and behavioral disturbance among epileptic children treated with barbiturate anticonvulsants. *Am J Psychiatry* 140: 112–113.

Garner E M, Kelly M W, Thompson D F (1993). Tricyclic antidepressant withdrawal syndrome. *Ann Pharmacother* 27: 1068–1072.

Goldstein T R, Frye M A (1999). Antidepressant discontinuation-related mania: critical prospective observation and theoretical implications in bipolar disorder. *J Clin Psychiatry* 60: 563–567.

Gravlin M A (1997). Serotonin syndrome: what causes it, how to recognise it and ways to avoid it. *Hosp Pharm* 32: 570–575.

Gray S L, Lai K V, Larson E B (1999). Drug-induced cognition disorders in the elderly: incidence, prevention and management. *Drug Safety* 21: 101–122.

Greenberg S M, Tennis M K, Brown L B et al. (2000). Donepezil therapy in clinical practice: a randomised crossover study. *Arch Neurol* 57: 94–99.

Griffiths P, Gossop M, Wickenden S et al. (1997). A transcultural pattern of drug use: qat (khat) in the UK. *Br J Psychiatry* 170: 281–284.

Hall W, Farrell M (1997). Comorbidity of mental disorders with substance abuse. *Br J Psychiatry* 171: 4–5.

Harrison R W, Ashton C H (1994). Do cholesterol-lowering agents affect brain activity? A comparison of simvastatin, pravastatin and placebo in healthy volunteers. *Br J Clin Pharmacol* 37: 231–236.

Hollister L E (1961). Current concepts in therapy. Complications from psychotherapeutic drugs. *N Engl J Med* 264: 291–293, 345–347, 399–400.

Hullett F J, Potkin S G, Levy A B, Ciasca R (1988). Depression associated with nifedipine-induced calcium channel blockade. *Am J Psychiatry* 145: 1277–1279.

Jacobsen F M, Comas-Diaz L (1999). Donepezil for psychotropic-induced memory loss. *J Clin Psychiatry* 60: 698–704.

Johns A R (1996). Management of withdrawal syndromes. In: Weatherall D J, Ledingham J G G, Warrell D A, eds. *Oxford Textbook of Medicine*, 3rd edn. Oxford: Oxford University Press, 4290–4294.

Joyce P R, Walsh J (1983). Nightmares during phenelzine withdrawal. *J Clin Psychopharmacol* 4: 121.

Kaplan J R, Muldoon M F, Manuck S B, Mann J J (1997). Assessing the observed relationship between low cholesterol and violence-related mortality. Implications for suicide risk. *Ann N Y Acad Sci* 836: 57–80.

Kay G G, Berman B, Mockoviak S H *et al.* (1997). Initial and steady state effects of diphenhydramine and loratadine on sedation, cognition, mood and psychomotor performance. *Arch Intern Med* 157: 2350–2356.

Knight Laird L, Benefield W H (1995). Mood disorders l: major depressive disorders. In: Young L Y, Koda-Kimble M A, eds. *Applied Therapeutics: The Clinical Use of Drugs*, 6th edn. Vancouver: Applied Therapeutics, 76.1–76.28.

Lane R, Baldwin D (1997). Selective serotonin reuptake inhibitor-induced serotonin syndrome: a review. *J Clin Psychopharmacol* 17: 208.

Larson E B, Kukull W A, Katzman R L (1987). Adverse drug reactions associated with global cognitive impairment in elderly persons. *Ann Intern Med* 107: 169–173.

Lim P O, MacDonald T M (1996). Antianginal and beta-adrenoceptor blocking drugs. In: Dukes M N G, ed. *Meyler's Side Effects of Drugs*, 13th edn. Amsterdam: Elsevier Science, chapter 18.

Lindberg G, Bingefors K, Ranstam J *et al.* (1998). Use of calcium channel blockers and risk of suicide: ecological findings confirmed in population based cohort study. *Br Med J* 316: 741–745.

Liskin B, Roose S P, Walsh B T, Jackson W K (1985). Acute psychosis following phenelzine discontinuation. *J Clin Psychopharmacol* 5: 46–47.

Longo V G (1966). Behavioural and EEG effects of atropine and related compounds. *Pharmacol Rev* 18: 965.

Lyndon R W, Johnson G, McKeough G (1991). Nifedipine induced depression. *Br J Psychiatry* 159: 447–448.

Mayou R A (1996). Organic (cognitive) mental disorders. In: Weatherall D J, Ledingham J G G, Warrell D A, eds. *Oxford Textbook of Medicine*, 3rd edn. Oxford: Oxford University Press, 4223–4226.

Meagher D J, O'Hanlon D, O'Mahoney E *et al.* (1996). The use of environmental strategies and psychotropic medication in the management of delirium. *Br J Psychiatry* 168: 512–515.

Menkes D B, Laverty R (1991). Hypnotics and sedatives. In: Davies D M, ed. *Textbook of Adverse Drug Reactions,* 4th edn. Oxford: Oxford University Press, chapter 5.

Moore A R, O'Keeffe S T (1999). Drug induced cognitive impairment in the elderly. *Drugs Aging* 15: 15–28.

Muldoon M F, Barger S D, Ryan C M *et al.* (2000). Effects of lovastatin on cognitive function and psychological well being. *Am J Med* 108: 538–546.

Murthy K K (1997). Psychosis during disulfiram therapy for alcoholism. *J Indian Med Assoc* 95: 80–81.

Naber D, Sand P, Heigl P (1996). Psychopathological and neuropsychological effects of 8 days' corticosteroid treatment: a prospective study. *Psychoneuroendocrinology* 21: 25–31.

Najib J (1997). Neuroleptic malignant syndrome: a case report and review of treatment. *Hosp Pharm* 32: 512–518.

Naylor M W, Grunhaus I, Cameron O (1987). Myoclonic seizures after abrupt withdrawal from phenelzine and alprazolam. *J Nerv Mental Dis* 175: 111–114.

Pacheco L, Malo P, Argues E *et al.* (1996). More cases of paroxetine withdrawal syndrome (letter). *Br J Psychiatry* 169: 384.

Partonen T, Haukka J, Vrtamo J *et al.* (1999). Association of low serum total cholesterol with major depression and suicide. *Br J Psychiatry* 175: 259–262.

Patten S B, Neutel C I (2000). Corticosteroid-induced adverse effects. *Drug Safety* 22: 111–122.

Peet M, Peters S (1995). Drug-induced mania. *Drug Safety* 12: 146–153.

Philips-Howard P A, ter Kuile F O (1995). CNS adverse events associated with antimalarial agents. Fact or fiction? *Drug Safety* 1995; 12: 370–383.

Poole R, Brabbins C (1996). Drug induced psychosis (editorial). *Br J Psychiatry* 168: 135–138.

Price J S, Waller P C, Wood S M *et al.* (1996). A comparison of the post-marketing safety of four selective serotonin reuptake inhibitors including the investigation of symptoms occurring on withdrawal. *Br J Clin Pharmacol* 42: 757–763.

Reckart M D, Eisendrath S J (1990). Exogenous corticosteroid effects on mood and cognition: case presentation. *Int J Psychosom* 37: 57–61.

Reynolds E H, Trimble M R (1985). Adverse neuropsychiatric effects of anticonvulsant drugs. *Drugs* 29: 570–581.

Rosenbaum J F, Fava M, Hogg S L *et al.* (1998). Selective serotonin reuptake inhibitor discontinuation syndrome: a randomized clinical trial. *Biol Psychiatry* 44: 77–87.

Routledge P A, Bialas M C (1997). Adverse reactions to drug withdrawal. *Adverse Drug React Bull* 187: 711–714.

Rundell J R, Wise M G (1989). Causes of organic mood disorder. *J Neuropsychiatry Clin Neurosci* 1: 398–400.

Saint-Cyr J A, Taylor A E, Lang A K (1993). Neuropsychological and psychiatric side effects in the treatment of Parkinson's disease. *Neurology* 43 (suppl 6): S47–S52.

Spencer C M, Noble S (1998). Rivastigmine. A review of its use in Alzheimer's disease. *Drugs Aging* 13: 391–411.

Sporer K A (1995). The serotonin syndrome. *Drug Safety* 13: 94–104.

Stockley I H (1999). *Drug Interactions*, 5th edn. London: Pharmaceutical Press, 743.

Sunderland T, Tariot P N, Newhouse P A (1988). Differential responsivity of mood behaviour and cognition to cholinergic agents in elderly neuropsychiatric population. *Brain Res* 13: 371–389.

Tyrer P (1984). Clinical effects of abrupt withdrawal from tricyclic antidepressants and monoamine oxidase inhibitors after long term treatment. *J Affect Disord* 6: 1–7.

Wardle J, Rogers P, Judd P *et al.* (2000). Randomised trial of the effects of cholesterol-lowering dietary treatment on psychological function. *Am J Med* 108: 547–553.

Young A H, Currie A, Ashton C H (1997). Antidepressant withdrawal syndrome (letter). *Br J Psychiatry* 170: 288.

11

Cardiovascular disorders

Fiona Maclean and Anne Lee

Adverse reactions affecting the cardiovascular system are common. There are many predictable type A reactions, for example the undesirable cardiac effects of cardioactive drugs such as digoxin and antiarrhythmics, but a considerable number of these reactions are less predictable and they are not unique to cardiovascular drugs. For example, the cytotoxic agent doxorubicin can cause heart failure and the appetite suppressants fenfluramine and dexfenfluramine can cause heart valve disorders.

Healthcare professionals should be aware of the drugs most likely to have adverse effects on the cardiovascular system and the patient groups at greatest risk of these problems. Factors predisposing to cardiovascular toxicity include heart disease, uncorrected electrolyte abnormalities and poor renal function. The potential contribution of over-the-counter medicines such as non-steroidal anti-inflammatory drugs (NSAIDs) and effervescent preparations with a high sodium content should also be considered. When taking a drug history it is important to include details of any self-medication.

Arrhythmias

There is increasing awareness of the problem of drug-induced cardiac arrhythmias (Doig, 1997; Thomas, 1997). In the UK the antihistamine terfenadine was returned to prescription only status in 1997 following reports of serious cardiac arrhythmias (Committee on Safety of Medicines, 1997a) and marketing of the antipsychotic sertindole was suspended in 1998 following concerns about reports of sudden death (Barnett, 1996; Committee on Safety of Medicines, 1999). There is concern about serious arrhythmias and sudden death with the motility stimulant cisapride, which has led to its withdrawal from the UK market.

A cardiac arrhythmia is defined as any abnormal cardiac rhythm, whether the abnormality is one of rate, regularity or origin of the impulse initiating each heart beat. Drug-induced arrhythmias may be an adverse effect of a non-cardiac drug, a proarrhythmic complication of an antiarrhythmic drug, or may arise from a drug overdose (Doig, 1997). The associated mortality is unknown. Predisposing factors include underlying rhythm disturbances (especially ventricular tachycardia or fibrillation), impaired left ventricular function, pre-existing heart disease, high plasma levels of antiarrhythmic drugs and electrolyte abnormalities, especially hypokalaemia, hypocalcaemia and hypomagnesaemia (Caron and Libersa, 1997).

All antiarrhythmic drugs may exacerbate pre-existing arrhythmias or cause new ones; they have been estimated to cause arrhythmias in 5–10% of patients. The risks of antiarrhythmic therapy in patients with one or more predisposing factors may be deemed too high; however, the clinical decision involves balancing therapeutic benefits against the potential risks. Patients should be carefully selected and monitored and doses should not be escalated rapidly.

Digoxin can cause almost any arrhythmia because it has two opposing effects; it enhances the automaticity of cells in the atria and ventricles and it slows conduction between them. Digoxin can cause dangerous bradyarrhythmias, ventricular bigeminy, and, rarely, ventricular arrhythmias. Digoxin-induced arrhythmias are generally associated with drug toxicity. Therapeutic and toxic ranges, however, overlap: a digoxin concentration therapeutic in one patient may be toxic for another. In general, provided the plasma potassium is normal, toxicity is unlikely with digoxin trough concentrations below 2 µg/l and very likely with values greater than 4 µg/l (Kearney et al., 1998). It is essential that samples are timed correctly. At least 6 hours should be allowed to elapse between dosing and sampling. The main factors influencing susceptibility to digoxin toxicity are renal impairment and hypokalaemia.

Prolonged QT interval and torsade de pointes

The QT interval on the electrocardiogram (ECG) is an indirect measure of the duration of the ventricular action potential and ventricular repolarisation. Ventricular repolarisation occurs by outward movement of potassium through specific channels in myocardial cell membranes. Prolongation of ventricular repolarisation can cause arrhythmias, the most characteristic of which is torsade de pointes (twisting of the points), a specific form of ventricular tachycardia. The name describes the characteristic twisting of the QRS complexes around the electrical axis on the ECG, which can appear as an intermittent series of rapid spikes lasting a few seconds during which the heart fails to pump effectively. This is usually a self-limiting arrhythmia that may cause dizziness or syncope, but it can lead to ventricular fibrillation which can cause sudden death (Committee on Safety of Medicines, 1996a; Thomas, 1997).

Prolongation of the QT interval, or long QT syndromes (LQTS), are due to malfunction of ion channels at the myocardial cell membrane that cause an intracellular surplus of positive charges (Viskin, 1999). Depending on which of the channels malfunction, inadequate outflow of potassium or excess sodium influx may result. The ensuing intracellular surplus of positive ions impairs ventricular repolarisation and can trigger torsade de pointes. The cause of malfunction may be genetic (congenital LQTS) or related to metabolic disturbance or drug therapy (acquired LQTS). Drugs are thought to prolong repolarisation either by blocking potassium channels and thus delaying potassium outflow, or by enhancing inward sodium or calcium currents. QT prolongation is usually assumed to be present when the QT interval corrected for changes in the heart rate (QTc) is greater than 440 msec, although arrhythmias are most often associated with values of 550 msec or more (Thomas, 1997). Drugs that are known to prolong the QT interval are shown in Table 11.1 and additional risk factors for this problem are shown in Table 11.2 (Thomas, 1997; Viskin, 1999).

Table 11.1 Some drugs that may cause QT interval prolongation

Antiarrhythmics	**Antimalarials** – *continued*
Amiodarone	Halofantrine
Disopyramide	
Procainamide	**Antipsychotics**
Propafenone	Chlorpromazine
Quinidine	Droperidol
Sotalol	Haloperidol
	Pimozide
Antihistamines	Sertindole
Astemizole	Thioridazine
Terfenadine	
	Antidepressants
Antibacterials	Tricyclic antidepressants
Clarithromycin	
Co-trimoxazole	**Others**
Erythromycin	Cisapride
	Pentamidine
Antifungals	Probucol
Ketoconazole	Tacrolimus
	Terodiline
Antimalarials	
Chloroquine	

Table 11.2 Some risk factors for torsade de pointes

Female sex
Hypokalaemia
Hypomagnesaemia
Diuretic use (independent of electrolyte serum concentrations)
Bradycardia (especially recent heart rate slowing)
Congestive heart failure or cardiac hypertrophy
Congenital long QT syndromes

Management of QT interval prolongation

Some patients with torsade de pointes may be asymptomatic while others experience dizziness, light-headedness, syncope, collapse, irregular heart beat and palpitations. Drugs that prolong the QT interval should be stopped immediately in patients developing any of these symptoms and an ECG recorded. The arrhythmia should be controlled by accelerating the heart rate, either by atrial pacing or by an isoprenaline infusion. Electrolyte abnormalities should be corrected and magnesium sulphate infusion may effectively terminate the arrhythmia, even in the presence of normal magnesium levels. Antiarrhythmic drugs may worsen the problem and should be avoided. Torsade de pointes that degenerates to ventricular fibrillation requires DC shock for termination.

Antiarrhythmic agents

Any antiarrhythmic drug can cause torsade de pointes, but it is most commonly associated with drugs that prolong action potential duration, i.e. class Ia and class III agents (see Table 11.1). The estimated frequency of torsade de pointes during quinidine therapy ranges from 2% to 8% and the risk is probably similar with other class Ia drugs (Viskin, 1999). With sotalol, the frequency is about 2–4%; the risk is dose-dependent and increased in the elderly and those with impaired renal function. Amiodarone also causes QT prolongation but, for reasons that are not completely understood, it causes torsade de pointes only rarely (Hohnloser *et al.*, 1994).

Psychotropic drugs

Reports of sudden unexplained death in patients taking antipsychotic drugs have raised the concern that drug-induced arrhythmias may be a factor. Many of these drugs are known to have cardiac electrophysiological effects similar to those of quinidine, but the prevalence of QT abnormalities in patients taking antipsychotic drugs is uncertain. However, a recent study in about 500 psychiatric patients found that tricyclic antidepressants, thioridazine and droperidol were robust predictors of QT interval prolongation (>456 msec), as was high antipsychotic dose (Reilly *et al.*, 2000). No significant association was found with lithium and QT prolongation but it was shown to increase QT dispersion. Before this study the risk associated with tricyclic antidepressants was only perceived to be a problem in overdose or in patients with pre-existing cardiac disease. Droperidol had been linked with ventricular arrhythmia after intravenous use in critically ill patients (Lawrence and Nasraway, 1997), but not recognised to prolong the QT interval when given orally to psychiatric patients. Of 61 patients prescribed thioridazine, 25% had QTc interval lengthening. Most of these patients were taking doses of less than 300 mg daily. These findings suggest that ECG monitoring may need to be considered in patients taking tricyclic antidepressants, droperidol and thioridazine, particularly if other risk factors are present.

Tricyclic antidepressants should be avoided if possible in patients with underlying cardiac disease (Kearney *et al.*, 1998).

The atypical antipsychotic sertindole has been associated with QT interval prolongation. Sertindole's marketing authorisation was suspended in the UK in 1998 following reports of sudden death and serious cardiac arrhythmia (Committee on Safety of Medicines, 1999).

Antihistamines

Torsade de pointes was first reported with terfenadine overdose in 1989 and subsequently after concomitant treatment with ketoconazole (Davies *et al.*, 1989; Monahan *et al.*, 1990; Cantilena *et al.*, 1991). Terfenadine is almost completely converted into the active metabolite, fexofenadine, in the liver. In patients with severe liver disease or those taking drugs inhibiting the metabolism of terfenadine (e.g. imidazole antifungals, protease inhibitors (e.g. ritonavir), and the macrolide antibiotics, erythromycin and clarithromycin), plasma levels of the parent drug can increase sufficiently to disturb ventricular repolarisation. Grapefruit juice, taken in large quantities, has also been shown to inhibit terfenadine's metabolism. Despite warnings about the seriousness of the reaction and the inclusion of precautions in product information, problems persisted, and in the UK the drug reverted to prescription-only status in 1997 (Committee on Safety of Medicines

1997a, 1997b; Anon 1997b). Terfenadine is still available in the UK but it is essential that the recommended dose is not exceeded. It should be avoided in significant hepatic impairment, hypokalaemia, patients with known or supected prolonged QT interval, and in those taking drugs that prolong the QT interval (see Table 11.1) or inhibit its metabolism. The active metabolite, fexofenadine, now a marketed antihistamine, does not prolong the QT interval.

Astemizole has also been shown to cause arrhythmias by the same mechanism (Simons *et al.*, 1988; Goss *et al.*, 1993). Predisposing factors include cardiac disease, liver dysfunction, electrolyte imbalance and overdose. It is no longer available in the UK.

Cisapride

Cisapride is a motility stimulant used to treat gastro-oesophageal reflux and other gastrointestinal disorders, including gastro-oesophageal reflux in children. It is metabolised by the cytochrome P450 CYP3A4 enzyme system. Inhibition of this enzyme by concomitant drug therapy can increase cisapride blood levels, leading to potentially fatal ventricular arrhythmias. Drugs known to increase cisapride blood levels include macrolide antibiotics, imidazole antifungals and protease inhibitors (Wysowski and Bakanyi, 1996; Committee on Safety of Medicines, 1996b). Warnings have been issued about the potential risks of cisapride, particularly in higher than recommended doses, in patients taking drugs known to inhibit its metabolism, those with conditions known to be associated with QT prolongation and in premature infants

Table 11.3 Prevention of QT interval prolongation

- Antiarrhythmic therapy should always be initiated with due caution (e.g. preferably in hospital and after plasma potassium and magnesium concentrations have been checked)
- The use of any drug that prolongs the QT interval should be avoided in patients with a personal or family history of QT prolongation
- The concurrent use of more than one drug that prolongs the QT interval should be avoided in all patients
- Patients should be advised not to take more than the recommended dose of any drug that can prolong the QT interval
- Patients taking terfenadine or cisapride should be advised to avoid concomitant grapefruit juice
- Patients should know that symptoms indicative of an arrhythmia (e.g. palpitations, irregular pulse, fainting) should be reported to their doctor

---

for up to 3 months after birth. However, serious reactions continued to occur, albeit rarely, and cisapride has recently had its UK marketing authorisation suspended pending a European safety investigation (Committee on Safety of Medicines, 2000).

Key points on the prevention of QT interval prolongation are shown in Table 11.3.

Atrial fibrillation

Atrial fibrillation is the most common sustained cardiac rhythm disorder and an important cause of morbidity and mortality. It is characterised by irregular, disordered and unsynchronised electrical activity of the atria, resulting in an irregular ventricular response (Nattel *et al.*, 1994; Lip and Kamath, 2000). Fatigue, angina, dyspnoea and palpitations are possible symptoms, although the condition may be asymptomatic and only discovered incidentally on ECG monitoring (Lip *et al.*, 1995; Drake *et al.*, 1997). There are many possible cardiac and noncardiac causes, including thyrotoxicosis, ischaemic heart disease, hypertension, rheumatic heart disease, infection and pneumonia. Drug therapy is an infrequent cause.

Alcohol is one of the commonest causes, accounting for 15–35% of hospital admissions of new-onset atrial fibrillation (Kearney *et al.*, 1998). Some of these patients have an overt alcohol-related heart disease but in others the arrhythmia is probably due to acute intoxication. It is well-established that alcoholic binges may induce episodes of atrial fibrillation. Attacks clustering at weekends and over holiday periods have been termed the 'holiday heart syndrome'. Excessive chronic alcohol consumption also leads to dilated cardiomyopathy (alcoholic heart muscle disease) (Lip *et al.*, 2000).

Drugs associated with atrial fibrillation include tricyclic antidepressants, trazodone and fluoxetine (Elphick, 1993). Serotonin reuptake inhibitors (SSRIs) are regarded as relatively safe with respect to the cardiovascular system. However, serotonin is involved in conduction processes in the heart and caution is still required when prescribing these antidepressants to patients with concomitant heart disease. Atrial fibrillation has also been reported after the administration of repeated large intravenous pulses of corticosteroids for conditions such as rheumatoid arthritis or systemic lupus erythematosus (Dukes, 1996).

Management depends on the type and cause of atrial fibrillation and may require hospital admission. If drug therapy is thought to be responsible, the suspected drug should be stopped. If alcohol excess is suspected, lifestyle intervention will be required. Restoration or maintenance of sinus rhythm may require electrical cardioversion or drug therapy.

Bradycardia

Bradycardia is a slowing of the heart rate to less than 60 beats/min. It is usually asymptomatic unless the rate is very low. Dizziness, syncope and fatigue are possible features. Drug-induced bradycardia has been extensively reported in the literature (Table 11.4). Mechanisms include effects on cardiac impulse generation and conduction. In some cases the underlying mechanism is not known (Kearney *et al.*, 1998).

Table 11.4 Some drugs that may cause bradycardia

Beta-blockers	Diltiazem
Carbamazepine	Histamine H$_2$-antagonists
Clonidine	Paclitaxel
Digoxin	Verapamil

Sinus bradycardia, where the rate of sinus node discharge is slowed, occurs with beta-blockers due to the blockade of sympathetic stimulation of the beta-receptors in the heart (Drake *et al.*, 1997). Atrioventricular block occurs when impulses are delayed as they pass through the atrioventricular node into the ventricles and can be caused by verapamil, diltiazem, digoxin and also beta-blockers. The interaction between beta-blockers and verapamil/diltiazem is well recognised and can result in serious bradycardia. If used together, the patient must be carefully monitored. An interaction between topical ophthalmic beta-blockers and verapamil has also been reported (Stockley, 1999). Treatment depends on the heart rate and may require discontinuation of the causative drug. Intravenous atropine or pacing may be required.

Prevention of drug-induced arrhythmias

Prevention of drug-induced arrhythmias is multifactorial. Polypharmacy should be avoided where possible and consideration given to potential adverse effects before initiating drug therapy. Drugs with known adverse effects on the cardiovascular system should be used with caution in patients with pre-existing heart disease and in those taking drugs which may cause electrolyte abnormalities. Treatment of drug-induced arrhythmias involves stopping the causative agent and correcting any electrolyte imbalance. Hospital admission is generally required to allow for intensive ECG monitoring and drug therapy or pacing if needed. Key points on the prevention of QT interval prolongation are shown in Table 11.3.

Cardiac failure

Cardiac failure is a syndrome which occurs when the heart fails to pump sufficient amounts of blood to meet the metabolic demands of the body (McDonagh and Dargie, 1998; Lip *et al.*, 2000). Features of acute cardiac failure include dyspnoea, tachycardia, hypotension and confusion. These arise due to a combination of salt and water retention, increased venous pressure and inadequate organ perfusion. Chronic cardiac failure is characterised by dyspnoea, fatigue, ankle oedema, dizziness, palpitations, wheeze, chest discomfort and cough (Coats, 1998). Alcohol is the identifiable cause of heart failure in 2–3% of cases (Lip *et al.*, 2000).

Drugs can induce or exacerbate cardiac failure. This can occur through an increase in preload (volume overload), an increase in afterload (resistance) or cardiac dysfunction (Lip *et al.*, 1995, 2000). Drugs that cause circulatory overload will increase the preload; intravenous infusion of excessive fluid is the most frequent iatrogenic cause. Drugs implicated include carbenoxolone, mineralocorticoid steroids such as fludrocortisone and NSAIDs. Clinically detectable oedema can be seen in 3–5% of patients treated with NSAIDs and this could exacerbate heart failure (Feenstra *et al.*, 1997). A recent case-control study investigating the relationship between recent NSAID use and hospitalisation with congestive heart failure found a doubling of the risk (Page and Henry, 2000). The risk was much greater in patients with a history of heart disease (odds ratio 10.5). Factors positively correlated with risk were high NSAID dose and long plasma drug half-life. These results add weight to the assertion that NSAIDs should be avoided in patients with left ventricular dysfunction. If an NSAID is considered essential in such patients, the lowest effective dose should be used and drugs with a long elimination half-life avoided.

Selective beta$_2$ adrenoceptor agonists used as tocolytics in the prevention of premature delivery may cause pulmonary oedema as a consequence of fluid overload (see Chapter 7). Prolonged treatment with high-dose ritodrine has been reported to cause cardiac failure (McCombs, 1995).

Drugs with negative inotropic, cardiotoxic or arrhythmogenic effects may cause cardiac dysfunction. Drug-induced arrhythmias have already been discussed.

The role of beta-blockers in cardiac failure has changed dramatically in recent years. Historically, the drugs have been contraindicated due to their negative inotropic action which weakens cardiac contractility and results in a reduced cardiac output. This has traditionally been thought to worsen existing cardiac failure or precipitate cardiac failure in patients who rely on a high sympathetic drive to maintain cardiac output (Dukes, 1996). The partial beta-agonist xamoterol was withdrawn after it was associated with increased mortality in severe heart failure (Committee on Safety of Medicines, 1990). Data from recent clinical trials involving metoprolol, bisoprolol and carvedilol have shown improvements in left ventricular function, suggesting that they may have a role in carefully selected patients.

Other drugs reported to cause or worsen cardiac failure include intravenous amiodarone and other antiarrhythmic drugs. Some calcium channel blockers have negative inotropic effects; verapamil is the most cardiodepressant, followed by nifedipine and diltiazem (Kearney *et al.*, 1998). The newer calcium antagonists such as felodipine and isradipine have a more selective vasodilator than cardiodepressant action. They may be used cautiously in patients who are unlikely to tolerate negative inotropism.

If cardiac failure is believed to be drug-induced, the agent responsible should be stopped. Management involves lifestyle modification and appropriate treatment with, for example, diuretics and angiotensin-converting enzyme (ACE) inhibitors. Over-the-counter medicines which should be discouraged in patients with heart failure include some antacids, effervescent preparations with a high sodium content and NSAIDs. Table 11.5 lists some drugs that may cause or worsen cardiac failure.

Table 11.5 Some drugs that may cause or worsen cardiac failure

Antacids (high sodium content)	Nifedipine
Anthracycline cytotoxic drugs	Non-steroidal anti-inflammatory drugs
Antiarrhythmic drugs	Thyroxine
Beta-blockers	Verapamil
Diltiazem	

Hypertension

Sympathomimetic drugs such as adrenaline (epinephrine), noradrenaline (norepinephrine), dobutamine, dopamine and phenylephrine can all cause systemic hypertension (Aziz, 1997). The most serious hypertensive emergency due to drugs is the crisis that can occur when patients taking monoamine oxidase inhibitors (MAOIs) also take sympathomimetic drugs or food or drink that contains a high concentration of tyramine. Healthcare professionals must ensure that patients taking MAOIs have been adequately counselled about these risks and carry a treatment card. The danger of interaction persists for up to 2 weeks after the MAOI is discontinued.

Ciclosporin causes hypertension (Textor *et al.*, 1994; Taler *et al.*, 1999). Arterial pressure rises within days of ciclosporin administration and is exacerbated by concomitant corticosteroid administration (Taler *et al.*, 1999). Neither the dose nor the serum concentration of ciclosporin correlates with the hypertension. The problem appears to be most severe in cases of heart and lung transplantation and in children. The mechanisms underlying this disorder are complex and include altered vascular endothelial function. Vasodilators such as prostacyclin and nitric oxide are suppressed, whereas vasoconstrictors, including endothelin, are increased. Changes in the kidney include vasoconstriction, reduced glomerular filtration and sodium retention. Effective therapy depends upon rigorous blood pressure control by administration of vasodilating agents. The dihydropyridine calcium channel blockers nifedipine, amlodipine, isradipine and felodipine have all been used successfully in transplant settings. Beta-blockers and ACE inhibitors may also be used (Taler *et al.*, 1999).

Drugs that may cause hypertension are shown in Table 11.6. Drugs that cause hypertension can precipitate heart failure.

Table 11.6 Some drugs that may cause hypertension

Ciclosporin	Naloxone
Corticosteroids	Non-steroidal anti-inflammatory drugs
Erythropoietin	Oestrogens
Interferon alfa	Sympathomimetics
Ketoconazole	Tacrolimus
Moclobemide	

Myocardial toxicity

Some drugs may cause direct injury to the heart, resulting in cardiomyopathy, contractile function abnormalities or conduction defects. Myocytolysis, in which the number of viable myocardial cells is reduced, can occur. Myocardial toxicity is difficult to diagnose and establishing causality can be difficult (Kearney *et al.*, 1998). Diagnosis may be based on histological identification of cellular changes; however, it is difficult to categorise injury into early, late, reversible or irreversible patterns.

Anthracycline cytotoxics

Anthracycline cytotoxics such as doxorubicin are among the most widely used anticancer drugs, yet long-term cardiac damage is a major adverse effect that limits their usefulness. Cardiotoxicity with these agents has been recognised for more than 30 years (Anon, 1999; Pai and Nahata, 2000). It has been described as three distinct types of cardiotoxicity: acute or subacute, early-onset chronic progressive or late-onset chronic progressive cardiotoxicity. Acute or subacute cardiotoxicity is a rare form of cardiotoxicity that may occur immediately after a single dose or course of anthracycline therapy, with clinical manifestations occurring within a week of treatment. These may be in the form of transient electrophysiological abnormalities, a pericarditis–myocarditis syndrome or acute left ventricular failure. Early-onset chronic progressive cardiotoxicity is a more common and clinically important type of cardiotoxicity. It usually presents within a year of treatment. It may persist or progress after discontinuation of anthracycline therapy and may evolve into a chronic dilated cardiomyopathy in adult patients and restrictive cardiomyopathy in paediatric patients. Late-onset chronic progressive anthracycline cardiotoxicity causes ventricular dysfunction years to decades after chemotherapy has been completed. More cases of late cardiac toxicity are now being observed with the prolonged survival and more frequent cure of patients treated for cancer.

Anthracycline-induced congestive heart failure is associated with a high reported incidence of morbidity and mortality. Many affected patients (about 60%) recover, but their cardiac reserve is limited and they may require careful medical or surgical management during other illnesses or surgical procedures. Several studies published beteen 1975 and 1980 and involving several thousands of patients described anthracycline cardiotoxicity occurring during the first year following treatment. These studies showed that the frequency of clinical heart failure was positively correlated with the cumulative treatment dose and identified several other risk factors. The cumulative lifetime dose of doxorubicin should not exceed 450–550 mg/m^2, although the problem has been reported with lower doses despite serial monitoring of cardiac function.

Predisposing factors to doxorubicin toxicity include mediastinal radiotherapy, female sex, the elderly or young, pre-existing heart disease and hypertension (Pai and Nahata, 2000). Severe doxorubicin toxicity is generally irreversible (Singal and Liskovic, 1998; Shan *et al.*, 1996). Doxorubicin's cardiotoxicity is thought to result from oxygen free radicals, production of which is catalysed by a doxorubicin–iron complex (Hellmann, 1999).

As anthracyclines are still widely used, the detection, prevention and treatment of cardiotoxicity remain a difficult problem. Careful monitoring of cardiac function is required during and after therapy, comprising physical examination, chest X-ray, ECG and echocardiograms. Monitoring should continue for a long time after chemotherapy is completed. There is currently much interest in the cardioprotective agent dexrazoxane, which is approved for use against anthracycline cardiotoxicity in the US and some European countries (Hellmann, 1999; Pai and Nahata, 2000). It acts by binding to intracellular iron and inhibiting the conversion of superoxide anions and hydrogen peroxide to superhydroxide free radicals. Current management of anthracycline cardiotoxicity consists of symptomatic treatment.

Several other cytotoxic drugs are known to be cardiotoxic (see Table 11.7).

Table 11.7 Some cytotoxic drugs that may cause cardiac toxicity

Amsacrine	Etoposide
Busulfan	Fluorouracil
Carmustine	Idarubicin
Cisplatin	Ifosfamide
Cyclophosphamide	Mitomycin
Cytarabine	Mitoxantrone (mitozantrone)
Daunorubicin	Paclitaxel
Doxorubicin	Vinca alkaloids
Epirubicin	

Interferon alfa

Dose-dependent cardiotoxicity has been reported with interferon alfa in 5–15% of patients within the first days of therapy. Severe but reversible cardiomyopathy has occurred in patients with no previous history of cardiac disease (Sacchi *et al.*, 1995). Interferon should be used with extreme caution in patients with cardiac disease, as further impairment in function may be critical.

Myocardial ischaemia or infarction

Ischaemia occurs when there is a mismatch in the cell between oxygen demand and supply. A metabolic disorder results in which anaerobic glycolysis produces lactic acid causing a lowered intracellular pH and impaired contractile function of the heart muscle. Angina is the pain resulting from myocardial ischaemia. It is typically described as choking or tightness and may radiate to the arms, back, neck or jaw. It is often confused with indigestion (Drake *et al.*, 1997). The mechanism of drug-induced myocardial ischaemia depends on the causative agent. Abrupt withdrawal of beta-blockers may lead to unstable angina, myocardial infarction and sudden death (Kearney *et al.*, 1998). Treatment withdrawal exposes the heart to greater sympathomimetic stimulation, partly because chronic receptor blockade leads to a compensatory increase in the number of beta-receptors. Removal of beta-blockade leads to an increased myocardial oxygen consumption due to the increase in heart rate. This effect is more commonly seen after short-acting beta-blockers are stopped.

All calcium channel blockers cause vasodilation. Short-acting nifedipine can cause abrupt vasodilation and exacerbation of angina has been widely reported with these formulations (Kearney *et al.*, 1998). The mechanism involves reflex tachycardia precipitated by vasodilation, increasing myocardial oxygen consumption. Concerns have been raised about the safety of short-acting nifedipine, as an increased mortality rate has been reported in some studies (Anon, 1997a). Nifedipine in capsule form should no longer be prescribed (Ramsay *et al.*, 1999).

Both levothyroxine (thyroxine) administration and hyperthyroidism have been reported to cause anginal pain. Sudden initiation of thyroid therapy in patients with hypothyroidism and cardiovascular disease may result in severe angina pectoris, myocardial infarction or sudden death (Dukes, 1996). The initial dose should be low (25 µg daily or 50 µg on alternate days) and increased every 4 weeks to the required maintenance dose. There is no increase in cardiovascular mortality or morbidity in patients on long-term thyroxine replacement. The antimigraine drug ergotamine can cause vasospasm which is potentially dangerous in patients with angina or ischaemic heart disease. Ergotamine can, in addition, cause generalised vasospasm with a corresponding increase in total peripheral resistance.

Fluorouracil

Myocardial ischaemia with the antimetabolite cytotoxic fluorouracil was first reported in 1969 (Anand, 1994). Cardiac events range from chest pain typical of mild angina to massive myocardial infarction culminating in cardiogenic shock and death. A retrospective review of 1083 patients receiving fluorouracil found a 1.6% incidence of clinically apparent cardiotoxicity. Other retrospective studies and anecdotal reports place this incidence at 24–68%. In up to 10% of patients cardiotoxicity was associated with high-dose therapy (>800 mg/m^2 per day). Fluorouracil cardiotoxicity frequently occurs during the first course of therapy, after the second or third dose. It is more common after continuous infusion than after bolus doses. The mean time to onset is 3 days, with the majority of patients experiencing angina within hours of administration. The symptoms may resolve at a mean of 48 hours after discontinuation of the infusion, but recur in 90% of cases when it is restarted and may be more severe than the previous episode. Prophylactic nitrates or calcium channel blockers have been ineffective. The overall mortality rate is estimated as between 2.2 and 13.3%. No delayed sequelae have been reported (Anand, 1994; Pai and Nahata, 2000). Predisposing factors include a history of coronary heart disease and radiotherapy. The mechanism underlying this reaction is not known.

Table 11.8 shows some drugs that may cause myocardial ischaemia.

Table 11.8   Some drugs that may cause myocardial ischaemia

Adenosine	Fluorouracil
Amfetamines	Nifedipine (short-acting)
Beta-agonists	Theophylline
Beta-blockers (withdrawal)	Levothyroxine (thyroxine)
Caffeine	Verapamil
Dipyridamole	Vinblastine
Ergotamine	Vincristine

Thromboembolic disorders

Thromboembolic disorders result from the sudden occlusion (embolism) of a blood vessel by a blood clot (thrombus) in the arterial or venous circulation. Venous thromboembolism is common and is associated with a mortality of 1–2%. Deep vein thrombosis (DVT) usually arises in the veins of the lower limbs or pelvis. Clinical features include pain involving the calf or thigh associated with swelling, redness and warmth. Management involves restoring normal circulation and anticoagulation. If part of a venous thrombus breaks off it can lodge in the pulmonary circulation, causing pulmonary embolism (PE). This can present with breathlessness, chest pain and collapse. In the arterial circulation, a thrombus may result in peripheral arterial occlusion, either in the lower limbs or in the cerebral circulation, where it may result in stroke (Chasan-Taber and Stampfer, 1998; Pritchard and Sandercock, 2000).

Oral contraceptives and venous thromboembolism

Epidemiological studies have demonstrated that combined oral contraceptives (COCs) increase the risk of cardiovascular disease. Oral contraceptives have complex effects on blood pressure, platelet function, blood coagulation, carbohydrate metabolism and lipid metabolism (Chasan-Taber and Stampfer, 1998; Anon, 2000). Since their introduction in the UK in the 1960s the presentations available and populations using them have changed dramatically. The first preparations contained at least 50 μg of oestrogen with a progestogen. Venous thromboembolism was subsequently identified as a serious unwanted effect of these preparations and doctors were advised to prescribe only pills containing 50 μg or less of oestrogen (Maling, 1998; Anon, 2000). Factors known to increase the risk of venous thromboembolism are smoking, obesity, a family history of DVT and the genetic factor known as factor V Leiden mutation.

The precise cardiovascular risk of oral contraceptives is poorly known because of a lack of reliable clinical studies and the numerous potential biases in epidemiological studies. Almost all epidemiological studies have shown an increased risk of DVT and/or PE in women on combined contraceptives, although the risk remains moderate. Case-control and cohort studies suggest that taking a norethisterone or levonorgestrel-containing combined oral contraceptive (second-generation) pill increases a woman's risk of developing venous thromboembolism from around five cases per 100 000 women per year to about 15 cases per 100 000 women per year (Anon, 1998, 2000).

Third-generation contraceptive pills are those containing newer progestogens, desogestrel, gestodene and norgestimate. The newer progestogens were introduced with the intention that they would be associated with a lower risk of arterial disease. However, in the mid-1990s four large case-control studies suggested that the risk of venous thromboembolism with desogestrel- and gestodene-containing pills was about twice that with second-generation pills (Weiss, 1995; Anon, 2000). These studies were criticised as being flawed by bias and confounding variables, but adjustment for several potentially confounding risk factors suggests that the initial assessment of risk is difficult to dismiss. The current consensus is that taking a third-generation pill containing desogestrel or gestodene increases the risk of venous thromboembolism to about 25 cases per 100 000 per year. More data are needed before the risks associated with pills containing norgestimate can be quantified. The absolute risk of venous thromboembolism in women using third-generation COCs remains very small and well below the risk associated with pregnancy. Provided that women are informed of and accept the relative risks of venous thromboembolism, the choice of oral contraceptive should be decided by the woman and her prescriber, taking her medical history and any contraindications into account.

Recent studies have shown a two- to fourfold increase in risk of venous thromboembolism in hormone replacement therapy (HRT) users (Committee on Safety of Medicines, 1996c). The absolute risk in current HRT users is believed to be small (estimated at 16–23 excess cases per 100 000 women per year for all venous thromboembolism). The studies indicated that the risk of venous thromboembolism disappears after HRT is stopped. There appears not to be any clinically significant differences between the different types of HRT preparations available. The risk of venous thromboembolism is thought to be greater in women with predisposing factors, including a history (personal or family) of DVT or PE, severe varicose veins, obesity, trauma, surgery or prolonged bed rest. The risks of therapy in these women may outweigh the benefits.

Antipsychotics

The antipsychotic clozapine has been linked with venous thromboembolic complications in a case series of twelve patients (Hägg et al., 2000). In eight patients symptoms occurred within the first three months of treatment; no predisposing factors were identified. A more recent case-control study concluded that current exposure to conventional antipsychotic drugs was associated with a significantly increased risk of venous thromboembolism compared with non-use (adjusted odds ratio 7.1 (95% CI 2.3–21.97)) (Zornberg and Jick, 2000). The association was strongest for the low potency antipsychotics chlorpromazine and thioridazine. Further study of this possible association is needed.

Stroke

Drugs are an uncommon but well-recognised cause of stroke (Pritchard and Sandercock, 2000). The literature contains many reports of stroke associated with drugs of abuse but there are no good epidemiological studies to determine the contribution of recreational drug use to ischaemic or haemorrhagic stroke. The agents most frequently implicated are cocaine, amphetamines and derivatives and phenylpropanolamine. Table 11.9 lists some therapeutic drugs that have been reported to cause stroke. Anticoagulants, thrombolytics and antiplatelet agents may cause haemorrhagic stroke when used in therapeutic dose or in excessive doses.

Table 11.9 Some drugs reported to cause stroke

Bromocriptine	Oral contraceptives
Danazol	Phenylpropanolamine
Desmopressin	Tranexamic acid
Hypoglycaemic agents	

Oral contraceptives and stroke

Oral contraceptives have been associated with both haemorrhagic and ischaemic stroke (Vessey *et al.*, 1984; Lidegeard, 1993; Hannaford *et al.*, 1994). Data from early studies relate to older COCs containing higher oestrogen doses than those now in use. Although the results of more recent studies have been conflicting, there is thought to be an up to threefold increase in the risk of ischaemic stroke in women taking COCs (Beral *et al.*, 1999; Anon, 2000; Pritchard and Sandercock, 2000). The risk is higher in women with other risk factors, particularly hypertension, but also diabetes and a history of thromboembolic events. The excess risk declines rapidly after ceasing to take oral contraceptives. Oral contraceptives probably account for no more than 10% of strokes in young women, an excess of between two and eight strokes per 100 000 woman years. In women aged under 35 years who do not smoke and are not hypertensive, taking the COC does not appear to increase the risk of haemorrhagic stroke. However, the pill appears to magnify the age-related increase in risk (Anon, 2000).

Bromocriptine and cerebrovascular events

There have been several reports of cerebrovascular events in patients taking bromocriptine for postpartum milk suppression (Comabella *et al.*, 1996; Iffy *et al.*, 1996). This may be due to vasospasm of cerebral blood vessels and may be associated with pre-existing hypertension and use in association with other ergot derivatives. Blood pressure should be carefully monitored in postpartum women taking bromocriptine, and particular care should be taken in those also on antihypertensives.

Valvular disorders

In 1988, cardiac murmurs suggestive of aortic valve disease were reported in a patient known to ingest excessive amounts of the serotonin antagonist ergotamine (Hendrikx *et al.*, 1996). Further reports described two patients who had taken ergotamine tartrate for migraine and who developed cardiac valve disease requiring surgery for valve replacement. More recently, valvular heart disease involving the mitral, aortic and/or tricuspid valves has been reported in association with appetite suppressants. Regurgitation and thickening of the valve leaflets was described in US patients who had been prescribed fenfluramine–phentermine in combination (Connolly *et al.*, 1997). The mitral valve was elongated, thickened, white and shiny and resembled the features of long-term ergotamine administration. The precise mechanism responsible for this type of cardiac injury has not been identified, although effects on serotonin are thought to be involved (Jick, 2000). Several studies have supported an association between anorectics and cardiac valve disease (Jick *et al.*, 1998; Khan *et al.*, 1998; Weissman *et al.*, 1998; Gardin *et al.*, 2000). The most recent of these showed that the prevalence of aortic regurgitation was greater in patients who had taken dexfenfluramine or phentermine–fenfluramine for longer periods of time (Gardin *et al.*, 2000). Both fenfluramine and dexfenfluramine have been withdrawn in the UK.

 CASE STUDY

Mrs L is a 56-year-old woman with chronic urticaria prescribed intermittent terfenadine by her dermatologist for symptom control. She requests advice after reading in a health magazine that grapefruit juice can interact with this drug, causing heart problems. The only other medication she takes is HRT. As part of a weight-reducing diet, Mrs L has recently been drinking lots of fruit juice and eating fresh and tinned grapefruit. She is anxious that she may have done some damage to her heart as she has noticed several episodes of palpitations over the past couple of months.

(continued overleaf)

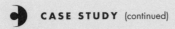

What is the mechanism for this potential interaction?

Grapefruit juice is known to interact with a number of medications. The effect seems to be mediated mainly by suppression of the cytochrome P450 enzyme system CYP3A4 in the small intestine wall. This results in a diminished first-pass metabolism with higher plasma concentrations of drugs which are substrates of this enzyme (Fuhr, 1998). The components of grapefruit juice which are the most probable cause of the interaction are psoralen derivatives, but the flavonoid naringenin may also contribute. Studies of the effect of grapefruit juice on terfenadine pharmacokinetics have shown an increase in plasma terfenadine concentrations. In addition, studies which monitored the QTc interval found that long-term intake of terfenadine with grapefruit juice resulted in QTc prolongation.

Should Mrs L be advised not to eat or drink anything containing grapefruit or is it sufficient to avoid grapefruit within a few hours of taking terfenadine?

Product literature for terfenadine states that the drug should not be taken with grapefruit juice. Studies suggest that the timing of juice intake relative to drug administration is important; taking both simultaneously is more likely to lead to increased plasma levels of terfenadine than allowing an interval of a few hours between drinking grapefruit juice and taking the drug (Spence, 1997; Fuhr, 1998). However, the duration of inhibition of metabolism is not known and it is unclear what time interval patients should allow between drinking grapefruit juice and taking terfenadine. There is no evidence that eating grapefruit (rather than drinking the juice) causes interactions (Committee on Safety of Medicines, 1997b). Although very few cases of problems have been described, it is simplest to advise patients to avoid drinking grapefruit juice while they are taking terfenadine.

Is it possible that the palpitations the patient describes could be a consequence of this interaction?

Palpitations are a possible symptom of a cardiac arrhythmia such as torsade de pointes. However, many healthy people taking no medication describe subjective problems like palpitations from time to time. In this case, it is unlikely that Mrs L has come to any harm through an interaction between terfenadine and grapefruit juice and it is probably unnecessary for specific investigations to be carried out unless she has other ongoing symptoms. Her general practitioner may have ECG facilities to check the QT interval, which would avoid hospital admission.

What other medicines interact with grapefruit juice? Would there be any merit in switching to another antihistamine?

Grapefruit juice can also interact with ciclosporin and most calcium channel blockers, leading to increased plasma levels. Other antihistamines (except astemizole, now withdrawn in the UK) would not be expected to cause any problems. However, there is probably no need to change Mrs L's medication as the interaction is easily avoided and it would be unwise to make a change without consulting her dermatologist.

References

Anand A J (1994). Fluorouracil cardiotoxicity. *Ann Pharmacother* 28: 374–377.

Anon. (1997a). Safety of calcium channel blockers. *Med Lett Drugs Ther* 39: 13–14.

Anon. (1997b). Torsades de pointes on terfenadine. *Prescrire Int* 6: 110–111.

Anon. (1998). Cardiovascular risk of oral contraceptives. *Prescrire Int* 7: 118–124.

Anon. (1999). Late cardiotoxicity of anthracyclines. *Prescrire Int* 8: 145–146.

Anon. (2000). Oral contraceptives and cardiovascular risk. *Drug Ther Bull* 38: 1–5.

Aziz E A (1997). Drug-induced cardiac failure. *Adverse Drug React Bull* 185: 703–706.

Barnett A A (1996). Safety concerns over antipsychotic drug, sertindole. *Lancet* 348: 256.

Beral V, Hermon C, Kay C *et al.* (1999). Mortality associated with oral contraceptive use: 25 year follow up of cohort of 46 000 women from Royal College of General Practitioners' oral contraception study. *Br Med J* 318: 96–100.

Cantilena L R, Ferguson C L, Monahan B P (1991). Torsades de pointes occurring in association with terfenadine use. *JAMA* 266: 2375–2376.

Caron J, Libersa C (1997). Adverse effects of class I antiarrhythmic drugs. *Drug Safety* 17: 8–36.

Chasan-Taber L, Stampfer M J (1998). Epidemiology of oral contraceptives and cardiovascular disease. *Ann Intern Med* 128: 467–477.

Coats A J S (1998). Investigation and medical treatment of heart failure. *Medicine* 26: 116–121.

Comabella M, Alverez-Sabin J, Rovira A *et al.* (1996). Bromocriptine and postpartum cerebral angiopathy: a causal relationship? *Neurology* 46: 1754–1756.

Committee on Safety of Medicines (1990). Xamoterol (Corwin) – revised indications, contra-indications, dose schedule and warnings. *Curr Probl Pharmacovigilance* 28: 1.

Committee on Safety of Medicines (1996a). Drug-induced prolongation of the QT interval. *Curr Probl Pharmacovigilance* 22: 2.

Committee on Safety of Medicines (1996b). Cisapride (Prepulsid, Alimix): interactions with antifungals and antibiotics can lead to ventricular arrhythmias. *Curr Probl Pharmacovigilance* 22: 1.

Committee on Safety of Medicines (1996c). Risk of venous thromboembolism with hormone replacement therapy. *Curr Probl Pharmacovigilance* 22: 9–10.

Committee on Safety of Medicines (1997a). Terfenadine: now only available on prescription. *Curr Probl Pharmacovigilance* 23: 9.

Committee on Safety of Medicines (1997b). Drug interactions with grapefruit juice. *Curr Probl Pharmacovigilance* 23: 2.

Committee on Safety of Medicines (1999). Suspension of availability of sertindole (Serdolect). *Curr Probl Pharmacovigilance* 25: 1.

Committee on Safety of Medicines (2000). Cisapride (Prepulsid) withdrawn. *Curr Probl Pharmacovigilance* 26: 9–10.

Connolly H M, Crary J L, McGoon M D (1997). Valvular heart disease associated with fenfluramine–phentermine. *N Engl J Med* 337: 581–588.

Davies A J, Harinda V, McEwan A *et al.* (1989). Cardiotoxic effect with convulsions in terfenadine overdose. *Br Med J* 298: 325.

Doig J C (1997). Drug-induced cardiac arrhythmias. Incidence, prevention and management. *Drug Safety* 17: 265–275.

Drake W M, Broadburst P A, Dymond D S (1997). *Cardiology Explained*. London: Chapman and Hall Medical.

Dukes M N G (1996). Corticotrophins and corticosteroids. In: Dukes M N G, ed. *Meyler's Side Effects of Drugs,* 13th edn. Amsterdam: Elsevier Science, chapter 39.

Elphick M (1993). Antidepressant drugs. In: Dukes M N G, Aronson J K, eds. *Side Effects of Drugs Annual 16.* Amsterdam: Elsevier, chapter 2.

Feenstra J, Grobbe D E, Mosterd A *et al.* (1997). Adverse cardiovascular effects of NSAIDs in patients with congestive heart failure. *Drug Safety* 17: 166–180.

Fuhr U (1998). Drug interactions with grapefruit juice: extent, probable mechanisms and clinical relevance. *Drug Safety* 18: 251–272.

Gardin J M, Schumacher D, Constantine G *et al.* (2000). Valvular abnormalities and cardiovascular status following exposure to dexfenfluramine or phentermine/fenfluramine. *JAMA* 283: 1703–1709.

Goss J E, Ramo B W, Blake K (1993). Torsades de pointes associated with astemizole (Histamal) therapy. *Arch Intern Med* 153: 2705.

Hägg S, Spigset O, Söderstrom T G (2000). Association of venous thromboembolism and clozapine. *Lancet* 355: 1155–1156.

Hannaford P C, Croft P R, Kay C R (1994). Oral contraceptives and stroke. Evidence from the Royal College of General Practitioners' oral contraceptive study. *Stroke* 25: 935–942.

Hellmann K (1999). Preventing the cardiotoxicity of anthracyclines by dexrazoxane. *Br Med J* 319: 1085–1086.

Hendrikx M, Van-Dorpe J, Flameng W *et al.* (1996). Aortic and mitral valve disease induced by ergotamine therapy for migraine: a case report and review of the literature. *J Heart Valve Dis* 5: 235–237.

Hohnloser S H, Klingenheben T, Singh B N (1994). Amiodarone-associated proarrhythmic effects. A review with special reference to torsade de pointes tachycardia. *Ann Intern Med* 121: 529–535.

Iffy L, Lindenthal J, McCardle J J *et al.* (1996). Severe cerebral accidents postpartum in patients taking bromocriptine for milk suppression. *Israel J Med Sci* 32: 309–312.

Jick H (2000). Heart valve disorders and appetite-suppressant drugs. *JAMA* 283: 1738–1740.

Jick H, Vasilakis C, Weinrauch L A *et al.* (1998). A population-based study of appetite suppressant drugs and the risk of cardiac valve regurgitation. *N Engl J Med* 339: 719–724.

Kearney M T, Wright D J, Tan L-B (1998). Cardiac disorders. In: Davies D M, Ferner R E, de Glanville H, eds. *Textbook of Adverse Drug Reactions*, 5th edn. London: Chapman and Hall Medical, 119–168.

Khan M A, Herzog C A, St Peter J V *et al.* (1998). The prevalence of cardiac valvular insufficiency assessed by transthoracic echocardiography in obese patients treated with appetite suppressant drugs. *N Engl J Med* 339: 713–718.

Lawrence K R, Nasraway S A (1997). Conduction disturbances associated with administration of butyrophenone antipsychotics in the critically ill: a review of the literature. *Pharmacotherapy* 17: 531–537.

Lidegeard O (1993). Oral contraception and risk of a cerebral thromboembolic attack: results of a case-control study. *Br Med J* 306: 956–963.

Lip G Y H, Kamath S (2000). Atrial fibrillation: the condition. *Pharm J* 264: 622–626.

Lip G Y H, Beevers D G, Singh S P (1995). ABC of atrial fibrillation. Aetiology, pathophysiology, and clinical features. *Br Med J* 311: 1425–1428.

Lip G Y H, Gibbs C R, Beevers D G (2000). ABC of heart failure. Aetiology. *Br Med J* 320: 104–107.

Maling T J B (1998). Oral contraceptives and venous thromboembolism – managing the uncertainty. *Adverse Drug React Bull* 191: 727–729.

McCombs J (1995). Update on tocolytic therapy. *Ann Pharmacother* 29: 515–522.

McDonagh T A, Dargie H (1998). Epidemiology and pathophysiology of heart failure. *Medicine* 26: 111–115.

Monahan B P, Ferguson C L, Killeavy E S *et al.* (1990). Torsades de pointes occurring in association with terfenadine use. *JAMA* 264: 2788–2790.

Nattel S, Hadjis T, Talejic M (1994). The treatment of atrial fibrillation. An evaluation of drug therapy, electrical modalities and therapeutic considerations. *Drugs* 48: 345–371.

Page J, Henry D (2000). Consumption of NSAIDs and the development of congestive heart failure in elderly patients. *Arch Intern Med* 160: 777–784.

Pai V B, Nahata M C (2000). Cardiotoxicity of chemotherapeutic agents. *Drug Safety* 22: 263–302.

Pritchard J, Sandercock P A G (2000). Drug-induced stroke. *Adverse Drug React Bull* 202: 771–774.

Ramsay L E, Williams B, Johnston D G *et al.* (1999). British Hypertension Society guidelines for hypertension management: summary. *Br Med J* 319: 630–635.

Reilly J G, Ayis S A, Ferrier I N *et al.* (2000). QTc-interval abnormalities and psychotropic drug therapy in psychiatric patients. *Lancet* 355: 1048–1052.

Sacchi S, Kantarjian H, O'Brien S *et al.* (1995). Immune-mediated and unusual complications during interferon alfa therapy in chronic myelogenous leukemia. *J Clin Oncol* 13: 2401–2407.

Shan K, Lincoff M, Young J B (1996). Anthracycline-induced cardiotoxicity. *Ann Intern Med* 125: 47–58.

Simons F E R, Kesselman M S, Giddins N G *et al.* (1988). Astemizole induces torsades de pointes. *Lancet* ii: 624.

Singal P K, Iliskovic N (1998). Doxorubicin-induced cardiomyopathy. *N Engl J Med* 339: 900–905.

Spence J D (1997). Drug interactions with grapefruit: whose responsibility is it to warn the public? *Clin Pharmacol Ther* 61: 395–400.

Stockley I H (1999). *Drug Interactions*, 5th edn. London: Pharmaceutical Press, 90.

Taler S J, Textor S C, Canzanello V J *et al.* (1999). Cyclosporin-induced hypertension. *Drug Safety* 20: 437–449.

Textor S C, Canzanello V J, Taler S J *et al.* (1994). Cyclosporine-induced hypertension after transplantation. *Mayo Clin Proc* 69: 1182–1193.

Thomas S H L (1997). Drugs and the QT interval. *Adverse Drug React Bull* 182: 691–694.

Vessey M P, Lawless M, Yeates D (1984). Oral contraceptives and stroke: findings in a large prospective study. *Br Med J* 289: 530–531.

Viskin S (1999). Long QT syndromes and torsade de pointes. *Lancet* 354: 1625–1633.

Weiss N (1995). Third generation oral contraceptives: how risky? *Lancet* 346: 1570.

Weissman N J, Tighe J F, Gottdiener J S *et al.* (1998). An assessment of heart-valve abnormalities in obese patients taking dexfenfluramine, sustained-release dexfenfluramine or placebo. *N Engl J Med* 339: 725–732.

Wysowski D, Bakanyi J (1996). Cisapride and fatal arrhythmias. *N Engl J Med* 335: 290–291.

Zornberg G L, Jick H (2000). Antipsychotic drug use and risk of first-time idiopathic venous thromboembolism: a case-control study. *Lancet* 356: 1219–1223.

12

Neurological disorders

Fiona Thomson

Drug-induced neurological effects are common. This chapter discusses the different types of disorders that can be produced, the drugs most commonly implicated and how the risk of reactions can be minimised. Many drugs have the potential to cause adverse effects on the central nervous system (CNS). This chapter discusses drug-induced neurological effects; drug-induced psychiatric effects are considered in Chapter 10.

Neurological adverse effects may mimic disease and it can be difficult to establish a drug's causative role. Some neurological disorders may be exacerbated or precipitated by drugs; for example, myasthenia gravis can be induced by penicillamine treatment and made worse by aminoglycoside antibiotics (Wittbrodt, 1997).

Drug-induced neurotoxicity may be minimised by identifying drugs that may be contributing to a patient's neurological symptoms or avoiding the use of inappropriate drugs in patients with neurological disorders. Often drug therapy can be optimised to reduce the risk of adverse effects, particularly in high-risk patients. For example, in a patient with Parkinson's disease requiring an antipsychotic, an agent with a relatively low incidence of extrapyramidal side-effects should be chosen.

Drugs used to treat neurological disorders, such as antiepileptics, may cause neurological adverse effects as a result of their mechanism of action (Wong and Lhatoo, 2000). These effects can occur at therapeutic doses. Sometimes these effects may be dose-limiting so that a balance between efficacy and side-effects in the individual patient is needed. Patients should be educated about the possibility of such adverse effects to ensure that they are identified at an early stage and managed appropriately.

Patients with liver or renal impairment may be at increased risk of neurological toxicity due to drug accumulation. For example, penicillin-induced neurotoxicity is associated with the use of high doses in patients with reduced renal function (Schliamser *et al.*, 1991). Drug abuse is associated with many neurological disorders and this should be considered as a possible aetiology in patients presenting with neurological symptoms.

Headache

Headache is a common symptom. The condition may be primary (e.g. migraine, tension headache) or secondary to factors such as systemic infection, head injury or drugs (Classification Committee of the International Headache Society, 1988). Drugs should always be considered as a possible cause as many can produce this symptom, although only about 3% of headaches are drug-induced (Burns and Schultz, 1993; Rassmussen, 1995).

Drug-induced headache may occur by the stretching of pain-sensitive cerebral blood vessel walls through vasodilatation or vasoconstriction or by chemical irritation of the meninges (Olesen, 1995). Vasodilators, such as calcium channel blockers, nitrates and hydralazine, may precipitate a vascular headache. If patients complain of headache at the start of treatment with these drugs they should be encouraged to persevere with the treatment as tolerance usually occurs with continued use. Anti-inflammatory drugs such as indometacin may also precipitate a vascular headache (Burns and Schultz, 1993). Headache is also a feature of the hypertensive crises induced by monoamine oxidase inhibitors when taken in combination with sympathetic agonists such as ephedrine, tricyclic antidepressants or foods containing tyramine.

Analgesic headache

Analgesic rebound headache is a problem which may be particularly difficult to manage (Ferrari, 1998). When taken daily, ergotamine, opioids and even simple analgesics may all aggravate tension headache and migraine (Silberstein and Young, 1995; Ferrari, 1998). Patients with frequent headaches often overuse analgesics. Overuse has been defined as the regular daily intake of simple analgesics more often than four times a week and opioids or ergotamine more often than twice a week (Silberstein and Young, 1995). Even a low dose used regularly is more likely to cause this problem than larger doses used intermittently. Concurrent consumption of caffeine either in drinks or in analgesic preparations may contribute to the effect (Ferrari, 1998). This regular use frequently produces chronic daily headache, or drug-induced rebound headache, leading to dependence on symptomatic medication. The problem is specific to use of analgesics for headache (i.e. it is not associated with their use for other indications) and the mechanisms involved are not clear. The problem is more likely with combination analgesics and it is unclear whether it occurs with simple aspirin or paracetamol. On stopping analgesics, the headache generally worsens before it resolves.

People with frequent headache often do not realise that excessive self-treatment can perpetuate the problem, and use of over-the-counter analgesics, as well as prescribed medicines, should be considered. Management of the problem requires gradual drug withdrawal, which can be very difficult. Many other treatments for this type of headache have been assessed, e.g. abrupt withdrawal of analgesics, the use of non-steroidal anti-inflammatory drugs (NSAIDs), dihydroergotamine, sumatriptan, amitriptyline, dexamethasone and valproate, but there is little published literature to support appropriate management of the condition (Zed *et al.*, 1999).

To minimise the problem, healthcare professionals should ensure that patients with frequent headaches are aware of this possibility. Such patients should never take analgesics every day; a proposed maximum is 15 days a month (Silberstein and Young, 1995). Simple analgesics are the drugs of choice; compound analgesics and opioids should be avoided.

Regular use of ergotamine and its derivatives may cause dependence. On drug withdrawal, rebound headache develops and this is only alleviated by ergotamine. This may occur even when treatment recommendations limiting its use to 2 days a week are followed. Ergotamine withdrawal under controlled conditions may be needed to break this cycle (Saper, 1987).

Although drug-induced headache associated with the use of serotonin (5-HT_1) agonists or 'triptans' has been reported, causality has not been established and the extent of any association is unknown (Kaube *et al.*, 1994; Dowson, 1999; Limmroth *et al.*, 1999).

Aseptic meningitis

Ibuprofen and other NSAIDs have occasionally been reported to cause aseptic meningitis, usually accompanied by severe headache (Committee on Safety of Medicines, 1991a; Seaton and France, 1999). The problem is most common in patients with systemic lupus erythematosus or other connective tissue disease. Patients develop classic symptoms of meningitis but an infective cause cannot be demonstrated, and the symptoms resolve rapidly on drug withdrawal. The two main mechanisms are thought to be direct chemical 'irritation' of the meninges by drugs introduced into the cerebrospinal fluid, or a hypersensitivity reaction involving the meninges (Jolles *et al.*, 2000). Patients who have previously experienced this reaction should be advised to avoid over-the-counter medicines containing ibuprofen. Aseptic meningitis has also been described following therapy with immunoglobulins, vaccines, ciprofloxacin, azathioprine, penicillin, isoniazid and co-trimoxazole and muromonab-CD3 (Kato *et al.*, 1988; Casteels-Van Daele *et al.*, 1990; Gordon *et al.*, 1990; Marinjac, 1992; Sekul *et al.*, 1994; Patey *et al.*, 1998; Seaton and France, 1999; Jolles *et al.*, 2000). Intrathecal drug administration may be followed by direct irritation of the meninges, occurring up to several weeks after intrathecal drug administration, but other factors such as pre-existing CNS disease or injection of contaminants should be considered when assessing causality (Jolles *et al.*, 2000). As this syndrome is difficult to distinguish from infective meningitis, the drug history should be considered in all meningitis cases (Moris and Garcia-Monco, 1999).

Benign intracranial hypertension (pseudotumour cerebri)

Drugs can also cause benign intracranial hypertension (pseudotumour cerebri). This syndrome is associated with headache and marked papilloedema (oedema of the optic nerve head), which usually arise from increased intracranial pressure (Rush, 1980). Nausea and vomiting, tinnitus and visual disturbances may also be present. It may be complicated by diplopia (double vision) due to sixth nerve paresis, visual blurring and visual field defects due to cerebral oedema. The mechanism may involve salt and water retention leading to intracranial fluid redistribution. Athough not usually life-threatening, optic nerve damage and loss of vision may develop. The diagnosis is confirmed by measurement of cerebrospinal fluid pressures. Symptoms develop between days and months after initiation of therapy and usually resolve once the causative agent is withdrawn, although there may be permanent visual loss in some patients. Table 12.1 lists some drugs that have been associated with benign intracranial hypertension (Rush, 1980; Cruz *et al.*, 1996; Blain and Lane, 1998; Chiu *et al.*, 1998; Riyaz *et al.*, 1998; Singh and Chye, 1998; Gurm and Farooq, 1999).

Table 12.1 Some drugs associated with benign intracranial hypertension

Amlodipine	Nalidixic acid
Corticosteroids (both oral and topical)	Nitrofurantoin
Danazol	Nitrous oxide
Etretinate	Oral contraceptives
Ketamine	Tetracyclines (e.g. minocycline)
Leuprorelin	Vitamin A (high doses and deficiency)

Seizures

Drugs may precipitate seizures, especially in patients with epilepsy or other risk factors. Risk factors include pre-existing cerebral or systemic disease (e.g. cerebrovascular disease or infection) or treatment with drugs known to reduce the seizure threshold. Drugs that act on the CNS or can cross the blood–brain barrier are most likely to cause this effect. As the consequences of loss of seizure control can be serious, healthcare professionals should be vigilant for use of drugs which may exacerbate epilepsy. As well as the morbidity and mortality associated with seizures, a seizure may have other consequences, such as the loss of a driving licence, even when precipitated by a drug. Anticonvulsants themselves may cause worsening of seizures (Wong and Lhatoo, 2000). Drugs which interact with antiepileptics may precipitate seizures through lowering of blood levels or may precipitate other neurological adverse effects through potentiation of the antiepileptic, leading to toxicity (see Table 12.2).

Table 12.2 Neurological toxicity of antiepileptics

Drug	Neurological adverse effect
Phenytoin	Ataxia, nystagmus, drowsiness, diplopia, dyskinesia
Carbamazepine	Ataxia, diplopia, drowsiness, headache, dyskinesia
Sodium valproate	Ataxia, drowsiness, tremor
Phenobarbital	Fatigue, listlessness, poor memory
Clonazepam	Fatigue, drowsiness, ataxia
Vigabatrin	Drowsiness, fatigue, dizziness, nervousness, headache, nystagmus, paraesthesiae, ataxia, tremor, diplopia, memory loss
Lamotrigine	Headache, fatigue, dizziness, drowsiness, insomnia, diplopia, blurred vision, headache
Gabapentin	Somnolence, dizziness, fatigue, nystagmus, headache, movement disorders, diplopia
Tiagabine	Dizziness, asthenia, nervousness, tremor, headache, paraesthesiae
Topiramate	Ataxia, dizziness, fatigue, paraesthesiae

Convulsions have occurred in patients taking quinolones (with or without a history of epilepsy), both in overdose and with normal doses (Committee on Safety of Medicines, 1991b). Isolated cases of neurological toxicity or convulsions have been described with ciprofloxacin taken together with theophylline or NSAIDs, but these appear to be rare. Nevertheless, the combination of a quinolone antibiotic with an NSAID should be avoided in patients at risk if a suitable alternative is available. Quinolones may inhibit theophylline's metabolism, leading to accumulation and a risk of seizures. The dose of theophylline may need to be reduced in patients who require a quinolone antibiotic. Animal models have shown that quinolones competitively inhibit the binding of gamma-aminobutyric acid (GABA), the inhibitory neurotransmitter, to its receptors. As GABA is implicated in the pathogenesis of seizures, this may account for their epileptogenic effect (Ball and Tillotson, 1995).

Post-marketing surveillance in the UK has highlighted a number of reports of seizure with donepezil (Babic and Zurak, 1999). It is unknown whether these are are due to the drug or to the underlying condition (Alzheimer's disease) being treated (Committee on Safety of Medicines, 1999). Convulsions have also been reported with tramadol, sometimes in association with other drugs which may reduce the seizure threshold (Committee on Safety of Medicines, 1996a). The UK Committee on Safety of Medicines has recommended that patients with a history of epilepsy or who are otherwise predisposed to seizures should only be treated with tramadol if there are compelling reasons, and that caution should be exercised when it is given to patients taking medication that can reduce the seizure threshold, particularly selective serotonin reuptake inhibitors (SSRIs) and tricyclic antidepressants.

Convulsions may also occur secondary to other medical causes precipitated by drugs. For example, desmopressin has been associated with convulsions secondary to hyponatraemia, and antiepileptic drugs have exacerbated seizures, where the underlying cause of seizures was later identified as porphyria (Committee on Safety of Medicines, 1996b; Schwab and Ruder, 1997).

Seizures may occur as part of a spectrum of toxicity known as the serotonin syndrome (see Chapter 10). It may occur with concurrent use of drugs that mimic or prolong the activity of serotonin, for example SSRIs and monoamine oxidase inhibitors (Mason *et al.*, 2000). Illicit drugs, such as cocaine, amphetamines, diamorphine and Ecstasy, may cause seizures, as well as other adverse neurological effects (Blain and Lane, 1998).

Abrupt withdrawal of antiepileptics may precipitate seizures, so treatment should be withdrawn gradually. Withdrawal syndromes associated with other drugs, including alcohol, benzodiazepines, barbiturates and baclofen, have also been implicated in causing seizures in non-epileptic patients (Hyser and Drake, 1984; Barker and Grant, 1992).

Table 12.3 lists some drugs that have been associated with seizures.

Table 12.3 Some drugs that may cause convulsions or exacerbate epilepsy

Amfebutamone	Non-steroidal anti-inflammatory
Antipsychotics	drugs
Baclofen	Oral contraceptives
Carbapenems	Penicillins
Chloroquine	Pethidine
Ciclosporin	Propofol
Donepezil	Quinolone antibiotics
Halothane	Selective serotonin reuptake
Isoniazid	inhibitors
Ketamine	Theophylline
Lidocaine (lignocaine)	Tramadol
Lithium	Tricyclic antidepressants
Mefloquine	Vaccines
Methylenedioxymethamfetamine	Vincristine
(MDMA or Ecstasy)	

Coma and encephalopathy

The clinical features of drug-induced coma are similar, regardless of the drug involved. Coma involves cortical dysfunction and features loss of brainstem reflexes, generalised flaccidity and depressed or absent tendon reflexes. Encephalopathy is a general term for cerebral dysfunction; the spectrum of symptoms includes tremor, myoclonus, confusion, lethargy, agitation, hallucination and seizures. Drug-induced coma can arise through a primary neurotoxic effect on the CNS, through indirect effects on cerebral metabolism, or through alterations in cerebral blood flow. Primary neurotoxic effects are usually dose-related. Most cases of drug-induced coma are caused by poisoning or overdose with drugs that act on the CNS, including benzodiazepines, antipsychotics, antidepressants and opioids (including those contained in over-the-counter cough medicines) (Cartlidge, 1981). Patient factors affecting metabolism or elimination may contribute to neurotoxicity as a result of drug accumulation.

Ciclosporin has been reported to cause coma as well as other neurological adverse effects, including seizures, encephalopathy and movement disorders (Vial and Descotes, 1996; Madan and Schey, 1997). The mechanism is unknown but may involve either a vasculopathy arising from ciclosporin's effect on the components of endothelial cells or specific enzyme inhibition (Hauben, 1996). Neurotoxicity is not always related to ciclosporin plasma concentrations. Possible risk factors include high-dose steroid therapy, hypocholesterolaemia, hypomagnesaemia and systemic hypertension.

Aciclovir and ganciclovir may cause neurotoxicity; symptoms usually occur within the first few days of treatment. Risk factors include intravenous administration, the use of high doses, renal impairment and old age (Ernst and Franey, 1998). Acute renal failure and neurotoxicity have also been associated with oral aciclovir administration in a patient with mild renal impairment, highlighting the importance of this risk factor (Johnson et al., 1994). Aciclovir may be used to treat suspected herpes simplex encephalitis and it may be difficult to distinguish between aciclovir neurotoxicity and encephalitis of other origin (Rashiq et al., 1993).

Coma and seizures have also been described with the immunosuppressants tacrolimus and muromonab-CD3 (Vial and Descotes, 1996). A number of cytotoxic drugs, including cisplatin, ifosfamide and high-dose methotrexate, may cause direct neurotoxicity, resulting in seizures and encephalopathy (Lindley et al., 1995).

Antiepileptics may cause encephalopathy, which is usually dose-related. Strategies to prevent this may include plasma concentration monitoring, where appropriate, and education of the patient to be aware of signs of toxicity. Valproate has recently been reported to cause coma in association with hyperammonaemia. The drug was being used to treat an affective disorder and symptoms of lethargy were initially interpreted as a therapeutic response, delaying treatment (Eze et al., 1998).

Severe and prolonged hypoglycaemia can cause coma; drugs which may precipitate hypoglycaemia include insulin, sulphonylureas, high-dose salicylates, ethanol, pentamidine and quinine (Ferner, 1996). Certain risk factors may contribute substantially to the morbidity and mortality of diabetic patients with drug-induced hypoglycaemic coma. These include age over 60 years, renal impairment, decreased energy intake and infection (Ben-Ami et al., 1999). Seizures may precede coma and permanent brain damage may result.

Neuropathies

Some drugs may have toxic effects on cranial and peripheral nerves.

Cranial neuropathies

Symptoms of cranial nerve toxicity depend on the nerve affected. These nerves are involved in vision and eye movements, smell, taste, hearing and balance. Cranial nerve toxicity, probably due to damage to the third cranial nerve, affects 1–10% of patients receiving vinca alkaloids. The main features are ptosis (drooping eyelids) and ophthalmoplegia (paralysis of the eye muscles) (Lindley *et al.*, 1995). Other cytotoxic agents which may cause cranial neuropathy include ifosfamide, platinum compounds and fluorouracil.

Ethambutol may cause optic neuropathy which is not always reversible (DeVita *et al.*, 1987). Patients should be advised to report changes in vision and should have regular eye examinations. Rare cases of optic neuritis have been reported with amiodarone but the association has not been proven. Desferrioxamine may cause visual and auditory neurotoxicity (Olivieri *et al.*, 1986). An association between omeprazole, particularly the intravenous preparation, with optic neuropathy, has been reported in Europe but causality has not been established (Schonhofer *et al.*, 1997; Lessell, 1998; Riorrdan-Eva and Sanders, 1998; Sachs, 1998).

Peripheral neuropathies

The pathological changes in drug-induced peripheral neuropathy usually consist of axonal degeneration with secondary breakdown of the myelin sheath. Depending on the type of damage to the nerve, several features can arise. The patient often complains of symmetrical numbness and tingling (paraesthesiae) in the hands and feet, often referred to as 'stocking-glove' neuropathy. There may also be muscle weakness and wasting and sensory loss. Tendon reflexes involving affected nerves are lost; ankle jerks are usually first affected. In most drug-induced peripheral neuropathies, investigations such as nerve conduction studies reveal axonal degeneration or secondary breakdown of the myelin sheath (demyelination). Neuropathies may be predominantly sensory, motor or a mixture of both.

Possible risk factors for drug-induced neuropathy are shown in Table 12.4. If possible, drugs suspected of causing a neuropathy should

Table 12.4 Risk factors for drug-induced peripheral neuropathy

Diabetes mellitus
Alcoholism
Vitamin deficiency/poor nutrition
Impaired renal/hepatic function (leading to drug accumulation)
Slow acetylator status (isoniazid, hydralazine)

be withdrawn, although the effect may not always be reversible. Early withdrawal of the causative agent may improve prognosis, so healthcare professionals should be alert for this problem. Several drugs are associated with peripheral neuropathy.

Alcoholic neuropathy is common, mainly arising from nutritional deficiency and a reduced capacity to absorb thiamine, although a direct toxic effect on peripheral nerves may also be involved. The clinical features are similar to those of beriberi, but there may be associated problems, such as Wernicke–Korsakoff encephalopathy. Thiamine is widely used to prevent and treat this problem in alcohol-dependent patients (Cook and Thomson, 1997).

Peripheral nerve toxicity is a common problem with vinca alkaloids. The problem is dose-related and mild sensory symptoms may have to be accepted to achieve a therapeutic response. If the neuropathy progresses, bilateral wrist and finger weakness may develop, followed by more widespread weakness. Other cytotoxic drugs associated with this problem are cisplatin, carboplatin, etoposide and taxanes (Lindley *et al.*, 1995; Fields Jones and Burris, 1996; Freilich *et al.*, 1996).

Isoniazid can cause a mixed motor and sensory neuropathy. Individuals who acetylate the drug slowly are more likely to be affected (Lennard, 1993). The neuropathy is due to interference with pyridoxine metabolism and can be prevented by adequate prophylactic doses of this vitamin. The dose of isoniazid given should take into account other patient factors that may predispose to neuropathy (e.g. poor nutrition, diabetes). Slow acetylators also have increased susceptibility to peripheral neuropathies caused by hydralazine and dapsone.

Some antiretroviral drugs, particularly the nucleoside reverse transcriptase inhibitors, including didanosine, stavudine, zidovudine and zalcitabine, may also cause peripheral nerve damage (Ellis, 1996). The most severe adverse effect of zalcitabine has been a painful peripheral neuropathy, mainly affecting the feet initially. The problem usually occurs in the first 6 months of treatment and is dose-related. It may resolve with dosage reduction but in some cases the drug may need to be discontinued (Blum *et al.*, 1996). The temporal association with drug initiation may help to distinguish drug-induced neuropathy from that associated with human immunodeficiency virus (HIV) infection itself. Patients at particular risk include those with low CD4 count, a prior history of an acquired immune deficiency syndrome (AIDS), defining illness or neoplasm, a history of peripheral neuropathy, use of other neurotoxic agents including high alcohol consumption and nutritional deficiencies such as low vitamin B_{12} levels (Moyle and Sadler, 1998). Clinicians may wish to avoid the use of neurotoxic nucleoside analogues in at-risk patients; otherwise they should ensure close monitoring during treatment.

Deficiency in vitamin B_{12} may also lead to peripheral neuropathy. Pyridoxine, if taken in very large doses, can cause a sensory neuropathy. Recent concern about this problem has led to revised UK recommendations for the use of pyridoxine, maximising the daily dose for general sale (in health food outlets, etc.) to 10 mg (Anon, 1997). There has been controversy over the evidence base supporting this recommendation; in the USA the daily dose considered safe for unrestricted sale is 100 mg (Anon, 1998; Chalmers and Barker, 1998; Marks, 1998).

Peripheral neuropathy with lipid-lowering drugs such as simvastatin has been reported, although this effect is less well established than the association of these drugs with myopathy (Ziajka and Wehmeier, 1998; Jeppesen *et al.*, 1999).

Some drugs that can cause peripheral neuropathy are shown in Table 12.5.

Table 12.5 Some drugs that may cause peripheral neuropathy

Alcohol	Perhexilene maleate
Amiodarone	Phenytoin
Dapsone	Platinum compounds
Didanosine	Pyridoxine (vitamin B_6)
Disulfiram	Quinolones
Ethambutol	Stavudine
Gold	Taxanes (paclitaxel, docetaxel)
Hydralazine	Thalidomide
Interferon alfa	Vinca alkaloids and other antimitotic
Isoniazid	cytotoxics
Metronidazole	Zalcitabine
Nitrofurantoin	Zidovudine

Guillain–Barré syndrome

The Guillain–Barré syndrome (GBS) is a rare immune-mediated disorder in which peripheral nerve myelin is damaged, with resultant peripheral nerve dysfunction that is frequently severe and fulminant. It occurs rarely as a consequence of drug exposure (Rees, 1995; Awong *et al.*, 1996). The syndrome usually starts with paraesthesiae of the toes or fingertips, followed by upper and lower limb and then total body weakness. Facial, ophthalmic and oropharyngeal muscles may be involved. These symptoms may develop within days to as long as 14 months after starting drug treatment. Recovery usually occurs over weeks to months. Many patients (85%) have residual impairment and up to 8% die. Management is mainly supportive, although corticosteroids, plasma exchange therapy and intravenous immunoglobulins may be of benefit.

Table 12.6 shows some drugs that have been associated with GBS (Dick and Raman, 1982; Knezevic *et al.*, 1984; Morris and Rylance, 1994; Arrowsmith *et al.*, 1985; Chakraborty and Ruddell, 1987; D'Cruz *et al.*, 1989; Awong *et al.*, 1996; Schonberger and Chen, 1998). Zimeldine, an SSRI, was withdrawn in the UK in 1983, after 200 000 prescriptions had been dispensed worldwide and 10 cases of GBS reported during that time.

Table 12.6 Some drugs associated with Guillain–Barré syndrome

Captopril	Measles, mumps and rubella (MMR) vaccine
Corticosteroids	Oxytocin
Gold	Penicillamine
Hepatitis B vaccine	Streptokinase
Influenza vaccine	Zimeldine

A possible association between vaccines and GBS has been suggested but causality has not been established. It appears that the magnitude of any risk is low (McMahon *et al.*, 1992; Rantala *et al.*, 1994; Rees and Hughes, 1994; Stricker *et al.*, 1994; Hughes *et al.*, 1996; da Silveira *et al.*, 1997; Ismail *et al.*, 1998; Kinnunen *et al.*, 1998; Lasky *et al.*, 1998; Ropper and Victor, 1998; Salisbury, 1998).

Myopathy

Drug-induced myopathy is discussed in Chapter 8.

Effects on the neuromuscular junction and myasthenia gravis

Some drugs can affect neuromuscular transmission (Table 12.7). Possible consequences of their effects include postoperative respiratory depression, the unmasking or exacerbation of myasthenia gravis and drug-induced myasthenic syndrome (Blain and Lane, 1998). Contributory factors include electrolyte disturbances (e.g. hyperkalaemia, hypocalcaemia) or high drug plasma concentrations due to impaired elimination.

Table 12.7 Some drugs that may affect the neuromuscular junction

Aminoglycoside antibiotics	Lithium
Beta-blockers	Penicillamine
Carnitine	Phenytoin
Chloroquine	Polymyxins (polymyxin B, colistin)
Clindamycin	Quinine
Interferon alfa	Tetracyclines

Some drugs with a neuromuscular-blocking effect, if used during the perioperative period, may prevent re-establishment of spontaneous respiration after the procedure. This problem, known as myasthenic crisis, occurs most commonly with aminoglycoside antibiotics, tetracyclines, lincomycin and clindamycin. Features include generalised weakness and paralysis of respiratory muscles. Treatment usually involves assisted respiration and use of anticholinesterase drugs, e.g. neostigmine (Blain and Lane, 1998).

Activation or exacerbation of myasthenia gravis

Myasthenia gravis is a disease of the neuromuscular junction in which normal transmission of impulses is impaired or prevented by acetylcholine receptor antibodies. Characteristic features include generalised muscle weakness, ptosis, dysphonia, dysphagia, difficulty chewing, dyspnoea and respiratory failure. Several classes of drugs have been associated with worsening of existing myasthenia gravis and a small number of drugs is thought to cause a variant of the disease.

Penicillamine can cause a syndrome almost identical to myasthenia gravis, mainly in patients with rheumatoid arthritis or Wilson's disease. In some reported cases, the diagnosis has been delayed as respiratory symptoms have been wrongly attributed to deteriorating chronic obstructive pulmonary disease (Adelman *et al.*, 1995). Nearly all patients with this syndrome have acetylcholine receptor antibodies but usually the condition remits within a year of discontinuing penicillamine. The exact mechanism of the problem has not been determined but an immunological basis seems likely.

Interferon alfa may cause development of autoantibodies and autoimmune diseases. Cases of myasthenia gravis either exacerbated by, or induced by this drug have been reported (Battochi *et al.*, 1995; Uyama *et al.*, 1996; Bori *et al.*, 1997).

High doses of corticosteroids may cause sudden deterioration of myasthenia gravis. Patients who are initiated on corticosteroids as immunosuppressive treatment for myasthenia are usually admitted to hospital, as up to 48% of patients will experience transient steroid-induced exacerbation in the first weeks of treatment (Johns, 1987). Other drugs that may exacerbate myasthenia gravis include phenytoin, aminoglycosides, ciprofloxacin and other quinolone antibiotics, beta-blockers, lithium, anticholinergics and neuromuscular-blocking agents. These drugs and those which affect neurotransmission (see Table 12.7) should preferably be avoided in myasthenic patients; even small amounts of quinine in tonic water should be avoided.

Drug-induced myasthenic syndrome

This is an uncommon syndrome in which the patient rapidly develops features of myasthenia gravis which remit promptly on drug withdrawal. In some cases, drug exposure appears to unmask myasthenia in predisposed patients. Again, factors such as electrolyte disturbances or impaired elimination of drugs often contribute. This syndrome can be distinguished from true myasthenia gravis by the absence of acetylcholine receptor antibodies. Drugs implicated include aminoglycoside antibiotics, polymyxins, beta-blockers and phenytoin (Blain and Lane, 1998).

Drug-induced movement disorders (extrapyramidal effects)

Drug-induced movement disorders include parkinsonism (tremor, rigidity, akinesia), neuroleptic malignant syndrome, acute dystonia, acute akathisia and tardive dyskinesia (American Psychiatric Association, 1994; Jimenez-Jimenez *et al.*, 1997; Anon, 1998). Neuroleptic malignant syndrome is discussed in Chapter 10.

The drugs most frequently implicated in movement disorders are those used for their therapeutic effect on the CNS, e.g. antipsychotics, antiemetics, antiepileptics, antiparkinsonian drugs and lithium (Jimenez-Jimenez *et al.*, 1997). It is not unusual for two or more types of drug-induced movement disorder to coexist in the same patient and single agents can cause more than one type of movement disorder.

In the last few years, there have been many reports of movement disorders associated with SSRIs and review of these suggests possible causality (Caley, 1997; Gerber and Lynd, 1998; Richard *et al.*, 1999). Drugs acting outside the CNS may also cause movement disorders, e.g. calcium channel blockers, and this may be less obvious when assessing the drug history of a patient presenting with symptoms suggestive of a movement disorder. Illicit drug use with cocaine, amphetamines and methylenedioxymethamfetamine (MDMA or Ecstasy) has been associated with various movement disorders.

Parkinsonism

Drugs may precipitate parkinsonism or exacerbate pre-existing parkinsonism. This is a frequent problem with drugs affecting dopaminergic neurotransmission in the basal ganglia. The mechanism may be depletion of presynaptic dopamine or blockade of postsynaptic dopamine receptors. The problem is particularly common in elderly patients, in whom dopamine receptor reserve may already be diminished. Major signs include resting tremor, cogwheel rigidity, akinesia and postural instability. The clinical signs are often indistinguishable from those of idiopathic Parkinson's disease, although in drug-induced cases postural tremor is more frequent and tardive dyskinesia or dystonia is often also present (Jimenez-Jimenez *et al.*, 1997). Although drug-induced parkinsonism is usually reversible, in some patients the symptoms do not resolve completely even when the drug is withdrawn; this may reflect an 'unmasking' of subclinical parkinsonism.

Antipsychotics such as haloperidol are the best recognised cause of iatrogenic parkinsonism but other drugs are implicated (Table 12.8; Committee on Safety of Medicines, 1994a). Naproxen, captopril, amiodarone, phenytoin, valproate and oral contraceptives have also been reported to cause or exacerbate parkinsonism but these cases are mainly anecdotal and causality has not been established (Anon, 1998). With antipsychotics, the adverse effect is dose-dependent and seems to be related to the extent of dopamine D_2-receptor blockade. Although it is difficult to quantify the prevalence of the problem with different

Table 12.8 Some drugs that may cause or exacerbate parkinsonism

Antiemetics, e.g. prochlorperazine, metoclopramide	Methyldopa
Antipsychotics	Selective serotonin reuptake inhibitors, e.g. paroxetine, fluoxetine
Calcium channel blockers, e.g. verapamil, amlodipine, flunarizine, cinnarizine, diltiazem	Tetrabenazine
	Tricyclic antidepressants
Lithium	Valproate

antipsychotics, the risk seems to be lower with newer atypical antipsychotics such as risperidone, olanzapine and clozapine. These agents have a lower affinity for D_2-receptors.

To avoid this problem, drugs implicated should be used with caution and antipsychotic doses should always be kept to a minimum. Where a drug is suspected to be the cause, it should be withdrawn. Most cases will resolve once the causative agent is removed. Antiparkinsonian therapy may be required but should not be started for at least 3 months. Anticholinergic drugs may be used to treat the effect but should not be given as prophylaxis as this may increase the risk of irreversible tardive dyskinesia (Barnes and McPhillips, 1996). In patients requiring antipsychotic therapy for schizophrenia, factors associated with an increased risk and severity of iatrogenic parkinsonism include early age at onset of schizophrenia, high ventricle : brain ratio and severity of negative symptoms (Jimenez-Jimenez et al., 1997).

In patients with a pre-existing extrapyramidal disorder, e.g. Parkinson's disease, drug choice will need to take into account potential benefit of the drug as well as risk. Patients with Parkinson's disease may experience psychosis as a result of levodopa or dopamine agonist therapy. Dose reduction may help psychosis but cause an unacceptable decrease in parkinsonian symptom control. An antipsychotic with low incidence of extrapyramidal effects, e.g. thioridazine, or newer agents such as risperidone, sulpiride, olanzapine or clozapine may be considered, but should be started at a low dose and titrated slowly.

Elderly patients with dementias are particularly susceptible to extrapyramidal reactions. In those with Lewy body dementia, which may account for up to one-fifth of cases of dementia diagnosed clinically, these reactions may be life-threatening (McKeith et al., 1992). Administration of a neuroleptic may result in the sudden onset of extrapyramidal rigidity, postural instability, profound confusion, immobility and reduced food and fluid intake. These reactions do not appear to be associated with any particular type of neuroleptic and may occur at doses within the recommended range for the elderly (Committee on Safety of Medicines, 1994b). The UK Committee on Safety of Medicines has advised that elderly patients with dementia should only be given neuroleptics at very low doses with cautious titration against the clinical state, and that particular care should be taken if features suggestive of Lewy body dementia are present.

Conversely, antipsychotic withdrawal may also preciptate or aggravate parkinsonism (Anon, 1998).

Acute dystonia

Acute dystonia is characterised by abnormal postures or muscle spasms. These may manifest as abnormal movements of the head and neck (e.g. torticollis), spasms of the jaw muscles (e.g. trismus), grimacing, dysphagia, laryngeal or pharyngeal spasm leading to breathing difficulty, dysphonia or tongue spasms leading to problems with speech, oculogyric crisis and opisthotonus (Launer, 1996; van Harten *et al.*, 1999). The onset of dystonia may be acute or chronic (tardive dystonia). The symptoms of tardive dystonia and acute dystonia are practically identical. However, tardive dystonia, which is much less frequent, occurs only after months or years of treatment (van Harten *et al.*, 1999).

Acute dystonia is often very frightening for the patient. Healthcare professionals, particularly those working in mental health, should be familiar with the risk factors for acute dystonia and should know how to prevent and treat the condition. Acute dystonia with antipsychotic drugs generally develops within 7 days of starting or increasing the dose of the antipsychotic, or of reducing medication used to prevent or treat extrapyramidal effects (e.g. anticholinergics). The reported prevalence varies widely and seems to depend on the presence of risk factors. Risk factors for antipsychotic drug-induced dystonia include younger age, male gender, previous instance of acute dystonia and recent cocaine use (van Harten *et al.*, 1999). In patients aged 10–19 years the risk of acute dystonia is high but it decreases linearly with age; in patients over 45 years of age acute dystonia is rare. Most studies have found that men are more likely to develop acute dystonia than women. A history of acute dystonia has been identified as the most powerful predictor of the likelihood of a patient developing the condition.

Dystonia is most commonly associated with antipsychotics, particularly high-potency drugs such as the butyrophenones, fluphenazine and pimozide. The frequency is less with low-potency drugs such as chlorpromazine and thioridazine. Atypical antipsychotics such as olanzapine and quetiapine are associated with a low incidence of acute dystonia. Clozapine is the only atypical antipsychotic thought not to induce acute dystonia (van Harten et al., 1999). Other drugs that may cause acute dystonia include metoclopramide and related drugs, antiparkinsonian drugs and SSRIs (Aryka, 1994; van Harten et al., 1999). Rarely, cases of dystonia following 5-HT$_1$ agonists (e.g. sumatriptan), calcium antagonists (e.g. verapamil, diltiazem and cinnarizine) and antiepileptic drugs (e.g. carbamazepine, phenytoin) have also been reported.

Metoclopramide is one of the most common agents implicated in acute dystonia (Bateman, 1991). The problem is more common in young adults than in the elderly and more common in women than men. A prospective study suggested that one in 80 patients under the age of 30 years given the drug in general practice would experience an extrapyramidal reaction. The dystonia usually resolves within 24 hours of drug withdrawal. Metoclopramide should be avoided in patients younger than 20 years old. In other patients, care should be taken to ensure that the recommended dose is not exceeded, particularly in the elderly and patients with renal impairment.

The treatment of acute dystonia is usually straightforward and nearly always effective. Anticholinergic agents, such as benzatropine or procyclidine, should be given by intramuscular or intravenous injection (Holloman and Marder, 1997; van Harten et al., 1999). Occasionally second or third injections are necessary. Tardive dystonia, however, is potentially irreversible and there is no established therapy, though treatment with tetrabenazine, reserpine or botulinum toxin may be tried (Raja, 1998).

Patients with Parkinson's disease treated with levodopa or dopamine agonists may experience painful dystonia of the lower extremities, particularly on waking in the morning. This may be managed by adjustment of the antiparkinsonian drug regimen or by the use of various agents including apomorphine, baclofen or benzodiazepines (Anon, 1998).

Acute akathisia

Akathisia is a subjective sensation of restlessness, often associated with an inability to keep still (Jiminez-Jiminez et al., 1997). It is the most common motor side-effect of antipsychotics, with an overall reported incidence of between 20 and 75% (Halstead et al., 1994). It has also been reported with SSRI antidepressants and with dopamine agonists (Anon, 1998). Treatment involves reducing the dose of the causative drug; if this is ineffective, diazepam or propranolol may be used (Launer, 1996). Other therapeutic options that have been investigated include amantadine, clonidine, sodium valproate and tricyclic antidepressants (Miller and Fleischhacker, 2000).

Tardive dyskinesia

Tardive dyskinesia is a chronic condition, consisting of choreiform (i.e. rapid and jerky), athetoid (i.e. slow and sinuous) or rhythmic stereotyped movements involving the tongue, jaw, trunk or extremities. The most common form presents as orofacial movements (buccolinguomasticatory syndrome). Tardive dyskinesia occurs during, or within a few weeks of stopping, long-term treatment (at least a month in someone aged over 60 years and at least 3 months in other patients) with a dopamine antagonist (Launer, 1996). It may occur at any age, but is more common in the elderly and particularly affects women. In some cases, tardive dyskinesia can be irreversible. Anticholinergic drugs may aggravate the symptoms. Treatment involves stopping or reducing the dose of the drug concerned and, if necessary, substituting a drug with less effect on dopamine D_2-receptors. If this is ineffective, an atypical antipsychotic such as clozapine or vitamin E may be effective. Other agents that may be useful include tetrabenazine, clonazepam and reserpine, although evidence of efficacy is limited (Anon, 1996; Gardos, 1999).

Other movement disorders

Other drug-induced movement disorders include tremor (seen with lithium and valproate), myoclonus (bismuth salts, dopamine antagonists, antidepressants, antiepileptics, antiparkinsonian agents and lithium) and tics and chorea (antiparkinsonian drugs and anticholinergic drugs). Most of these have also been associated with antipsychotic use (Anon, 1998).

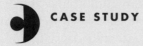

Miss A is a 23-year-old woman with epilepsy. Over the last few months she has had symptoms of depression, and therapy with an antidepressant is now being considered. Miss A has been taking carbamazepine 800 mg sustained-release twice a day for the last few years. She has not previously been prescribed an antidepressant.

What factors should be considered when choosing an antidepressant for this patient?

All antidepressants may lower the seizure threshold and precipitate seizures in susceptible patients (Rosenstein *et al.*, 1993). A history of epilepsy is considered a risk factor, though the incidence of the problem is unknown. However, where there is a clinical indication for treatment of depression, an antidepressant agent may be given with caution. Potential consequences of loss of seizure control (e.g. loss of driving licence) should be considered and weighed against the need to treat depression and the consequences of untreated depression.

Adverse effects can be minimised by choosing an antidepressant with minimal effects on the seizure threshold. However, other drug factors (e.g. interactions with current medication) and patient factors (e.g. patient compliance, previous seizure control, possibility of pregnancy) should be considered when choosing therapy.

Is dosulepin (dothiepin) an appropriate choice of drug for Miss A?

Convulsions induced by tricyclic antidepressants represent a substantial risk in susceptible patients and the drugs should be used cautiously in patients with pre-existing seizure disorders (Zaccara *et al.*, 1990). Dosulepin (dothiepin) may have a higher rate of convulsions in overdose than other tricyclic antidepressants (Buckley *et al.*, 1994), although it is unclear whether this can be extrapolated to use at therapeutic doses. The newer antidepressants, such as the SSRIs, are thought to be safer than older antidepressants in patients with epilepsy (Rosenstein *et al.*, 1993). Unless there are specific contraindications to an SSRI, one of these agents would generally be considered as first-line therapy in epilepsy. Dosulepin (dothiepin) would not, therefore, be a first-line choice as safer drugs are available.

How should Miss A be managed?

The choice of therapy and relative risks and benefits should be discussed with the patient. One of the SSRIs could be recommended. Fluoxetine may interact with carbamazepine and would not be the most appropriate choice. SSRIs have been associated with seizures, although causality is not established. In

→

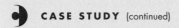

CASE STUDY (continued)

addition, SSRIs may have some antiepileptic activity although the extent of this is not fully established (Favale *et al.*, 1995; Dailey and Naritoku, 1996). Drugs such as paroxetine, fluvoxamine or sertraline may be preferable to newer drugs such as citalopram for which fewer safety data are available. As seizures have been associated with high plasma levels of antidepressants, low doses should be used initially and titrated slowly upwards if necessary (Preskhorn and Fast, 1992).

Miss A should be told of the small possibility of precipitation of seizures. Epilepsy is listed as a caution in patient information leaflets for antidepressants, and this may alarm patients or result in non-compliance if they are not informed of this in advance. However, she should be reassured that the risk is very low, and the benefits of antidepressant treatment should be explained. Any exacerbation of seizures should be reported immediately to her doctor. Case reports suggest that seizures are most likely in the first week of therapy or immediately after an increase in the dose (Dailey and Naritoku, 1996). The healthcare professional could, therefore, take the opportunity to provide additional reassurance at the patient's next visit if no adverse events have occurred.

References

Adelman H M, Winters P R, Mahan S C *et al.* (1995). D-penicillamine-induced myasthenia gravis: diagnosis obscured by co-existing chronic obstructive pulmonary disease. *Am J Med Sci* 309: 191–193.

American Psychiatric Association (1994). *Diagnostic and Statistical Manual of Mental Disorders* (DSM-IV), 4th edn. New York: American Psychiatric Association, 737–751.

Anon. (1996). No easy solution to antipsychotic-induced tardive dyskinesia. *Drugs Ther Perspect* 7: 13–16.

Anon. (1997). Sale of high-dose vitamin B_6 products restricted following reports of toxicity. *Pharm J* 259: 46.

Anon. (1998). Which drugs cause movement disorders? *Drugs Ther Perspect* 11: 9–13.

Arrowsmith J B, Milstein J B, Kuritsky J N *et al.* (1985). Streptokinase and the Guillain–Barré syndrome. *Ann Intern Med* 103: 302.

Aryka D K (1994). Extra-pyramidal symptoms with selective serotonin reuptake inhibitors. *Br J Psychiatry* 164: 177–183.

Awong I E, Dandurand K R, Keeys C A *et al.* (1996). Drug-associated Guillain–Barré syndrome: a literature review. *Ann Pharmacother* 30: 173–180.

Babic T, Zurak N (1996). Convulsions induced by donepezil (letter). *J Neurol Neurosurg Psychiatry* 66: 410.

Ball P, Tillotson G (1995). Tolerability of quinolone antibiotics. Past, present and future. *Drug Safety* 13: 343–358.

Barker I, Grant I S (1992). Convulsions after abrupt withdrawal of baclofen. *Lancet* ii: 556–557.

Barnes T R E, McPhillips M A (1996). Antipsychotic-induced extrapyramidal symptoms. Role of anticholinergic drugs in treatment. *CNS Drugs* 6: 315–330.

Bateman N (1991). Selected side effects: 4. Metoclopramide and acute movement disorders. *Prescribers' J* 31: 213–215.

Battochi A P, Evoli A, Servidei S *et al.* (1995). Myasthenia gravis during interferon alfa therapy. *Neurology* 45: 382–383.

Ben-Ami H, Nagachandran P, Mendelson A *et al.* (1999). Drug-induced hypoglycaemic coma in 102 diabetic patients. *Arch Intern Med* 159: 281–284.

Blain P G, Lane J M (1998). Neurological disorders. In: Davies D M, ed. *Textbook of Adverse Drug Reactions*, 5th edn. Oxford: Oxford Medical Publications, 585–629.

Blum A S, Dal Pan G J, Feinberg J *et al.* (1996). Low-dose zalcitabine-related toxic neuropathy: frequency, natural history and risk factors. *Neurology* 46: 999–1003.

Bori I, Karli N, Bakar M *et al.* (1997). Myasthenia gravis following IFN-alpha-2a treatment. *Eur Neurol* 38: 68.

Buckley N A, Dawson A H, Whyte I M *et al.* (1994). Greater toxicity in overdose of dothiepin than of other tricyclic antidepressants. *Lancet* 343: 159–162.

Burns R J, Schultz D W (1993). Drug-induced neurological disorders. *Med J Aust* 159: 624–626.

Caley C F (1997). Extrapyramidal reactions and the selective serotonin-reuptake inhibitors (review). *Ann Pharmacother* 31: 1481–1489.

Cartlidge N E F (1981). Drug-induced coma. *Adverse Drug React Bull* 88: 320–323.

Casteels-Van Daele M, Wijndaele L, Hanninck K *et al.* (1990). Intravenous immune globulin associated and acute aseptic meningitis. *N Engl J Med* 323: 614–615.

Chakraborty T K, Ruddell W S (1987). Guillain–Barré neuropathy during treatment with captopril. *Postgrad Med J* 63: 221–222.

Chalmers C, Barker W (1998). Evidence on vitamin B_6 questioned (letter). *Lancet* 352: 655–656.

Chiu A M, Chuenkongkaew W L, Cornblath W T *et al.* (1998). Minocycline treatment and pseudotumour cerebri syndrome. *Am J Opthalmol* 126: 116–121.

Classification Committee of the International Headache Society (1988). Classification and diagnostic criteria for headache disorders, cranial neuralgias and facial pain. *Cephalalgia* 8 (suppl 7): 1–96.

Committee on Safety of Medicines (1991a). Convulsions due to quinolone antimicrobial agents. *Curr Probl Pharmacovigilance* 32: 2.

Committee on Safety of Medicines (1991b). NSAID-related aseptic meningitis. *Curr Probl Pharmacovigilance* 32: 3.

Committee on Safety of Medicines (1994a). Drug-induced extrapyramidal reactions. *Curr Probl Pharmacovigilance* 20: 15–16.

Committee on Safety of Medicines (1994b). Neuroleptic sensitivity in patients with dementia. *Curr Probl Pharmacovigilance* 20: 6.

Committee on Safety of Medicines (1996a). Tramadol (Zydol, Tramake and Zamadol). *Curr Probl Pharmacovigilance* 22: 11.

Committee on Safety of Medicines (1996b). Hyponatraemic convulsions in patients with enuresis treated with vasopressin. *Curr Probl Pharmacovigilance* 22: 4.

Committee on Safety of Medicines (1999). Donepezil (Aricept). *Curr Probl Pharmacovigilance* 25: 7.

Cook C C H, Thomson A D (1997). B complex vitamins in the treatment of Wernicke–Korsakoff syndrome. *Br J Hosp Med* 57: 461–465.

Cruz O A, Fogg S G, Roper-Hall G (1996). Pseudotumour cerebri associated with cyclosporin use. *Am J Opthalmol* 122: 436–437.

Dailey J W, Naritoku D K (1996). Antidepressants and seizures: clinical anecdotes overshadow neuroscience. *Biochem Pharmacol* 52: 1323–1329.

da Silveira C M, Salisbury D M, DeQuadros C A (1997). Measles vaccination and Guillain–Barré syndrome. *Lancet* 349: 14–16.

D'Cruz O F, Shapiro E D, Spiegelman K N *et al.* (1989). Acute inflammatory demyelinating polyradiculoneuropathy (Guillain–Barré syndrome) after immunization with *Haemophilus influenzae* type b conjugate vaccine. *J Pediatr* 115: 743–746.

DeVita E G, Miao M, Sadun A A (1987). Optic neuropathy in ethambutol-treated renal tuberculosis. *J Clin Neuro-opthalmol* 7: 77–83.

Dick D J, Raman D (1982). The Guillain–Barré syndrome following gold therapy. *Scand J Rheumatol* 11: 119–123.

Dowson A (1999). Drug-induced headaches. *Lancet* 353: 378.

Editorial (1998). Still time for rational debate about vitamin B_6. *Lancet* 351: 1523.

Ellis C J (1996). Adverse drug reactions in patients with HIV infection. *Adverse Drug React Bull* 178: 675–678.

Ernst M E, Franey R J (1998). Acyclovir- and ganciclovir-induced neurotoxicity. *Ann Pharmacother* 32: 111–113.

Eze E, Workman M, Donley B (1998). Hyperammonemia and coma developed by a woman treated with valproate for affective disorder. *Psychiatr Serv* 49: 1358–1359.

Favale E, Rubino V, Mainardi P *et al.* (1995). Anticonvulsant effect of fluoxetine in humans. *Neurology* 45: 1926–1927.

Ferner R E (1996). Drug-induced hypoglycaemia. *Adverse Drug React Bull* 179: 679–682.

Ferrari M D (1998). Migraine. *Lancet* 351: 1043–1051.

Fields Jones S, Burris H A (1996). Vinorelbine: a new antineoplastic drug for the treatment of non-small-cell lung cancer. *Ann Pharmacother* 30: 501–506.

Freilich R J, Balmaceda C, Seidman A D *et al.* (1996). Motor neuropathy due to docetaxel and paclitaxel. *Neurology* 47: 115–118.

Gardos G (1999). Managing antipsychotic-induced tardive dyskinesia. *Drug Safety* 20: 187–193.

Gerber P E, Lynd L D (1998). Selective serotonin-reuptake inhibitor-induced movement disorders (review). *Ann Pharmacother* 32: 692–698.

Gordon M F, Allon M, Coyle P K (1990). Drug-induced meningitis. *Neurology* 40: 163–164.

Gurm H S, Farooq M (1999). Calcium channel blockers and benign hypertension. *Arch Intern Med* 159: 1011.

Halstead S M, Barnes T R, Speller J C (1994). Akathisia: prevalence and associated dysphoria in an in-patient population with chronic schizophrenia. *Br J Psychiatry* 164: 177–183.

Hauben M (1996). Cyclosporine neurotoxicity. *Pharmacotherapy* 16: 576–583.

Holloman L C, Marder S R (1997). Management of acute extrapyramidal effects induced by antipsychotic drugs. *Am J Health System Pharmacy* 54: 2461–2477.

Hughes R, Rees J, Smeeton N *et al.* (1996). Vaccines and Guillain–Barré syndrome (letter). *Br Med J* 312: 1475–1476.

Hyser C L, Drake M E Jr (1984). Status epilepticus after baclofen withdrawal. *J Natl Med Assoc* 76: 533–538.

Ismail E A, Shabani I S, Badawi M *et al.* (1998). An epidemiologic, clinical, and therapeutic study of childhood Guillain–Barré syndrome in Kuwait: is it related to the oral polio vaccine? *J Child Neurol* 13: 488–492.

Jeppesen U, Gaist D, Smith T *et al.* (1999). Statins and peripheral neuropathy. *Eur J Clin Pharmacol* 54: 835–838.

Jimenez-Jimenez F J, Garcia-Ruiz P J, Molina J A (1997). Drug-induced movement disorders. *Drug Safety* 16: 180–204.

Johns T R (1987). Long term corticosteroid treatment of myasthenia gravis. *Ann NY Acad Sci* 505: 568–583.

Johnson G L, Limon L, Trikha G, Wall H (1994). Acute renal failure and neurotoxicity following oral acyclovir. *Ann Pharmacother* 28: 460–463.

Jolles S, Sewell W A C, Leighton C (2000). Drug-induced aseptic meningitis. *Drug Safety* 22: 215-226.

Kato E, Shindo S, Eto Y *et al.* (1988). Administration of immune globulin associated with aseptic meningitis. *JAMA* 259: 3269–3271.

Kaube H, May A, Pfaffenrath V *et al.* (1994). Sumatriptan misuse in daily chronic headache. *Br Med J* 308: 1573–1574.

Kinnunen E, Junttila O, Haukka J *et al.* (1998). Nationwide oral poliovirus vaccination campaign and the incidence of Guillain–Barré syndrome. *Am J Epidemiol* 147: 69–73.

Knezevic W, Quuntner J, Matagha F L *et al.* (1984). Guillain–Barré syndrome and pemphigus foliaceus associated with D-penicillamine therapy. *Aust NZ J Med* 14: 50–52.

Lasky T, Terracciano G J, Magder L *et al.* (1998). The Guillain–Barré syndrome and the 1992–1993 and 1993–1994 influenza vaccines. *N Engl J Med* 339: 1797–1802.

Launer M (1996). Selected side-effects:17. Dopamine receptor antagonists and movement disorders. *Prescribers' J* 36: 37–41.

Lennard M S (1993). Genetically determined adverse drug reactions involving metabolism. *Drug Safety* 9: 60–77.

Lessell S (1998). Omeprazole and ocular damage. Concerns on safety of drug are unwarranted (letter). *Br Med J* 316: 67.

Limmroth V, Kazarawa Z, Fritsche G *et al.* (1999). Headache after frequent use of serotonin agonists zolmitriptan and naratriptan. *Lancet* 353: 1363–1364.

Lindley C M, Finley R S, LaCivita C L (1995). Adverse effects of chemotherapy. In: Young L Y, Koda-Kimble M A, eds. *Applied Therapeutics: The Clinical Use of Drugs,* 6th edn. Vancouver: Applied Therapeutics, chapter 91.

Madan B, Schey A S (1997). Reversible cortical blindness and convulsions with cyclosporin A toxicity in a patient undergoing allogenic peripheral stem cell transplantation. *Bone Marrow Transplant* 20: 793–795.

Marinjac J S (1992). Drug- and chemical-induced aseptic meningitis: a review of the literature. *Ann Pharmacother* 26: 813–822.

Marks J (1998). Evidence on vitamin B6 questioned (letter). *Lancet* 352: 656.

Mason P J, Morris V A, Balcezak T J (2000). Serotonin syndrome: presentation of 2 cases and review of the literature. *Medicine (Baltimore)* 79: 201–209.

McKeith I, Fairbairn A, Perry R *et al.* (1992). Neuroleptic sensitivity in patients with senile dementia of Lewy body type. *Br Med J* 305: 673–678.

McMahon B J, Helminiak C, Wainwright R B *et al.* (1992). Frequency of adverse reactions to hepatitis B vaccine in 43 618 persons. *Am J Med* 92: 254–256.

Miller C H, Fleischhacker W W (2000). Managing antipsychotic-induced acute and chronic akathisia. *Drug Safety* 22: 73–81.

Moris G, Garcia-Monco J C (1999). The challenge of drug-induced aseptic meningitis (review). *Arch Intern Med* 159: 1185–1194.

Morris K, Rylance G (1994). Guillain–Barré syndrome after measles, mumps and rubella vaccine. *Lancet* 343: 60.

Moyle G J, Sadler M (1998). Peripheral neuropathy with nucleoside antiretrovirals: risk factors, incidence and management (review). *Drug Safety* 19: 481–494.

Olesen J (1995). Analgesic headache. *Br Med J* 310: 479–480.

Olivieri N F, Buncic J R, Chew E *et al.* (1986). Visual and auditory neurotoxicity in patients receiving subcutaneous desferrioxamine infusions. *N Engl J Med* 314: 869–873.

Patey O, Lacheheb A, Dellion S *et al.* (1998). A rare case of cotrimoxazole-induced eosinophilic aseptic meningitis in an HIV-infected patient. *Scand J Infect Dis* 30: 530–531.

Preskhorn S H, Fast G A (1992). Tricyclic antidepressant-induced seizures and plasma drug concentration. *J Clin Psychiatry* 53: 160–162.

Raja M (1998). Managing antipsychotic-induced acute and tardive dystonia. *Drug Safety* 19: 57–72.

Rantala H, Cherry J D, Shields W D *et al.* (1994). Epidemiology of Guillain–Barré syndrome in children: relationship of oral polio vaccine administration to occurrence. *J Pediatr* 124: 220–223.

Rashiq S, Briewa L, Mooney M *et al.* (1993). Distinguishing aciclovir neurotoxicity from encephalomyelitis. *J Intern Med* 234: 507–511.

Rassmussen B K (1995). Epidemiology of headache. *Cephalalgia* 15: 45–68.

Rees J (1995). Guillain–Barré syndrome. Clinical manifestations and directions for treatment. *Drugs* 49: 912–920.

Rees J, Hughes R (1994). Guillain–Barré syndrome after measles, mumps and rubella vaccine. *Lancet* 343: 733.

Richard I H, Maughn A, Kurlan R (1999). Do serotonin reuptake inhibitor antidepressants worsen Parkinson's disease? A retrospective case control series. *Movement Disord* 14: 155–157.

Riorrdan-Eva P, Sanders M D (1998). Omeprazole and ocular damage. Facts of case are unclear (letter). *Br Med J* 316: 67–68.

Riyaz A, Aboobacter C M, Sreelatha P R (1998). Nalidixic acid induced psudotumour cerebri in children. *J Indian Med Assoc* 96: 304–314.

Ropper A H, Victor M (1998). Influenza vaccination and the Guillain–Barré syndrome (editorial). *N Engl J Med* 339: 1845–1846.

Rosenstein D L, Nelson J C, Jacobs S C (1993). Seizures associated with antidepressants: a review. *J Clin Psychiatry* 54: 289–299.

Rush M A (1980). Pseudotumour cerebri: clinical profile and visual outcome in 63 patients. *Mayo Clin Proc* 55: 541.

Sachs G (1998). Omeprazole and ocular damage. Lack of causality holds true (letter). *Br Med J* 316: 67–68.

Salisbury D M (1998). Association between oral poliovaccine and Guillain–Barré syndrome? *Lancet* 351: 79–80.

Saper J R (1987). Ergotamine dependency – a review. *Headache* 27: 435–438.

Schliamser S E, Cars O, Norrby S R (1991). Neurotoxicity of beta-lactam antibiotics: predisposing factors and pathogenesis. *J Antimicrob Chemother* 27: 405–425.

Schonberger L B, Chen R T (1998). The Guillain–Barré syndrome and the 1992–1993 and the 1993–1994 influenza vaccines. *N Engl J Med* 339: 1797–1802.

Schonhofer P, Werner B, Troger U (1997). Ocular damage associated with proton pump inhibitors. *Br Med J* 314: 1805.

Schwab M, Ruder H (1997). Hyponatraemia and cerebral convulsion due to DDAVP administration in patients with enuresis nocturna or urine concentration testing (letter; comment). *Eur J Pediatr* 156: 668.

Seaton R A, France A J (1999). Recurrent aseptic meningitis following non-steroidal anti-inflammatory drugs – a reminder. *Postgrad Med J* 75: 771–772.

Sekul E A, Cupler E J, Dalakas M C (1994). Aseptic meningitis associated with high-dose intravenous immunoglobulin therapy: frequency and risk factors. *Ann Intern Med* 121: 259–262.

Silberstein S D, Young W B (1995). Analgesic rebound headache. How great is the problem and what can be done? *Drug Safety* 13: 133–144.

Singh K, Chye G C (1998). Adverse effects associated with contraceptive implants: incidence, prevention and management. *Adv Contraception* 14: 1–13.

Stricker B H, van der Klauw M M, Ottervanger J P *et al.* (1994). A case-control study of drugs and other determinants as potential causes of Guillain–Barré syndrome. *J Clin Epidemiol* 47:1203–1210.

Uyama E, Fujiki N, Uchino M (1996). Exacerbation of myasthenia gravis during interferon-alpha treatment (letter). *J Neurol Sci* 144: 221–222.

van Harten P N, Hoek H W, Kahn R S (1999). Acute dystonia induced by drug treatment. *Br Med J* 319: 623–626.

Vial T, Descotes J (1996). Drugs acting on the immune system. In: Dukes M N G, ed. *Meyler's Side Effects of Drugs*, 13th edn. Amsterdam: Elsevier, chapter 37.

Wittbrodt E T (1997). Drugs and myasthenia gravis. An update. *Arch Intern Med* 157: 399–408.

Wong I C K, Lhatoo S D (2000). Adverse reactions to new anticonvulsant drugs. *Drug Safety* 23: 35–56.

Zaccara G, Muscas G C, Messori A (1990). Clinical features, pathogenesis and management of drug-induced seizures. *Drug Safety* 5: 109–151.

Zed P J, Loewen P S, Robinson G (1999). Medication-induced headache: overview and systematic review of therapeutic approaches. *Ann Pharmacother* 33: 61–72.

Ziajka P E, Wehmeier T (1998). Peripheral neuropathy and lipid-lowering therapy (review). *South Med J* 91: 667–668.

13

Sexual dysfunction and infertility

Fiona Maclean

The issue of sexual health, once regarded as a taboo subject, has been widely debated recently, provoked by the introduction of sildenafil, the first licensed oral treatment for male erectile dysfunction. It is now generally accepted that good sexual health is an important aspect of physical well-being and the possibility that drug therapy can cause sexual dysfunction is increasingly recognised (Forman *et al.*, 1996; Tomlinson, 1998). Although sexual dysfunction is not life-threatening, it can have a major impact on personal relationships, quality of life and the ability to conceive. It is also an important factor in non-compliance; studies have confirmed that many patients with hypertension, depression and schizophrenia discontinue their medication because of sexual side-effects (Bateman, 1998; Collaborative Working Group on Clinical Trial Evaluations, 1998). Patient information leaflets may alert patients to the possibility that their sexual function may be affected by medicines. Healthcare professionals should have some knowledge of the types of problem that can occur in case questions arise.

The overall incidence of drug-induced sexual dysfunction is difficult to quantify. Patients are often unwilling to raise the issue of sexual health with healthcare professionals, leading to under-reporting of problems. In addition, many diseases can affect sexual function, making it difficult to establish causality with a drug rather than concurrent illness. Antihypertensive medication, for example, is associated with erectile dysfunction but it is often prescribed for patients with diabetes, which itself may cause impotence. Other factors that can influence sexual function in men and women are age, alcohol consumption, smoking, drugs of abuse, over-the-counter medicines and exposure to environmental or occupational toxins (Bateman, 1998). Most of the published literature relates to the adverse effects of drugs on male sexual function. It is more difficult to assess these effects in women and this aspect of drug safety has seldom been considered in clinical studies.

Sexual dysfunction as a consequence of drug therapy has been reported with a range of drugs, notably antihypertensives, antipsychotics and antidepressants. Some types of reproductive dysfunction should be regarded as serious (e.g. infertility, congenital abnormalities and some pregnancy complications) and if these problems are suspected to be due to drug therapy they should always be reported to the appropriate regulatory authority. This chapter reviews the most frequently reported drug-induced sexual problems, including infertility. The effects of environmental toxins and drugs of abuse will not be discussed.

Infertility

Infertility is one element of a spectrum of reproductive disorders that includes miscarriage, congenital abnormality, premature delivery and stillbirth. Infertility, defined as the failure to conceive after 2 years of unprotected intercourse, is fairly common, affecting one in six couples at some time during their reproductive lives (Cooke, 1996). It is generally only detected when a couple is actively trying to conceive. It can be difficult to draw firm conclusions about trends in infertility rates but the number of couples seeking treatment for infertility is increasing each year (Healy 1994; Cooke, 1996). Although the prevalence of infertility does not seem to be increasing, the spectrum of disorders is changing and there is good evidence that sperm quality is falling throughout the developed world (Ledger, 1997).

Causes of infertility in women include failure of ovulation, tubal damage, endometriosis and hostile cervical mucus. In men, sperm defects, coital factors such as impotence or retrograde ejaculation and hypogonadism may be implicated (Healy, 1994; Wu, 1996). In about 20% of couples the cause of the problem cannot be found. Drugs and environmental toxins may be responsible in a small proportion of cases but, in general, the effects of drugs on fertility have been poorly studied.

The activity of the gonads (testes or ovaries) is regulated by the pituitary gonadotrophins, follicle-stimulating hormone (FSH) and luteinising hormone (LH). Secretion of both hormones is controlled by gonadotrophin-releasing hormone (GnRH) from the hypothalamus. FSH regulates the development of Sertoli cells (which are involved in sperm maturation) in the testes, and the Graafian follicle in females (Buchanan and Davis, 1984; Forman et al., 1996). LH controls formation of the corpus luteum in females and testosterone production by the Leydig cells in males. Both FSH and LH regulate oestrogen production and ovulation. Decreased amounts of FSH and/or LH reaching the testes can inhibit spermatogenesis (Cooke, 1996; Forman *et al.*, 1996).

Primary drug-induced infertility results from a direct toxic effect of the drug on the gonads or an indirect effect on pituitary gonadotrophin secretion (Table 13.1). Secondary drug-induced infertility results from drug effects on erection, libido or performance which may compromise the ability to conceive.

Table 13.1 Some drugs that may cause primary infertility

Alkylating agents (e.g. chlorambucil, cyclophosphamide, melphalan)	Non-steroidal anti-inflammatory drugs (women)
Anabolic steroids	Procarbazine
Colchicine	Sulfasalazine (males)
Diethylstilbestrol	Vincristine
Methotrexate	

Cytotoxic chemotherapy

Cytotoxic chemotherapy can cause infertility by a direct effect on the gonads. The effects differ in men, women and children and depend on the patient's stage of reproductive life at the time of treatment. The dose and duration of drug exposure are also important (Beeley, 1984; Bateman, 1998). The potential effect of chemotherapy on reproductive function is an important consideration in cancer treatment, particularly of young patients. Now that a number of cancers are curable, the long-term effects of chemotherapy on fertility may influence the choice of therapy. Men may be offered sperm banking before treatment is begun but for many reasons this may not be possible or successful. As cryopreservation of female ova is not yet established, women may be faced with the prospect of premature menopause and/or drug-induced infertility. Advances in the techniques used to preserve ovarian and testicular tissue have been reported recently but more research is required before these are adopted into practice (Radford and Shalet, 1999).

Alkylating agents are highly toxic to the testes. Cyclophosphamide and chlorambucil have been most extensively studied. The extent of gonadal damage depends on the dose and duration of treatment. Typically there is a progressive decline in sperm numbers, leading to azoospermia (absence of sperm) within several months, and this may be irreversible. Damage may be avoided if low doses are used (Lenz and Valley, 1996). There is often partial recovery of spermatogenesis after cyclophosphamide treatment and with chlorambucil recovery can occur even after many years.

Methotrexate is thought to be less toxic than the alkylating agents but it still causes a reduction in sperm count. Reversible reductions in sperm count have been reported with the use of low doses of methotrexate in the treatment of psoriasis (Sussman and Leonard, 1980). Vincristine and cisplatin have been reported to cause azoospermia (Aubier et al., 1989; Wallace et al., 1989).

In general, combination chemotherapy, at least in males, appears to produce more persistent effects on reproductive function than single-agent treatment.

It is more difficult to determine how chemotherapy affects female reproductive function as there is no direct way of monitoring toxic effects on the ovaries. Gonadal damage is often manifest by amenorrhoea, low oestrogen levels and increased concentrations of FSH and LH, which resemble the hormonal changes seen at menopause. As in men, alkylating agents appear to be the most toxic. Primary ovarian failure has been reported with both melphalan and cyclophosphamide (Lenz and Valley, 1996).

Other drugs

Sulfasalazine was reported to cause oligospermia (subnormal concentration of sperm) and infertility in men with inflammatory bowel disease over 20 years ago (Drife, 1987). The effects on sperm become apparent within 2 months of starting treatment. Sperm motility is reduced, abnormal forms develop and sperm density is decreased (Birnie et al., 1981; Korelitz, 1985). These effects are reversible within 2–3 months of stopping treatment. The effects on sperm function are probably due to the sulfapyridine component of sulfasalazine; slow acetylators of the drug are more likely to be affected. Return to normal fertility has been reported when treatment was changed to mesalazine (Cann and Holdsworth, 1984; Riley et al., 1987).

Diethylstilbestrol (DES) is a synthetic oestrogen that was given to some pregnant women between 1940 and 1970; it was used to prevent threatened and recurrent abortion. DES is now known to have caused a number of reproductive tract abnormalities in the offspring of exposed women (Forman et al., 1996). These include clear-cell adenocarcinoma of the vagina, anatomical abnormalities of the uterus and increased risk of ectopic pregnancy, miscarriage and premature delivery. Fertility rates appear to be reduced in the daughters, but not sons, of exposed women (Anon, 1996).

Anovulation and amenorrhoea

About 30% of infertile women have anovulatory infertility. They may present with amenorrhoea (primary or secondary), oligomenorrhoea (infrequent or irregular periods) or occasionally with regular menstrual cycles but low or undetectable serum progesterone concentrations in the putative luteal phase. Secondary amenorrhoea is defined as the absence of menstruation for at least 6 months in a woman with previously normal and regular menses (McIver *et al.*, 1997). Hyperprolactinaemia is a common finding in women with amenorrhoea or oligomenorrhoea; occasionally this is drug-induced (see Chapter 6). Drugs known to increase prolactin include methyldopa, metoclopramide, cimetidine and oestrogens. All traditional neuroleptics and risperidone are capable of elevating serum prolactin (Dickson and Glazer, 1999; Kim *et al.*, 1999). This problem is less common with more 'prolactin-sparing' antipsychotics such as clozapine, olanzapine and quetiapine (Dickson and Glazer, 1999).

Amenorrhoea has been associated with high-dose corticosteroids, danazol and isoniazid therapy (Forman *et al.*, 1996). There has in the past been concern about a high incidence of amenorrhoea shortly after stopping combined oral contraceptives. However, studies have shown that the incidence of amenorrhoea in such women is no greater than in the general population and that the use of oral contraceptives does not impair subsequent fertility (Guillebaud, 1993). Spironolactone has been reported to cause amenorrhoea at daily doses of 100–200 mg. Normal menstrual periods usually return within 2 months of it being stopped. The mechanism is believed to involve inhibition of dihydrotestosterone binding to androgen receptors (Potter *et al.*, 1992).

Evidence is accumulating that non-steroidal anti-inflammatory drugs (NSAIDs) taken in the middle of the menstrual cycle may inhibit ovulation (Killick and Elstein, 1987; Kennedy *et al.*, 1991; Akil *et al.*, 1996; Smith *et al.*, 1996). It has been suggested that the NSAID prevents rupture of the ovarian follicle which has developed normally. Progesterone levels measured in the second half of the menstrual cycle may be compatible with ovulation having occurred, which can obscure the diagnosis.

This problem has been reported with indometacin, diclofenac and naproxen. NSAIDs should preferably be avoided around the time of ovulation in women trying to conceive and should be withdrawn in women undergoing investigation of infertility.

Table 13.2 lists some drugs that may cause anovulation or amenorrhoea.

Table 13.2 Some drugs that may cause anovulation or amenorrhoea

Anabolic steroids	Risperidone
Danazol	Spironolactone
Isoniazid	

Sexual dysfunction

Sexual function may be divided into three categories reflecting the sexual response cycle: firstly, libido or sexual desire; secondly, arousal, including erectile function in men and lubrication in women; and thirdly, release (ejaculation in men and orgasm in women) (Bateman, 1998; Woodrum and Brown, 1998). Drugs can affect one or more areas of the response cycle. Understanding of the sexual response remains incomplete but there is evidence of dopaminergic, adrenergic, muscarinic and serotonergic involvement. In general, dopamine increases sexual behaviour and serotonin inhibits it. Libido is influenced by reproductive hormones and the emotional and physical health of the individual. Testosterone is necessary for normal sexual arousal, probably in both men and women, and in men testosterone deficiency is associated with impotence.

Erectile dysfunction and ejaculatory disorders

Erectile dysfunction, or impotence, is the inability to achieve or maintain an erection sufficient for satisfactory sexual performance. It is the most common form of male sexual dysfunction. The prevalence of erectile dysfunction is up to 10% across all ages, rising to over 50% in men between 50 and 70 years old (Feldman *et al.*, 1994; Ernst and Pittler, 1998; Wagner and Saenz de Tejada, 1998; Dinsmore, 1999). The aetiology is often vascular but other contributory factors include drug therapy, endocrine disease and neurological dysfunction. Erectile dysfunction often occurs with diabetes, heart disease, hypertension and peripheral vascular disease. It may also be a consequence of spinal cord injuries and pelvic or perineal radiotherapy or surgery (Korenman, 1995). Smoking and alcohol intake are important contributing factors (Anon, 1998; Gregoire, 1999).

Male sexual function depends on the co-ordination of neurogenic, hormonal and psychological mechanisms; disruption of one or more of these may result in erectile dysfunction. The penile blood vessels and smooth muscle receive both sympathetic and parasympathetic innervation and erection is primarily a parasympathetic function (Rousseau, 1988). In the flaccid state the smooth muscle is contracted, preventing inflow of blood. Parasympathetic nerve stimuli, mediated by nitric oxide, relax the smooth muscle of the arterioles in the corpora cavernosa, allowing blood to flow rapidly into the penis. Venous outflow from the penis is reduced, blood is trapped within the corpora cavernosa and rigid erection ensues (Wagner and Saenz de Tejada, 1998).

About 25% of cases of erectile dysfunction are believed to be drug-induced (Anon, 1998; Keene and Davies, 1999). The classes of drugs most frequently implicated are antihypertensives, antidepressants, antipsychotics and antiepileptics (see Table 13.3).

Table 13.3 Some drugs that may cause erectile dysfunction

Anabolic steroids	Digoxin
Antiandrogens (e.g. finasteride)	Gabapentin
Anticholinergics	Methyldopa
Antidepressants (tricyclics, monoamine oxidase inhibitors, selective serotonin reuptake inhibitors)	Metoclopramide
	Omeprazole
	Phenothiazines
Benzodiazepines	Phenytoin
Beta-blockers	Prazosin
Carbamazepine	Spironolactone
Cimetidine	Thiazide diuretics

Ejaculation describes the expulsion of seminal fluid from the posterior urethra. This is achieved via stimulation of alpha-adrenergic receptors, leading to contraction of the smooth muscle of the prostate, seminal vesicles and vas deferens (Duncan and Bateman, 1993). Disorders of ejaculation comprise ejaculatory failure and retrograde ejaculation in which semen passes into the bladder. A number of drugs have been implicated in these disorders.

Antihypertensives

The prevalence of both erectile dysfunction and ejaculatory disorders is significantly greater in untreated hypertensive men than in matched normotensive controls, so caution is needed when assessing whether medication is likely to be the cause of such problems. Most epidemiological studies addressing this issue were carried out over 10 years ago when the types of drugs used did not reflect those in use today. More recent studies confirm that the rate of erectile dysfunction depends on the class of antihypertensive (Bateman, 1998; Bulpitt *et al.*, 1989). The effects of treatment on quality of life are particularly important in the management of hypertension, which can require lifelong therapy despite being asymptomatic. Evidence suggests that many hypertensive patients experiencing sexual side-effects will stop taking their medication.

Most classes of antihypertensive agent have been reported as causing erectile dysfunction, with centrally acting agents, non-selective beta-blockers, potassium-sparing and thiazide diuretics most often implicated. High rates of erectile dysfunction and ejaculatory failure are associated with the older adrenergic blockers reserpine and guanethidine, which are no longer used. Clonidine and methyldopa have also caused loss of libido, erectile dysfunction and ejaculatory failure. The alpha-adrenergic blockers indoramin and prazosin can cause ejaculatory failure and retrograde ejaculation.

The incidence of sexual dysfunction in men taking diuretics is between two and six times higher than in men taking placebo (Chang *et al.*, 1991). Thiazides may cause reduced libido, erectile dysfunction and problems with ejaculation. The underlying mechanism is unclear as thiazides lack significant hormonal, autonomic or central nervous system effects; a direct effect on smooth muscle is thought to be responsible.

Erectile dysfunction is well documented with propranolol and can occur with other beta-blockers. The problem is more likely with lipid-soluble beta-blockers but has also been reported with atenolol and with ophthalmic timolol (Katz, 1986; Lim and MacDonald, 1996). Reduced perfusion pressure caused by a drop in blood pressure or a direct effect on smooth muscle may be responsible.

In a recent study which directly compared five different antihypertensive classes (the Treatment of Mild Hypertension Study, TOMHS) most problems were associated with the thiazide chlortalidone (TOMHS study group, 1997). The rate of erectile failure in patients taking chlortalidone was 17% versus 8% in controls. The incidence with amlodipine, acebutolol and enalapril was similar to that in controls and doxazosin was associated with the lowest rate of erectile dysfunction.

Although there are several published case reports of erectile dysfunction with calcium channel blockers and angiotensin-converting enzyme inhibitors, these classes of antihypertensive seem to cause fewer problems with sexual function than diuretics or beta-blockers (Keene and Davies, 1999).

Psychotropic drugs

As sexual dysfunction is a common feature of psychiatric illness, particularly depression, it can be difficult to assess the relative contribution of the disease and drug therapy. Both antidepressants and antipsychotics have recognised adverse effects on sexual function in men and women (Mitchell and Popkin, 1983; Clayton and Shen, 1998).

Erectile dysfunction has been described with all classes of antidepressant. Numerous case reports have implicated tricyclic antidepressants but the association has not been confirmed in the few published controlled trials (Segraves, 1998). There is consistent evidence that serotonergic antidepressants (e.g. selective serotonin reuptake inhibitors (SSRIs), monoamine oxidase inhibitors (MAOIs) and clomipramine) are associated with high rates of decreased libido, ejaculatory disturbance, delayed orgasm and anorgasmia (Woodrum and Brown, 1998; Rosen *et al.*, 1999). Serotonin appears to have a mainly inhibitory effect on sexual function. The mechanism of orgasm has not been confirmed but it is thought to be regulated by a balance of cholinergic and adrenergic influences and that serotonin receptor stimulation inhibits adrenergically mediated ejaculation (Segraves, 1998).

Evidence that SSRIs cause sexual dysfunction is accumulating as their use increases. The reported incidence varies widely, mainly because of differences in methodology between studies, but is probably at least 20% (Segraves, 1998; Rosen *et al.*, 1999). Problems may occur with all SSRIs. Delayed orgasm or ejaculation appears to be the most frequent problem and this has been observed in controlled studies. As a consequence of this effect, the SSRIs are now used in the treatment of premature ejaculation (Clayton and Shen, 1998; Woodrum and Brown, 1998). Newer antidepressants such as nefazodone and mirtazapine may be less likely to interfere with sexual function, perhaps as a consequence of their post-synaptic 5-HT$_2$ blocking properties (Hirschfeld, 1999; Gutierrez and Stimmel, 1999).

MAOIs can also cause delayed ejaculation (Clayton and Shen, 1998). The phenothiazines, particularly thioridazine, have caused changes in ejaculation (no ejaculate or a reduced volume) and pain on orgasm. Chlorpromazine is also associated with dose-related ejaculatory failure. Newer antipsychotics, such as olanzapine, may be less likely to cause these problems.

Priapism

Priapism is a prolonged penile erection that is usually unrelated to sexual stimulation. The problem occurs when the regulatory mechanisms which initiate and maintain penile flaccidity are disturbed and venous drainage from the corpora cavernosa is obstructed (Harmon and

Nehra, 1997). It is a medical emergency requiring immediate treatment to prevent fibrosis or even gangrene. Management involves the aspiration of blood and administration of a vasoconstrictor sympathomimetic such as phenylephrine or metaraminol. Drug therapy is an important cause of priapism, accounting for up to 40% of cases (see Table 13.4; Thompson *et al.*, 1990). Alpha-adrenoceptor antagonism is the most likely mechanism; constriction of the blood vessels supplying erectile tissue is prevented and detumescence does not occur. Prazosin is the drug most frequently associated with the problem (Banos *et al.*, 1989; Clayton and Shen, 1998). Among psychotropic drugs, the phenothiazines and the antidepressant trazodone are most commonly implicated. Trazodone-induced priapism may affect patients at any age and is most likely to occur in the first month of treatment. Priapism has also been attributed to hydralazine, nifedipine, anticoagulants and risperidone. Drugs given by intracavernosal injection in the treatment of erectile dysfunction (e.g. papaverine, phentolamine, alprostadil) may cause priapism and patients should be warned of this and advised to seek prompt medical attention should it occur.

Table 13.4 Some drugs that may cause priapism

Anticoagulants	Phenothiazines
Haloperidol	Phentolamine
Hydralazine	Prazosin
Nifedipine	Risperidone
Olanzapine	Trazodone
Papaverine	

Female orgasm dysfunction

In women, sexual dysfunction has not been thoroughly investigated and the underlying mechanisms are not fully understood. Most reported problems relate to orgasm dysfunction, reduced vaginal lubrication or loss of libido. Female orgasm involves involuntary rhythmic vaginal and pelvic muscle contractions; it can be assumed that the neurovascular control is similar to that in males (Forman *et al.*, 1996). Thioridazine has been known since 1961 to inhibit ejaculation in men but it was not until over 20 years later that the first report of inhibition of female orgasm was published (Clayton and Shen, 1998). Failure to achieve orgasm (anorgasmia) is one of the most common sexual adverse effects of psychotropic drugs in women. This problem has been described with SSRIs. Delayed orgasm or anorgasmia has been reported with MAOIs, tricyclic antidepressants, clozapine and risperidone (Clayton and Shen, 1998; Segraves, 1998). The antihypertensives clonidine and methyldopa have also been linked with anorgasmia (see Table 13.5).

Table 13.5 Some drugs that may affect female sexual function

Antidepressants (tricyclics, monoamine oxidase inhibitors, selective serotonin reuptake inhibitors)	Methyldopa
	Oestrogens
	Propranolol
Benzodiazepines	Spironolactone
Cimetidine	Thiazide diuretics
Clonidine	Trazodone
Gonadorelin analogues	

Multiple spontaneous orgasms have been described in women treated with fluoxetine (Morris, 1991; Garcia-Campayo et al., 1995). There have also been occasional case reports of spontaneous orgasm induced by yawning caused by clomipramine (McLean et al., 1983) and by fluoxetine (Modell, 1989).

Altered libido

Loss of libido or sexual desire is frequently attributed to medication in both men and women. For example, all drugs causing central nervous system depression can potentially decrease libido. In women, loss of libido is the commonest reported form of sexual dysfunction; it is extremely difficult to quantify and manage (Butcher, 1999). Changes in desire may be due to illness (e.g. gynaecological disorders causing pain on intercourse), stress or fatigue, or may be drug-induced (Duncan and Bateman, 1993). In controlled studies women have rarely been questioned about the effect of medication on sexual function and therefore most reports of altered libido are anecdotal or case reports.

Several antihypertensives, including clonidine and methyldopa, reduce female libido. Studies of both men and women taking methyldopa report an incidence of decreased libido ranging from 7 to 14% (Duncan and Bateman, 1993). Spironolactone has antiandrogenic effects and is clearly linked with decreased libido. Propranolol, thiazide diuretics and calcium antagonists are believed to have mild effects (if any) while captopril appears to have no effect. Psychotropic drugs affect sexual desire in men and women by several possible mechanisms, including sedation, effects on central or peripheral neurotransmitters or effects on hormones (e.g. prolactin). Antidepressants have been reported to decrease sexual desire. MAOIs, particularly phenelzine, are frequently implicated (Clayton and Shen, 1998). The SSRIs have all been reported to decrease libido, possibly as a consequence of an indirect effect on dopamine; the incidence in men and women may be as high as 40% (Gitlin, 1994; Segraves, 1998).

In general, rates of sexual dysfunction appear to be greatest with the SSRIs, followed by MAOIs, then tricyclic antidepressants. Rates of sexual dysfunction appear to be similar for all the SSRIs and it is not known if switching between them will diminish sexual side-effects. Case reports of decreased libido with anxiolytics have been published; centrally mediated sedation and muscle relaxation are thought to be responsible (Gitlin, 1994).

Cimetidine has been reported to cause loss of libido, possibly because of its antiandrogen activity (Pierce and Rush, 1983). This is likely to be dose-related. The problem is not seen with ranitidine (Beeley, 1984). The influence of testosterone on libido is well recognised and any drug that reduces serum testosterone may lead to a loss of sexual desire. In men, this includes drugs such as oestrogens, antiandrogens and gonadorelin analogues (Kirschenbaum, 1995). There are preliminary data linking protease inhibitors with loss of libido and also with erectile dysfunction and problems with ejaculation (Colebunders *et al.*, 1999; Martinez *et al.*, 1999).

Increased sexual desire is a rare adverse effect. Trazodone has been reported to increase libido in both men and women, possibly by decreasing prolactin levels or by increasing dopamine (Gartrell, 1986; Sullivan, 1988). Levodopa has caused hypersexuality in men with Parkinson's disease. The reversible inhibitor of monoamine oxidase A, moclobemide, has been reported to increase sexual desire in some patients.

Management

The management of drug-induced sexual dysfunction can be difficult. Occasionally these problems may remit spontaneously over time. In some situations it may be possible to change therapy to a drug in another class which is less likely to cause problems, e.g. changing from a thiazide to an angiotensin-converting enzyme inhibitor in hypertension. There may not always be an effective or tolerated alternative, however. Other possible options may include dose reduction, delaying dosing until after sexual intercourse or advocating 'drug holidays'.

Pharmacological management of drug-induced sexual dysfunction with agents such as cyproheptadine or sildenafil is seldom indicated (Woodrum and Brown, 1998; Gutierrez and Stimmel, 1999; Shen *et al.*, 1999).

Sexual dysfunction due to medication is relatively uncommon and probably not an issue that healthcare professionals will be consulted about very often. If approached by a patient or partner about the possibility that a sexual problem may be drug-related, a sympathetic and non-judgemental attitude should be adopted. Complex and sensitive issues surround sexual dysfunction but consideration should be given to possible drug causes. In most cases the individual should be advised to discuss the matter with his or her GP.

 CASE STUDY

Mr J is a 42-year-old man with depression. He showed a good response to flu-oxetine during a previous episode about 3 years ago. However, he stopped treatment abruptly when he noticed that he had difficulties with erection and ejaculation. Mr J has now told the psychiatrist that he would rather be depressed than take another drug that will ruin his sex life.

How common is sexual dysfunction with SSRIs? Are both men and women affected?
The exact incidence of these problems is unknown. The reported frequency ranges between 2 and 75% but data from controlled clinical studies are lacking. It is likely that at least 20% of patients will experience problems (Taylor, 1998; Rosen *et al.*, 1999). The reported frequency is usually higher in men, who complain of decreased libido, delayed ejaculation, erectile difficulty or anorgasmia. There is also evidence that women may experience loss of libido or orgasm dysfunction.

Would another SSRI or a newer antidepressant be less likely than fluoxetine to cause problems?
Of the SSRIs, there are limited data to suggest that paroxetine may be associated with an increased rate of sexual difficulties compared with fluoxetine, fluvoxamine and sertraline (Rosen *et al.*, 1999). The newer antidepressants nefazodone and mirtazapine are thought to be associated with a lower incidence of sexual side-effects (Clayton and Shen, 1998; Farah, 1999).

(continued overleaf)

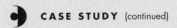 **CASE STUDY** (continued)

If problems do develop, might they remit during continued treatment?
There have been reports of tolerance to sexual side-effects developing, sometimes after months of treatment. If the antidepressant is effective it may be
worth continuing it for a period of time to see whether the problem resolves, if
this is acceptable to the patient and his or her partner. Some patients may find
that the effect diminishes but does not disappear entirely.

How else could this problem be managed? Would sildenafil be of benefit?
The preferred approach is to find a medication that is effective without
causing sexual adverse effects. These problems are generally dose-related so
it is important to ensure that the minimum effective dose is given. In a patient
who experiences problems it is not clear whether switching from one SSRI to
another is helpful but it may be tried. There are reports of a 'drug holiday'
being used to allow patients to time sexual intercourse with a medication-free
period. However, this is not a very practical option and is only appropriate
with short half-life drugs.

Sildenafil is of benefit in erectile failure but there is limited evidence of efficacy in drug-induced sexual dysfunction (Clayton and Shen, 1998; Rosenberg, 1999). A number of specific treatment strategies have been reported to
be effective in reversing SSRI-induced sexual dysfunction, including cyproheptadine (an antihistamine with serotonin-blocking properties), yohimbine (a
presynaptic alpha-blocker), amantadine, buspirone, granisetron and ginkgo
biloba. Adding a medication to treat the adverse effect of another should
always be avoided if possible because of the potential for additional adverse
effects and drug interactions.

References

Akil M, Amos S, Stewart P (1996). Infertility may sometimes be associated
    with NSAID consumption. *Br J Rheumatol* 35: 76–78.
Anon. (1996). Late sequelae of DES. *Prescrire Int* 5: 149.
Anon. (1998). Sildenafil for erectile dysfunction. *Drug Ther Bull* 36: 81.
Aubier F, Flamant F, Brauner R *et al.* (1989). Male gonadal function after
    chemotherapy for solid tumours in childhood. *J Clin Oncol* 7: 304–309.
Banos J E, Bosch F, Farre M (1989). Drug-induced priapism. Its aetiology,
    incidence and treatment. *Med Toxicol* 4: 46–58.
Bateman D N (1998). Drug-induced sexual dysfunction and infertility. In:
    Davies D M, Ferner R E, de Glanville H, eds. *Textbook of Adverse
    Drug Reactions*, 5th edn. London: Chapman and Hall Medical,
    875–887.

Beeley L (1984). Drug-induced sexual dysfunction and infertility. *Adv Drug React Acute Pois Rev* 3: 23–42.

Birnie G G, McLeod T I F, Watkinson G (1981). Incidence of sulphasalazine-induced male infertility. *Gut* 22: 425.

Buchanan J F, Davis L J (1984). Drug-induced infertility. *Drug Intell Clin Pharm* 18: 122–132.

Bulpitt C J, Beevers G, Butler A *et al.* (1989). The effects of anti-hypertensive drugs on sexual function in men and women: a report from the DHSS Hypertension Care Computing Project. *J Hum Hypertens* 3: 53.

Butcher J (1999). Female sexual problems I: loss of desire – what about the fun? *Br Med J* 318: 41–43.

Cann P A, Holdsworth C D (1984). Reversal of male infertility on changing treatment from sulphasalazine to 5-aminosalicylic acid. *Lancet* ii: 1189.

Chang S W, Fine R, Siegel D *et al.* (1991). The impact of diuretic therapy on reported sexual function. *Arch Intern Med* 141: 2402.

Clayton D O, Shen W W (1998). Psychotropic drug-induced sexual function disorders. Diagnosis, incidence and management. *Drug Safety* 19: 299–312.

Colebunders R, Smets E, Verdonck K *et al.* (1999). Sexual dysfunction with protease inhibitors. *Lancet* 353: 1802.

Collaborative Working Group on Clinical Trial Evaluations (1998). Adverse effects of atypical antipsychotics. *J Clin Psychiatry* 59 (suppl 12): 17–22.

Cooke S (1996). Treatment of infertility: the general approach to the infertile couple. *Prescribers' J* 36: 42–45.

Dickson R A, Glazer W M (1999). Neuroleptic-induced hyperprolactinemia. *Schizophr Res* 35: S75–S86.

Dinsmore W (1999). ABC of sexual health. Erectile dysfunction. *Br Med J* 318: 387–390.

Drife J O (1987). The effects of drugs on sperm. *Drugs* 33: 610–622.

Duncan L, Bateman D N (1993). Sexual function in women. Do antihypertensive drugs have an impact? *Drug Safety* 8: 225–234.

Ernst E, Pittler M H (1998). Yohimbine for erectile dysfunction: a systematic review and meta-analysis of randomised clinical trials. *J Urol* 159: 433–436.

Farah A (1999). Relief of SSRI-induced sexual dysfunction with mirtazapine treatment. *J Clin Psychiatry* 60: 260–261.

Feldman H A, Goldstein I, Hatzichristou D G *et al.* (1994). Impotence and its medical and psychosocial correlates: results of the Massachusetts Male Aging Study. *J Urol* 151: 54–61.

Forman R, Gilmour-White S, Forman N (1996). *Drug-induced Infertility and Sexual Dysfunction*. Cambridge: Cambridge University Press.

Garcia-Campayo J, Sanz-Carillo C, Lobo A (1995). Orgasmic sexual experiences as a side effect of fluoxetine: a case report. *Acta Psychiatr Scand* 91: 69–70.

Gartrell N (1986). Increased libido in women receiving trazodone. *Am J Psychiatry* 143: 781–782.

Gitlin M J (1994). Psychotropic medications and their effects on sexual function: diagnosis, biology and treatment approaches. *J Clin Psychiatry* 55: 406–413.

Gregoire A (1999). ABC of sexual health. Male sexual problems. *Br Med J* 318: 245–247.

Guillebaud J (1993). Oral contraception – the combined oral contraceptive. In: *Contraception: Your Questions Answered*, 2nd edn. Edinburgh: Churchill Livingstone, 127–128.

Gutierrez M A, Stimmel G L (1999). Management of and counselling for psychotropic drug-induced sexual dysfunction. *Pharmacotherapy* 19: 823–831.

Harmon W J, Nehra A (1997). Priapism: diagnosis and management. *Mayo Clin Proc* 72: 350–355.

Healy D L (1994). Female infertility: causes and treatment. *Lancet* 343: 1539–1544.

Hirschfeld R M A (1999). Management of sexual side effects of antidepressant therapy. *J Clin Psychiatry* 60 (suppl 14): 27–30.

Katz I M (1986). Sexual dysfunction and ocular timolol. *JAMA* 255: 37–38.

Keene L C, Davies P H (1999). Drug-related erectile dysfunction. *Adverse Drug React* 18: 5–24.

Kennedy S H, Forman R G, Barlow D H (1991). Non-steroidal anti-inflammatory drugs and infertility. *J Obstet Gynaecol* 11: 151–152.

Killick S, Elstein M (1987). Pharmacological production of luteinized unruptured follicles by prostaglandin synthetase inhibitors. *Fertil Steril* 47: 773–777.

Kim Y K, Kim L, Lee M S (1999). Risperidone and associated amenorrhea: a report of 5 cases. *J Clin Psychiatry* 60: 315–317.

Kirschenbaum A (1995). Management of hormonal treatment effects. *Cancer Suppl* 75: 1983–1986.

Korelitz B I (1985). Pregnancy, fertility and inflammatory bowel disease. *Am J Gastroenterol* 80: 365–370.

Korenman S G (1995). Advances in the understanding and management of erectile dysfunction. *J Clin Endocrin Metab* 80: 1985–1988.

Ledger W L (1997). Female infertility. *Medicine* 25: 48–52.

Lenz K L, Valley A W (1996). Infertility after chemotherapy: a review of the risks and strategies for prevention. *J Oncol Pharm Pract* 2: 75–100.

Lim P O, MacDonald T M (1996). Antianginal and beta-adrenergic blocking drugs. In: Dukes M N G, ed. *Meyler's Side Effects of Drugs*, 13th edn. Amsterdam: Elsevier, 488–535.

Martinez E, Collazos J, Mayo J *et al.* (1999). Sexual dysfunction with protease inhibitors. *Lancet* 353: 810–811.

McIver B, Romanski S A, Nippoldt T B (1997). Concise review for primary-care physicians. Evaluation and management of amenorrhea. *Mayo Clin Proc* 72: 1161–1169.

McLean J D, Forsythe R G, Kapkin I A (1983). Unusual side effects of clomipramine associated with yawning. *Can J Psychiatry* 28: 569–570.

Mitchell J E, Popkin M K (1983). Antidepressant drug therapy and sexual dysfunction in men: a review. *J Clin Psychopharmacol* 3: 76.

Modell J G (1989). Repeated observations of yawning, clitoral engorgement and orgasm associated with fluoxetine administration. *J Clin Psychopharmacol* 9: 63–65.

Morris P L (1991). Fluoxetine and orgasmic sexual experiences. *Int J Psychiatry Med* 4: 379–382.

Pierce J R Jr (1983). Case report. Cimetidine-associated depression and loss of libido in a woman. *Am J Med Sci* 286: 31–34.

Potter C, Willis D, Sharp H L *et al.* (1992). Primary and secondary amenorrhoea associated with spironolactone therapy in chronic liver disease. *J Pediatr* 121: 141–143.

Radford J A, Shalet S M (1999). Fertility after treatment for cancer. *Br Med J* 319: 935–936.

Riley S A, Lecarpentier J, Mani T *et al.* (1987). Sulphasalazine-induced seminal abnormalities in ulcerative colitis: results of mesalazine substitution. *Gut* 28: 1008–1012.

Rosen R C, Lane R M, Menza M (1999). Effects of SSRIs on sexual function: a critical review. *J Clin Psychopharmacol* 19: 67–85.

Rosenberg K P (1999). Sildenafil citrate for SSRI-induced sexual side effects. *Am J Psychiatry* 156: 157.

Rousseau P (1988). Impotence in elderly men. *Postgrad Med* 83: 212–219.

Segraves R T (1998). Antidepressant-induced sexual dysfunction. *J Clin Psychiatry* 59 (suppl 4): 48–54.

Shen W W, Urosevich Z, Clayton D O (1999). Sildenafil in the treatment of female sexual dysfunction induced by selective serotonin reuptake inhibitors. *J Reprod Med* 44: 535–542.

Smith G, Roberts R, Hall C *et al.* (1996). Reversible ovulatory failure associated with the development of luteinized unruptured follicles in women with inflammatory arthritis taking non-steroidal anti-inflammatory drugs. *Br J Rheumatol* 35: 458–462.

Sullivan G (1988). Increased libido in three men treated with trazodone. *J Clin Psychiatry* 49: 202–203.

Sussman A, Leonard J M (1980). Psoriasis, methotrexate and oligospermia. *Arch Dermatol* 116: 215.

Thompson J W, Ware M R, Blashfield R K (1990). Psychotropic medication and priapism: a comprehensive review. *J Clin Psychiatry* 51: 430–433.

TOMHS study group (1997). Long-term effects on sexual function of five antihypertensive drugs and nutritional hygienic treatment in hypertensive men and women. Treatment of Mild Hypertension Study (TOMHS). *Hypertension* 29: 8–14.

Tomlinson J (1998). ABC of sexual health. Taking a sexual history. *Br Med J* 317: 1573–1576.

Wagner G, Saenz de Tejada I (1998). Update on male erectile dysfunction. *Br Med J* 316: 678–682.

Wallace W H B, Shalet S M, Crowne E C *et al.* (1989). Gonadal dysfunction due to cisplatinum. *Med Pediatr Oncol* 17: 409.

Woodrum S T, Brown C S (1998). Management of SSRI-induced sexual dysfunction. *Ann Pharmacother* 32: 1209–1215.

Wu F C-W (1996). Treatment of infertility: infertility in men. *Prescribers' J* 36: 55–61.

Index